T0200738

Polio Across the Iron Curtain

By the end of the 1950s Hungary became an unlikely leader in what we now call global health. Only three years after Soviet tanks crushed the revolution of 1956, Hungary became one of the first countries to introduce the Sabin vaccine into its national vaccination programme. This immunisation campaign was built on years of scientific collaboration between East and West, in which scientists, specimens, vaccines and iron lungs crossed over the Iron Curtain. Dóra Vargha uses a series of polio epidemics in communist Hungary to understand the response to a global public health emergency in the midst of the Cold War. She argues that despite the antagonistic international atmosphere of the 1950s, spaces of transnational cooperation between blocs emerged to tackle a common health crisis. At the same time, she shows that epidemic concepts and policies were influenced by the very Cold War rhetoric that medical and political cooperation transcended. Also available as Open Access.

DÓRA VARGHA is Lecturer in Medical Humanities at the University of Exeter. Her research has been awarded the J. Worth Estes Prize by the American Association for the History of Medicine, and the Young Scholar Book Prize by the International Committee for the History of Technology.

Global Health Histories

Series editor:
Sanjoy Bhattacharya, University of York

Global Health Histories aims to publish outstanding and innovative scholarship on the history of public health, medicine and science worldwide. By studying the many ways in which the impact of ideas of health and well-being on society were measured and described in different global, international, regional, national and local contexts, books in the series reconceptualise the nature of empire, the nation state, extra-state actors and different forms of globalisation. The series showcases new approaches to writing about the connected histories of health and medicine, humanitarianism, and global economic and social development

Polio Across the Iron Curtain

Hungary's Cold War with an Epidemic

Dóra Vargha

University of Exeter

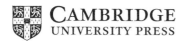

CAMBRIDGE
UNIVERSITY PRESS

University Printing House, Cambridge CB2 8BS, United Kingdom

One Liberty Plaza, 20th Floor, New York, NY 10006, USA

477 Williamstown Road, Port Melbourne, VIC 3207, Australia

314–321, 3rd Floor, Plot 3, Splendor Forum, Jasola District Centre, New Delhi – 110025, India

79 Anson Road, #06–04/06, Singapore 079906

Cambridge University Press is part of the University of Cambridge.

It furthers the University's mission by disseminating knowledge in the pursuit of education, learning, and research at the highest international levels of excellence.

www.cambridge.org
Information on this title: www.cambridge.org/9781108420846
DOI: 10.1017/9781108355421

© Dóra Vargha 2018

First published 2018

Printed and bound in Great Britain by Clays Ltd, Elcograf S.p.A.

A catalogue record for this publication is available from the British Library

Library of Congress Cataloging-in-Publication Data
Names: Vargha, Dóra, 1979- author.
Title: Polio across the Iron Curtain : Hungary's Cold War with an epidemic / Dóra Vargha.
Description: Cambridge ; New York, NY : Cambridge University Press, 2018. | Series: Global health histories | Includes bibliographical references.
Identifiers: LCCN 2018026566 | ISBN 9781108420846 (hardback : alk. paper) | ISBN 9781108431019 (pbk. : alk. paper)
Subjects: LCSH: Poliomyelitis–Hungary–History. | Poliomyelitis vaccine, Oral–History. | World health–History–20th century.
Classification: LCC RC181.H9 V37 2018 | DDC 616.8/35009439–dc23
LC record available at https://lccn.loc.gov/2018026566

ISBN 978-1-108-42084-6 Hardback

For my father

Contents

List of Figures

Acknowledgements

Throughout my journey to this book, I was privileged to share my work with and receive insightful comments, suggestions and guidance from multiple academic communities. Working with such an exceptional collection of scholars made writing this book a most rewarding experience.

I express gratitude to Paul Hanebrink, Julie Livingston, Bonnie Smith, Keith Wailoo and Jessica Reinisch for their advice, their continuous and tireless efforts in reading and re-reading countless versions of the manuscript, and the inspiring conversations that pushed my research forward. Temma Kaplan, Dina Fainberg, Bridget Gurtler, Anita Kurimay, Yvette Florio Lane, Tal Zalmanovich, Marissa Mika and Tamar Novick offered their friendship and critical reading in formulating the project from its early stages. I thank Friederike Kind-Kovacs for introducing me to the richness of European scholarship on the history of childhood. Gergely Baics pointed out sources and archives to me that became central elements of this book. I greatly benefited from a wide group of wonderful historians who enriched this work with their comments over coffees, dinners or through discussions in workshops, conferences and working groups. I thank Sandra Eder, Jeremy Greene, David Jones, Naomi Rogers, Paul Theerman, Nancy Tomes, Daniel Wilson, Alex Mold, Martin Gorsky, Gareth Millward, Robert Aronowitz, Susan Gross Solomon, Sandrine Kott, Claudia Stein, Roger Cooter, Anne-Emanuelle Birn, Melissa Feinberg, Mary Brazelton, Waqar Zaidi, Mat Savelli, Jim Mills, Yong-an Zhang, María-Isabel Porras, Rosa Ballester, Marcos Cueto, Sanjoy Bhattacharya, Paul Greenough, Christine Holmberg, Stuart Blume, Niels Brimnes, Emese Lafferton, Csaba Békés, Gábor Egry, Elidor Mehilli, Brigid O'Keeffe, Heidi Tworek, Davide Rodogno and Thomas David.

At the Center for Race and Ethnicity at Rutgers University, Mia Bay, Jeffrey Dowd, Anantha Sudhakar and Melissa Stein introduced me to the benefits of interdisciplinary work. A wonderful and generous group of scholars at Department II of the Max Planck Institute for the History of Science in Berlin was always available to make time and read and comment on several chapters of the book, among them Christine von Oertzen, Elena Aronova, Etienne Benson,

Dan Bouk, Markus Friedrich, Yulia Frumer, Courtney Fullilove, Harun Kucuk, András Németh, Skúli Sigurdsson, Kathleen Vongsathorn and Oriana Walker. I would especially like to thank Lorraine Daston for creating and welcoming me to this community. At Birkbeck, the Reluctant Internationalist research group, Jessica Reinisch, Ana Antic, David Brydan, Johanna Conterio, and the monthly writing group with Marcie Holmes, Francesca Piana and Sarah Marks gave me an opportunity to polish my arguments and complete the manuscript. A virtual writing group with Jenny Bangham and Boris Jardine, conducted entirely through video conferencing with plenty of freezing, blurring and helloing, shaped the final chapters of this work. In Exeter, Luna Dolezal and Arthur Rose offered a hand in the final touches of the manuscript.

Many friends and colleagues provided a roof over my head as I followed sources around the world. Catarina Pizzigoni and Gergely Baics took me in and supplied me with wonderful coffee and inspiration in New York. Joanna Radin's brilliant mind and insight kept surpassing my expectations whenever we crossed paths in New Haven, Philadelphia, London and Budapest, and her own work on Cold War biotechnologies and generous comments on my research are much present on the pages of this book. My sister, Zsuzsanna Vargha, and Martin Giraudeau always opened their home to me, whether in London, New York or Cambridge, MA, and provided me with meals, wine and great STS perspectives. The amazing Clare Mac Cumhaill and Rob Leach offered their golden couch, their culinary magic and warm friendship in Geneva and the UK, for which I am eternally grateful. Gergely Szöllősi and Ágnes Drosztmér always made space and time for me in their lives in Lyon and Budapest, with long nights of intense conversation over elaborate meals, good wine and undeground music from the 1980s. Many others helped me keep an anchor in Hungary over the years through stories, laughter and lively dinners. Thank you Anna Breuer, Fanni Kadocsa, Attila Keresztes, Lilla Zakariás, Ágnes Vargha, Péter Keresztes, Márton Matkó, Gabi Pajna, Lea Kőszeghy, Dániel Kőrösi, Gábor Csuday, Kinga Eszes, Bori Bacsó, Gábor Kiricsi, Zsófia Jávor, Viola Fátyol, Zoltán Juhász, Vanda Kozma, Éva Bujalos and István Kun, for keeping it real.

Members of the National Federation of Disabled Persons' Association (MEOSZ) of Hungary, and the Hungarian Polio Foundation have most generously committed their time and stories, for which I am very grateful. The advice and knowledge of the archivists at the National Archives of Hungary, especially Piroska Kovács, were invaluable for my work. At the Budapest City Archives András Lugosi offered his expertise to guide me in my search for hospital papers and party documents. Furthermore, I would like to thank archivists Marie Villemin and Reynald Erard, and librarian Thomas Allen at the World Health Organization, and Daniel Palmieri historical research officer at the International Committee of the Red Cross for helping my research. This book benefited greatly from generous awards. I thank Rutgers University; the Andrew W. Mellon Foundation; the Karen Johnson Freeze Fellowship Fund; the Max Planck Institute for the History of Science; the Consortium for the History of Science, Technology and Medicine; Birkbeck, University of London; and The Wellcome Trust for supporting my research.

I am indebted to my family for their continued presence in my scholarly adventures and their readiness to keep up with my haphazard travels as I was pursuing my research. I am grateful to Filomena Moura, Zé Luís Matías, São Salavessa, Isabella Salavessa and Paulo Mota, who provided support in countless ways over the years. My sister, Zsuzsi, never failed to make time from her own academic work to read portions of my manuscript and to affront me with astute questions. My father, György Vargha, and my grandmother, Irén Lázok, have been the inspiration that brought me to this project in the first place, while my mother, Etelka Fátyol, has served as a role-model in balancing professional and personal life. Oscar and Zsigmond Vargha Rangel de Almeida, both of whom were born into the writing process, kept me grounded in this endeavour through Lego sessions and never-ending Kisvakond stories, and most sweetly endured my late nights of writing and absences due to research trips.

None of this would have been possible without my best friend, partner, most thorough reader and critic, João Rangel de Almeida, who commented on more versions of this work than I could possibly care to count and gave me laughter in the most difficult times of writing.

Introduction

In early November 1956 Katalin Parádi emerged from the shelter beneath her house near Corvin Köz, Budapest. Surrounded by buildings peppered with bullet holes, the remainders of a barricade, a broken-down tank and dead bodies scattered on the ground, she was shocked by the scene, where one of the most notorious bloodbaths in the revolution had taken place. The alley that was once known for its lively cinema was now a battlefield. However, the young girl was determined to make her way through the destruction. The 17-year-old Katalin had an appointment for post-operative physical therapy treatment in the nearby children's hospital. She was recovering from polio.

It had started one morning in the summer of 1945 in Budapest, when the six-year-old Katalin became feverish. Her parents suspected the flu as their daughter became weaker and weaker. The next day, however, Katalin could not move her arm. It became suddenly clear: she had contracted polio. Her parents rushed her to the district paediatrician, who directed them to the nearby infectious disease hospital, where she spent a couple of weeks, the acute phase of her illness. Over ten years later she became an outpatient in the paediatric hospital for physical therapy and orthopaedic treatment, under the care of Dr László Lukács, who operated on her arm in August 1956. However, her treatment was soon interrupted: a revolution that broke out on 23 October prevented her usual visits. Living at the very centre of the armed conflict, Katalin spent weeks in the underground shelter of her house, along with her family and neighbours, while soldiers and civilians fought a desperate battle with tanks, machine guns and Molotov cocktails. During this period, she tried to maintain a certain routine and continued to perform exercises prescribed by her orthopaedist. The conditions were definitely not optimal for managing a disease that debilitated her muscles and required constant work to avoid atrophy. She did manage to progress in her 'treatment', though, when a nearby bomb explosion blasted the cellar door and slammed her into the wall in a very fortunate position, making up for lost physical therapy in the process.[1]

---

[1] Katalin Parádi, interview by Dora Vargha, 27 January 2010.

1

Katalin's treatment was not just an individual affair; it embodied the personal and political realities of the Cold War.

Her trip to the physiotherapist in the wake of the revolution was the last time she visited the paediatric hospital ward. A couple of weeks after gunfire stopped interrupting her days, in mid-November 1956, she became one of the first patients of the new Heine-Medin Post Treatment Hospital in the elegant and elitist district of Rózsadomb. Created during the most turbulent days of 1956, the hospital was founded on the direct orders of Imre Nagy, prime minister of the revolution.[2] Nagy would never see the result of his orders, as he was soon imprisoned then executed as the leader of the 'counter-revolution' by the communist government. Despite Nagy's ill fate, the hospital was not closed down. It survived and even flourished in the early 1960s as a major Hungarian centre for polio treatment.

Katalin's history with the disease was not over. As part of a national immunisation plan and as a high school student, she received the Salk vaccine in 1957. This vaccine had been imported, after much deliberation by the communist government in 1957, from the West. Shortly after the injection she contracted another strain of the poliovirus that paralysed her yet untouched legs. It is unclear if the disease was directly introduced by the vaccine (this had happened before in the United States, in the infamous Cutter incident[3]) or if the vaccine failed to provide the desired immunisation.[4] She was not the only one who came down with polio well after the introduction of the Salk vaccination programme. In fact, just two years later in 1959, the new hospital's wards were filled with new polio patients in the second largest epidemic in the country's history.

Only in 1960 did polio epidemics finally stop. A new vaccine from the East was introduced in Hungary: the Sabin drops. As case incidence dwindled in the

[2] László Lukács, 'Feljegyzés a Fővárosi Heine-Medin Kórház és Rendelőintézet Alapításáról, Működéséről, Eredményeiről és Ezzel Kapcsolatos Tevékenységéről.' Budapest: Personal archives of Dr. Prof. Ferenc Péter, 1993.

[3] In April 1955 almost 200 patients in the United States (mostly children and family members) contracted paralytic polio from a faulty batch of Salk vaccine produced by Cutter Laboratories. Neal Nathanson and Alexander D. Langmuir, 'The Cutter Incident Poliomyelitis Following Formaldehyde-Inactivated Poliovirus Vaccination in the United States during the Spring of 1955', *American Journal of Epidemiology* 78, no. 1 (1964): 16–28. See also Paul A. Offit, *The Cutter Incident: How America's First Polio Vaccine Led to the Growing Vaccine Crisis* (New Haven: Yale University Press, 2005).

[4] While in polio epidemics preceding 1957 the dominant strains were Type II and III, in 1957 Type I caused the most paralysis in children who contracted the virus. Therefore, the immunity acquired with illness caused by one type would not protect the body against another. This is why it is possible, although very rare for one person to become ill with polio several times. István Dömök, 'A Hazai Járványügyi Helyzet az Élő Poliovírus Vakcina Bevezetése Előtt', in *A Gyermekbénulás Elleni Küzdelem. Beszámoló a Ma Már Múlttá Vált Betegség Ellen Folytatott Hősies Küzdelemről és Felszámolásának Lehetőségéről*, ed. Rezső Hargitai and Ákosné Kiss (Budapest: Literatura Medicina, 1994), 41–45, at 42.

new hospital, now Katalin's workplace, polio ceased to be an important issue in the eyes of the state. What the failure of a revolution did not manage, the success of a vaccine did – the hospital's polio treatment centre was closed down in 1963 and was transformed into a general children's hospital.

Katalin was one of thousands of children who contracted polio or received specialised care in the 1950s in Hungary. Her story is but one of many that this book tells: lives with and around polio in Hungary entangled with global Cold War politics through their encounter with vaccination, treatment and the long-term effects of a debilitating disease. This book uses the series of polio epidemics in communist Hungary to understand the response to a global public health emergency in the midst of an international political crisis. Despite the antagonistic international atmosphere of the 1950s, spaces of transnational cooperation between blocs emerged to tackle a common health crisis. At the same time, epidemic concepts and policies were largely influenced by the very Cold War rhetoric that this medical and political cooperation transcended.

Spread by a virus and potentially causing permanent paralysis, poliomyelitis (or infantile paralysis, as it was also known in the era) in the 1950s became a major public health concern across the globe – and the Iron Curtain. However, international cooperation in polio control and treatment has been little investigated,[5] as the history of the disease has mostly been explored through national histories, primarily in an American context.[6] Equally scarce is the literature on

---

[5] Saul Benison, 'International Medical Cooperation: Dr. Albert Sabin, Live Poliovirus Vaccine and the Soviets', *Bulletin of the History of Medicine* 56, no. 4 (1982): 460–83; David M. Oshinsky, *Polio: An American Story* (Oxford and New York: Oxford University Press, 2005), 237–54; Rosa Ballester and María Isabel Porras, 'La Lucha Europea Contra La Presencia Epidémica De La Poliomielitis: Una Reflexión Histórica', *Dynamis* 32, no. 2 (2012): 273–85; Naomi Rogers, *Polio Wars: Sister Kenny and the Golden Age of American Medicine* (Oxford: Oxford University Press, 2014).

[6] Dilene Raimundo do Nascimento, 'Poliomyelitis Vaccination Campaigns in Brazil Resulting in the Eradication of the Disease (1961–1994)', *Hygiea Internationalis* 11, no. 1 (2015): 130–44; Enrique Beldarraín, 'Poliomyelitis and Its Elimination in Cuba: An Historical Overview', *MEDICC Review* 15, no. 2 (2013): 30–36; Bernardino Fantini, 'Polio in Italy', *Dynamis* 32, no. 2 (2012): 329–61; Per Axelsson, 'The Cutter Incident and the Development of a Swedish Polio Vaccine', ibid.: 311–28; Elisha P. Renne, *The Politics of Polio in Northern Nigeria* (Bloomington: Indiana University Press, 2010); Pietro Crovari, 'History of Polio Vaccination in Italy', *Italian Journal of Public Health* 7, no. 3 (2010): 322–24; Juan Antonio Rodríguez Sánchez and Jesús Seco Calvo, 'Las Campañas De Vacunación Contra La Poliomielitis en España en 1963', *Asclepio. Revista de Historia de la Medicina y la Ciencia* 61, no. 1 (2009): 81–116; Ulrike Lindner and Stuart Blume, 'Vaccine Innovation and Adoption: Polio Vaccines in the UK, the Netherlands and West Germany, 1955–1965', *Medical History* 50, no. 4 (2006): 425–46; Luis Barreto, Rob Van Exan, and Christopher J. Rutty, 'Polio Vaccine Development in Canada: Contributions to Global Polio Eradication', *Biologicals*, no. 34 (2006): 91–101; D. Slonim et al., 'History of Poliomyelitis in the Czech Republic – Part III', *Central European Journal of Public Health* 3, no. 3 (1995): 124–6; Jean C. Ross, 'A History of Poliomyelitis in New Zealand' (MA thesis, University of Canterbury, 1993).

4   Introduction

the history of medicine and health in Eastern Europe during the Cold War, especially regarding Hungary.[7]

From a Hungarian perspective, the book explores the Cold War history of polio on three registers of analysis that move from global politics, governmental and institutional concerns, to the patient–doctor level. On an international level, it asks how Cold War divisions can be re-evaluated when viewed through the lens of a disease that disregarded borders and ideologies. On a national level, the book investigates how post-war societies and nascent political systems dealt with an epidemic that worked against their modernist projects. On an individual level, it raises questions about definitions of treatment and authority of care, and investigates the boundary between professional and lay knowledge.

The unique geopolitical situation of Hungary on the boundary of the Iron Curtain and the construction of a new communist regime makes the country an ideal ground to understand the influence of the Cold War in forming global health responses to epidemic crises.[8] With a vaccine first arriving from the West, followed by a new serum from the East, the Hungarian story highlights issues of international politics, experimentation and standardisation in epidemic prevention. Furthermore, focus on Hungary allows linking of the intimate world of families with national and international agendas through care for disabled children with polio.

Major polio epidemics struck the country in 1952, 1954, 1956, 1957 and 1959, becoming more and more severe as the decade progressed. By the

---

[7] See for instance Lily M. Hoffman, 'Professional Autonomy Reconsidered: The Case of Czech Medicine under State Socialism', *Comparative Studies in Society and History* 39, no. 2 (1997): 346–72; Bradley Matthys Moore, 'For the People's Health: Ideology, Medical Authority and Hygienic Science in Communist Czechoslovakia', *Social History of Medicine* 27, no. 1 (2014): 122–43; Sarah Marks and Mat Savelli, *Psychiatry in Communist Europe*, Mental Health in Historical Perspective (Houndmills, Basingstoke, Hampshire; New York, NY: Palgrave Macmillan, 2015); Ana Antic, 'Heroes and Hysterics: "Partisan Hysteria" and Communist State-Building in Yugoslavia after 1945', *Social History of Medicine* 27, no. 3 (2014): 349–71; Carsten Timmermann, 'Americans and Pavlovians: The Central Institute for Cardiovascular Research at the East German Academy of Sciences and Its Precursor Institutions as a Case Study of Biomedical Research in a Country of the Soviet Bloc (c. 1950–1980)', in *Medicine, the Market and Mass Media*, ed. Virginia Berridge and Kelly Loughlin (London: Routledge, 2005); Donna Harsch, 'Medicalized Social Hygiene? Tuberculosis Policy in the German Democratic Republic', *Bulletin of the History of Medicine* 86, no. 3 (2012): 394–423. Several non-historical studies can give an insight into Eastern European medicine in the 1950s and 1960s: see Richard E. Weinerman and Shirley B. Weinerman, *Social Medicine in Eastern Europe: The Organization of Health Services and the Education of Medical Personnel in Czechoslovakia, Hungary, and Poland* (Cambridge, Mass.: Harvard University Press, 1969); Zdenek Stich, *Czechoslovak Health Services* (Prague: Ministry of Health, Czechoslovak Socialist Republic, 1962).
[8] Conversely, many historians have argued for the importance of borderlands and border crossings in the study of state socialist and communist regimes, see for instance the special section Libora Oates-Indruchová and Muriel Blaive, 'Border Visions and Border Regimes in Cold War Eastern Europe', *Journal of Contemporary History* 50, no. 3 (2015): 656–59.

mid-1960s one in 500 out of the population of 10 million had become permanently disabled because of the disease, a rare documentary film from 1967 claimed.[9] As Katalin's story shows, children with polio had to deal not only with the consequences of their disease but also with the challenges of a difficult decade: an over-zealous but in many ways inefficient Stalinist regime, a violent revolution, bloody retributions and gradual consolidation of the Kádár government. Their treatment was affected by and continued through tumultuous times and was shaped by the meagre resources of a post-war society in a world divided by Cold War barriers.

Polio, in its worst decade, afflicted a relatively small number of people in Hungary, just as elsewhere in the world, compared to other contemporary health issues. For example, in the year of the second largest epidemic in Hungary, nearly four times as many people fell ill with influenza and its complications, resulting in a death toll 140 times larger than that of polio.[10] Polio is a disease that is rather difficult to diagnose in its early phases. Many children got through the disease without even knowing it, as if fighting a common flu. Due to this diagnostic difficulty, paired with inaccurate registry and belated reporting,[11] it is hard to tell how many children needed to be hospitalised, and if all registered cases were paralytic. However, one thing is quite clear: polio became a priority in the eyes of the communist state, regardless of changing governments.

The disease symbolised a destructive threat to communist and modernist projects. Thus, it became a major global concern in the 1950s, and one of the most important public health issues by the end of the decade. It affected children in post-war societies, leaving crippled bodies behind at a time of heightened industrial production and recuperation from the war. Epidemics hit Hungary at a time when, together with most of Europe and a good part of the world, the country was recovering from the shock of the Second World War. In the course of the war, Hungary, which fought on the side of Nazi Germany, lost 40 per cent of its national wealth and over 10 per cent of its population, around 1 million people. This was devastating, given that the country was already among the poorer half of European nations in the interwar era.[12]

---

[9] 'Minden Ötszázadik', Hungary, 1967. This film is unique in actually portraying disability. Children who lived with permanent paralysis due to the disease were otherwise invisible and were physically and socially secluded.

[10] Központi Statisztikai Hivatal, 'Egészségügyi Helyzet 1963', Statisztikai időszaki közlemények, no. 5 (1964): 86.

[11] Dr. Tibor Bakács. 'Poliomyelitis Betegek Védőoltására Vonatkozó Adatgyűjtés'. Budapest: National Archives of Hungary, Országos Közegészségi Intézet Járványügyi és Mikrobiológiai Főosztályának iratai, XXVI-C-3-e/1959, 5587, 1959.

[12] This number includes military and civil casualties, and the Jewish population that was deported to concentration camps and civilians and soldiers deported to Siberian work camps. Ignác Romsics, Hungary in the Twentieth Century (Budapest: Osiris, 1999). The loss of military

6 Introduction

A battle that lasted almost a year left Budapest, the capital, in ruins and claimed the lives of thousands. It took decades to rebuild houses, bridges and transportation systems and for the new communist regime that took exclusive power in 1949 to build and consolidate a whole new administrative, social and economic system. It is into this context that polio made an entrance, continuing to place challenges in front of international organisations, governments and society until the early 1960s.

To understand the significance of polio in the Cold War, we must stop for a moment to consider the social, economic and political history of the era in question. In a wider context of the history of science, the looming threat of nuclear war overshadowed the era. Military and strategic considerations contributed to the formation of Big Science and affected research funding structures and research practices all over the world.[13] While the potential threat of destruction was pervasive, other effects of the Second World War were equally important to how the politics of polio played out in the 1950s – on the economy, on concepts of citizens' roles, on beliefs in progress in medicine and science, on concerns over ethical issues in medicine. Moreover, this was also a time of formation of international agencies like the World Health Organisation; decolonisation; the establishment of new regimes; and the emergence of ideas of modern societies.

One of the key sites for new regimes that worked with particular ideas of modernity was Eastern Europe, where, in accordance with the Soviet Union, communist governments emerged to gain exclusive political control between 1945 and 1952. Soon after the war, countries of the emerging Eastern Bloc embarked on a project of socialist modernity in dialogue with the West's liberal modernity. In many ways exhibiting hallmarks of Western variants, the state socialist 'alternative modernity' encompassed the goal of a complete reshaping of state, society and economy; rapid industrialisation; a developing welfare state, an extensive surveillance and scientific state administration; together with a non-public public sphere and a depoliticised polity.[14] It is no

troops was about 300,000; civilians killed in air raids and military campaigns 80,000–100,000; Jews destroyed in death camps, labour battalions and atrocities during the reign of the Arrow Cross Party 480,000 (200,000–210,000 for Trianon Hungary); and about 200,000–250,000 of people captured in battle or collected for forced labor perished in Gulags. Gábor; Kövér Gyáni, György; Valuch, Tibor, ed. *Social History of Hungary from the Reform Era to the End of the Twentieth Century*, Atlantic Studies on Society in Change (New York: Columbia University Press, 2004), 522–23.
[13] See for instance Naomi Oreskes and John Krige, eds., Science and Technology in the Global Cold War (Transformations: Studies in the History of Science and Technology) (Cambridge, Mass.: MIT Press, 2014); Paul Erickson, 'The Politics of Game Theory: Mathematics and Cold War Culture' (University of Wisconsin, 2006).
[14] Katherine Pence and Paul Betts, 'Introduction', in *Socialist Modern: East German Culture and Politics* ed. Katherine Pence and Paul Betts (Ann Arbor: University of Michigan Press, 2008), 1–37.

wonder, then, that public health campaigns, disease surveillance, medical research and epidemic management were very much part of the Hungarian socialist modern project, where disorganised and unruly reporting practices and vaccination campaigns coexisted with the oppressive practices of the post-1956 regime and the surveillance of citizens. The interaction of children, parents, virologists and physicians with the socialist modern state in the epidemic years reveals the way this modern project was co-constructed in a tumultuous time of political upheaval.

Hungary in the 1950s faced a decade that saw the establishment of a Stalinist dictatorship, reform, revolution and early consolidation. Four successive governments followed each other in a dynamically changing political, economic and social scene. After an initial attempt to restore parliamentary democracy between 1945 and 1947, the Hungarian Communist Party gained more and more power and started laying down the foundations of state socialism. The communist takeover was a mix of failed negotiations, planned strategy and election fraud, rather than part of a uniform process in Eastern Europe controlled wholly by the Soviet Union, as recent scholarship has pointed out.[15] Regardless of historiographical interpretations, the merge of the Communist Party and the Social Democrat Party to form the Hungarian Workers' Party, HWP (Magyar Dolgozók Pártja, MDP), in 1948 marked the beginning of a one-party system that lasted until 1989.

The peculiarity of the Hungarian political system was its dual structure. Every level of the state administration was paired with a counterpart in the party administration. The dual structure resulted in the creation of a cobweb of hierarchies and dependencies.[16] As Ivan T. Berend put it, 'the monolithic party, in a paradoxical way, was itself an institution of a fragmentary pluralism'.[17] This does not mean that the political system was not oppressive – it was a dictatorship and as the communist government's grip on power became more and more firm, the repression of the opposition intensified. Based on the foundations of anti-fascist retribution, the regime split society into 'supporters' and 'enemies'. The State Security Agency (ÁVO, later ÁVH) expanded with escalating speed from 1948 and former political allies were put on show trials to underline the image of the enemy within.[18] The Catholic Church, whose

---

[15] See e.g. Peter Kenez, 'The Hungarian Communist Party and the Catholic Church 1945–1948', *The Journal of Modern History* 75, no. 4 (2003).

[16] Mária Csanádi, 'Honnan Tovább? A Pártállam És Az Átalakulás', in *Magyarország Társadalomtörténete (1945–1989)*, ed. Nikosz Fokasz and Antal Örkény (Budapest: Új Mandátum, 1998), 147–73.

[17] Ivan T. Berend, *Central and Eastern Europe, 1944–1993: Detour from the Periphery to the Periphery*, Cambridge Studies in Modern Economic History (Cambridge: Cambridge University Press, 1996), 54.

[18] Mark Pittaway, *Eastern Europe 1939–2000*, ed. Jeremy Black, Brief Histories (London: Hodder Arnold, 2004), 51–55.

head, Cardinal József Mindszenty, was an emblem of conservative criticism, also found itself in a difficult situation. In fact, the figure of Mindszenty remained a sensitive point in Cold War domestic and foreign politics for many years to come.[19]

In terms of economics, Hungary operated a centralised, planned economy. Economic planning of this sort was not particular to Eastern Europe, nor was it unique to communist regimes.[20] The first three-year plan was launched in 1947 and targeted economic reconstruction from the effects of the war. The first five-year plan followed in 1950, with the goals of industrialisation and agricultural collectivisation, based on Stalinist policies. The darkest days of Hungarian communism followed, now termed the Rákosi dictatorship after Mátyás Rákosi, the General Secretary of the HWP. In the process of collectivisation, all produce found in random searches of peasants' homes was confiscated, including seeds intended for planting next year's crop (colloquially called 'sweeping the attics'); about 130,000 people were banned from Budapest and forced to resettle in villages; and rationing was introduced to combat the shortage of food supplies.[21]

Stalin's death in 1953 resulted in political change across the Eastern Bloc and Hungary was no exception: Rákosi was removed and Imre Nagy became prime minister. Reforms followed, mainly regarding the economic structure; victims of show trials were rehabilitated; the hated head of ÁVH, Gábor Péter, was imprisoned; and a thaw in cultural life permitted many writers and poets to publish again. However, taking advantage of a frost in international relations (West Germany joining NATO and the foundation of the Warsaw Pact) and change in Soviet politics, Rákosi succeeded in removing Nagy in the spring of 1955 and regained control of Hungarian politics once more. The efforts of the Nagy government and the renewed thaw signalled by Khrushchev's famous speech did not strengthen Rákosi's position. In the summer of 1956 he emigrated to the Soviet Union, never to return. On 23 October 1956 a mass demonstration of university students turned into a desperate and bloody revolution, and soon a new government was set up with Nagy as prime minister and prominent politicians and intellectuals such as György Lukács. The revolution lasted a little over two weeks. Soviet tanks rolled into the streets of Budapest on 4 November and in a few days broke all resistance. While the uprising was short-lived, it became a key moment in the Cold War. The Hungarian revolutionary became 'The Man of the Year' on the cover of

[19] Kenez, 'The Hungarian Communist Party and the Catholic Church 1945–1948'.

[20] Martha Lampland, 'The Technopolitical Lineage of State Planning in Mid-Century Hungary (1930–1956)', in *Entangled Geographies: Empire and Technopolitics in the Global Cold War*, ed. Gabrielle Hecht (Cambridge, Mass: MIT Press, 2011), 155–84.

[21] Ivan T. Berend, 'The First Phase of Economic Reform in Hungary: 1956–1957', *Journal of European Economic History* 12, no. 3 (1983): 523–71.

TIME magazine and the events of October became significant in shaping the international relations and domestic politics of the new János Kádár regime for decades to come. Overall, the successive communist regimes in the 1950s set out to establish a new society that positioned itself against the pre-war bourgeois world. The proclaimed aim of socialism was to create a classless society and to do away with social inequality. One of the methods in achieving this goal was to widen access to education. The number of children entering and finishing eight years of primary schooling grew significantly compared to the pre-war era, as did the number of students entering secondary schools.[22] However, inequalities based on social connections, prestige, urban and rural spaces, and gender prevailed.

For the most part, the inequalities of the pre-war era were replaced by new inequalities, based on political position and influence, or hierarchy in work.[23] Moreover, there was no clean break with the pre-war society – about 60–70 per cent of professionals in 1956 occupied a similar position as before the war.[24] As this book demonstrates, one of these groups comprised physicians, who, despite becoming a predominantly conservative or outright right-wing profession in the interwar era (after doctors of Jewish origin were removed), retained their status and were able to secure some political independence simply based on the grave need for doctors. Additionally, bourgeois families that were marginalised in the early 1950s gradually adapted and regained their social status.[25]

Inequalities in society mapped onto the urban structure of the country as well. The emphasis on industrialisation affected where and how people lived, as well as the services and resources to which they had access. Budapest remained the disproportionately large urban and administrative centre of the country,[26] but other industrial centres also emerged, like the new city of Sztálinváros, founded in 1951, which was meant to be a model socialist settlement with model working-class citizens.[27] Hamlets were to be abolished,

---

[22] Gyáni et al., *Social History of Hungary from the Reform Era to the End of the Twentieth Century*, 572–73.

[23] Szonja Szelényi, *Equality by Design: The Grand Experiment in Destratification in Socialist Hungary* (Stanford: Stanford University Press, 1998).

[24] Pittaway, *Eastern Europe 1939–2000*, 57.

[25] Gyáni et al., *Social History of Hungary from the Reform Era to the End of the Twentieth Century*, 579. For a detailed discussion of the bourgeoisie in post-war Hungary, see James Mark, 'Discrimination, Opportunity and Middle-Class Success in Early Communist Hungary', *The Historical Journal* 48, no. 2 (2005): 499–521.

[26] This was partially the result of the Treaty of Trianon of 1920, when the boundaries of Hungary were redrawn, reducing the country's size by two-thirds. Other large cities and administrative centers now fell outside the border, leaving Budapest to account for about a tenth of the population.

[27] Sándor Horváth, 'Everyday Life in the First Hungarian Socialist City', *International Labor and Working-Class History* 68 (2005): 24–46.

since their inhabitants could not be closely monitored for the sake of collectivisation. Development in villages that were not cooperative production centres was barred until the 1960s, also in order to encourage the peasantry to participate in collectives. The infrastructure of these settlements did not change much in the first decades of the communist regime, as most roads were not paved and houses were left without electricity and running water.[28]

Faced with the effects of the war, as well as the economic goals and ideals of the new era, the state enforced a strict pro-natalist policy in the early 1950s in the hope of increasing live births and thereby the number of productive workers. However, a short increase was soon followed by a decrease in live births after the 1956 revolution, paired with a massive emigration of dissidents. Demography mattered to this nascent communist state – as did able bodies.

The epidemic waves of polio came to Hungary at the time of this demographic shock and challenged the process of social, political and economic reorganisation. The relatively new communist government, which positioned itself as the answer to a bright and productive future, had to deal with the traumatic effects of polio epidemics, which threatened communist ideals at their foundations. Therefore, during the 1950s, the state took numerous steps to fight the disease. Besides promoting poliomyelitis research,[29] the government educated the public about prevention and treatment of polio through propaganda films[30] and issued a weekly report during epidemics detailing the geographical spread of the disease and the number of people affected. To curb the spread of the disease, regulations controlled the public travel of children under 14 years old, requiring a medical examination before departure.[31]

Despite education and restrictions on travel, many children contracted the virus and required urgent care. Iron lungs were an extremely important technology in saving and treating children with polio in hospitals. A forerunner of the modern respirator and a cutting-edge and costly technology, the iron lung mechanically breathed for paralysed children who were unable to breathe for themselves. The first iron lung arrived in Hungary in 1948, with the cooperation of the American embassy. In the first half of the 1950s, iron lungs began to be produced in Czechoslovakia and the GDR, and finally, in the mid-1950s, in Hungary as well.[32] A number of devices arrived

---

[28] Gyáni, *Social History of Hungary from the Reform Era to the End of the Twentieth Century*, 537–39.

[29] The State Hygienic Institute, which cooperated with the Epidemics Department of the Health Ministry, led the research beginning in 1953, Tibor Dr Bakács, *Az Országos Közegészségügyi Intézet Működése 1927–1957* (Budapest: Országos Közegészségügyi Intézet 1959), 82.

[30] 'Bemutatták a Gyermekparalízisről Készült Filmet', *Népszabadság*, 9 August 1957, 9; 'Szülők, Vigyázzatok!', Health Ministry, Hungary, 1957.

[31] A Magyar Forradalmi Munkás-Paraszt Kormány 1027/1958 (VIII. 3.) számú határozata a gyermekbénulás elleni védekezésről (1958).

[32] Domokos Boda, *Sorsfordulók* (Budapest: Harmat, 2004), 60.

during the epidemic years as a result of a lending system orchestrated by the Red Cross. By 1959, over 100 Hungarian iron lungs were in use in the country, a considerable amount if one takes into account the high cost and constant care that these machines required.

The effort against polio in Hungary crossed borders in other ways as well, all of which appear to have been surprisingly cooperative. Hungarian scientists were regular participants in Western conferences on polio. Experts in Hungary could keep an eye on global trends in virology and treatment, occasionally publishing in Western journals as well. The professional situation of sciences, especially medicine, remained relatively autonomous in comparison to humanities, which were placed under strict state control.[33]

Iron lungs were not the only medical technology crossing the Iron Curtain – vaccines also made their way through the seemingly impenetrable wall in numerous ways. Nationwide vaccination began in Hungary in 1957, first with the killed virus vaccine developed by Jonas Salk and followed by Albert Sabin's live virus vaccine in 1959. Vaccines containing dead and live viruses appeared to be solutions to contagion, but also had the potential power to cause disease instead of fighting it and thus to inflict serious damage on the most innocent and pure members of society, the promise of the future: children. Therefore, questions about the source of the vaccine, where and from what it was made, who produced it and who distributed it became important political problems. However, the fact that there was, indeed, cooperation between the two sides of the Iron Curtain implies that at the same time, vaccination was perceived as a goal above politics and Cold War tensions.

Effective vaccination in Hungary was attained only with the introduction of the live virus Sabin vaccine on 14 December 1959, this time making its way from the Soviet Union. After 1963 the number of cases was reduced to 0–4 in the whole population, and since 1972 there have been no recorded wild polio cases.[34] Once free vaccination with the Sabin vaccine put an end to epidemics, it also put an end to the existence of specialised polio hospitals, although vaccination made little difference to those already disabled by the disease. With the threat of the epidemics gone, the productive bodies of Hungary's future generation were no longer considered physically in danger of becoming disabled, and therefore the state was no longer politically invested in polio. As

---

[33] For example in Poland, East Germany and the Czech Republic, see John Connelly, *Captive University: The Sovietization of East German, Czech and Polish Higher Education, 1945–1956* (Chapel Hill: University of North California Press, 2000).

[34] István Dömök, A kampányoltások időszaka (1959–1991), in Rezső Hargitai and Ákosné Kiss, eds., *A Gyermekbénulás Elleni Küzdelem: Beszámoló egy Ma Már Múlttá Váló Rettegett Betegség Ellen Folytatott Hősies Küzdelemről és Felszámolásának Lehetőségéről: a Szent László Kórház Centenáriumára Készült Összeállítás* (Budapest: Literatura Medica, 1994), 169–78, at 169.

the disease vanished entirely from public discourse and centres for polio treatment and care were dispersed, disabled polio patients disappeared from the medical gaze as well.

While the 'official' history of polio in Hungary ends with the eradication of the disease, the story of the people, knowledge and institutions affected by it does not. Certain professional and patient groups, which had become the centre of social and political focus during the time of the epidemics, disappeared along with lay and medical knowledge of prevention and treatment as the 'heroic struggle' came to an end. At the same time, other groups such as disabled civil societies arose, beginning new stories of their own.

To explore this complex Cold War history of polio, this study relies on extensive, original research, in the archives of international organisations such as the World Health Organisation and the International Committee of the Red Cross; The National Archives of the Hungarian government and the Hungarian Red Cross Society; the City Archives of Budapest; institutional archives of the Hungarian Film Institute, Yale University, the Sabin archives at the University of Cincinnati, the College of Physicians and the American Philosophical Society in Philadelphia. The book also draws heavily on published sources such as newspapers, magazines, medical journals, hospital newsletters, memoirs, conference proceedings, interviews and documentaries. Written sources were complemented with oral history interviews with health professionals and former polio patients, conducted by the author between 2007 and 2012.

Through the movement of people, technologies and ideas that frame the Hungarian narrative of polio, this work particularly focuses on international cooperation and exchange in the Cold War. Traditionally, Cold War scholarship has focused on high politics and security studies. Cold War relations between East and West have been analysed through military, political and socio-economic rivalries, as conflicts between socialism and capitalism. These considerations are no doubt crucial parts of the story, as the book demonstrates. However, mostly through the study of material culture and modernity, histories that approach the Cold War divide and the Iron Curtain itself in more dynamic ways have begun to move this scholarship towards the investigation of interaction and collaboration. György Péteri's 'nylon curtain' concept,[35] or Michael David-Fox's idea of the Iron Curtain as a semipermeable membrane,[36] are indicative of this turn in Cold War scholarship.

---

[35] György Péteri, *Nylon Curtain: Transnational and Transsystemic Tendencies in the Cultural Life of State-Socialist Russia and East-Central Europe*, Trondheim Studies on East European Cultures & Societies (Trondheim: Program on East European Cultures and Societies, 2006).

[36] Michael David-Fox, 'The Iron Curtain as a Semipermeable Membrane: Origins and Demise of the Stalinist Superiority Complex', in *Cold War Crossings: International Travel and Exchange across the Soviet Bloc, 1940s–1960s*, ed. Patryk Babiracki and Kenyon Zimmer (College Station: Texas A&M University Press, 2014), 14–40.

Indeed, new dimensions of interaction between the two sides can be traced when looking at the Cold War from different perspectives[37] – in this case from the experience of polio in Hungary. One of the approaches that argue for a broadening of geographical focus and scope of historical investigation comes from recent studies in the fields of history of science, and science and technology studies.[38] This book shifts attention from the two superpowers to an Eastern European state and focuses on the circulation of medical knowledge and technology rather than on the competition between the Soviet Union and the United States. Instead of Cold War intransigence, the case of polio in Hungary shows surprising flexibility in foreign and domestic policies and demonstrates the circumstances under which the Iron Curtain was drawn to let people, vaccines and practices through.

On the national level of investigation, the book takes a closer look at the relationship between the communist state and Hungarian society. Polio struck in the formative years of the communist government, when the new regime was striving to establish a new political, economic and social order. I investigate the limits and possibilities of the paternal state[39] and the fluctuation of parental duties to the health of children between state and parents.

---

[37] See for instance approaches in Sari Autio-Sarasmo and Brendan Humphreys, eds., *Winter Kept Us Warm: Cold War Interactions Reconsidered*, Aleksanteri Cold War Series (Helsinki: University of Helsinki, 2010); Zuoyue Wang, 'Transnational Science during the Cold War: The Case of Chinese/American Scientists', *Isis* 101, no. 2 (2010): 367–77; Nikolai Krementsov, *The Cure. A Story of Cancer and Politics from the Annals of the Cold War* (Chicago and London: University of Chicago Press, 2002).

[38] See David A. Hounshell, 'Rethinking the Cold War; Rethinking Science and Technology in the Cold War; Rethinking the Social Study of Science and Technology', *Social Studies of Science* 31, no. 2 (2001): 289–97; Marcos Cueto, *Cold War, Deadly Fevers: Malaria Eradication in Mexico, 1955–1975* (Washington, D.C.; Baltimore: Woodrow Wilson Center Press; Johns Hopkins University Press, 2007); Gabrielle Hecht, ed. *Entangled Geographies: Empire and Technopolitics in the Global Cold War*, Inside Technology (Cambridge, Mass.: MIT Press, 2011). Hunter Heyck and David Keiser, 'Focus: New Perspectives on Science and the Cold War. Introduction', *Isis* 101, no. 2 (2010): 362–66; Rachel Rotschild, 'Détente from the Air: Monitoring Air Pollution during the Cold War', *Technology and Culture* 57, no. 4 (2016): 831–65; Simo Mikkonen and Pia Koivunen, eds., *Beyond the Divide: Entangled Histories of Cold War Europe* (New York and Oxford: Berghahn Books, 2015); Kate Brown, *Plutopia: Nuclear Families, Atomic Cities, and the Great Soviet and American Plutonium Disasters* (Oxford: Oxford University Press, 2013).

[39] On the paternal state in Eastern Europe see Gail Kligman, *The Politics of Duplicity: Controlling Reproduction in Ceausescu's Romania* (Berkeley: University of California Press, 1998); Lynne Haney, *Inventing the Needy: Gender and the Politics of Welfare in Hungary* (Berkeley, Los Angeles and London: University of California Press, 2002); Catriona Kelly, *Children's World: Growing up in Russia 1890–1991* (New Haven: Yale University Press, 2007); Katherine Verdery, 'From Parent-State to Family Patriarchs: Gender and Nation in Contemporary Eastern Europe', *East European Politics and Societies* 8, no. 2 (1994): 225–55.

14   Introduction

Following new historical approaches that concentrate on features of communist regimes that are neglected by traditional analysis[40] and aim to deconstruct Cold War narratives, the involvement of society and questions of agency are central to this book. I do not consider the state to be a monolithic entity,[41] nor communist Hungary to be totalitarian in the way that it is often portrayed in Hungarian historiography[42] and public history collections.[43] Eventual failure to control the reproductive rights of women in the early 1950s, as detailed in Chapter 1, or the inefficiency of disease reporting and vaccination organisation, shown in Chapter 3, point to a possible understanding of Hungarian communism as an unsuccessful effort at totalitarianism.

While I show inefficient bureaucratic structures, internal conflicts and wavering positions through the history of polio, in the majority of the study I refer to the respective governments in this era as the 'state'. In the story that unfolds through the prevention and treatment of the disease, most of the actors

[40] E.g. Katherine A. Lebow, 'Public Works, Private Lives: Youth Brigades in Nowa Huta in the 1950s', *Contemporary European History* 10, no. 2 (2001): 199–219; Gail Kligman and Katherine Verdery, 'Social Dimensions of Collectivization: Fomenting Class Warfare in Transylvania', in *World Order after Leninism: Essays in Honor of Ken Jowitt*, ed. Vladimir Tismaneanu, Marc Morjé Howard, and Rudra Sil (Seattle: Herbert J. Ellison Center for Russian, East European, and Central Asian Studies, University of Washington, 2006). 'Malgorzata Fidelis, 'Equality through Protection: The Politics of Women's Employment in Postwar Poland, 1945–1956', *Slavic Review* 63, no. 2 (2004): 301–24; Eagle Glassheim, 'Ethnic Cleansing, Communism, and Environmental Devastation in Czechoslovakia's Borderlands, 1945–1989', *Journal of Modern History* 78, no. 1 (2006): 65–92.

[41] On the fluidity and multiplicity of the Hungarian communist state, see Haney, *Inventing the Needy*.

[42] On the historiography of totalitarianism, see Michael Geyer and Sheila Fitzpatrick, 'After Totalitarianism – Stalinism and Nazism Compared', in *Beyond Totalitarianism: Stalinism and Nazism Compared*, ed. Michael Geyer and Sheila Fitzpatrick (New York: Cambridge University Press, 2008), 1–41. The totalitarian approach to the communist state, as represented by Arendt and Brzezinski has seen a revival after 1989. As Claudia Koonz notes in her chapter *Between Memory and Oblivion* (1994), there was a shift in the appliance of the totalitarian concept after the Berlin Wall fell. Previously, Western rhetoric presented Nazism and Communism as equal, while after the *Wende*, Eastern countries took on this view in order to get their suffering acknowledged. This shift is most apparent in commemorations. Claudia Koonz, 'Between Memory and Oblivion: Concentration Camps in German Memory', in *Commemorations: The Politics of National Identity*, ed. John R. Gillis (Princeton: Princeton University Press, 1994), 258–80. Hannah Arendt, *The Origins of Totalitarianism* (Orlando: Harcourt, 1973); Carl Friedrich and Zbigniew Brzezinski, *Totalitarian Dictatorship and Autocracy* (Cambridge, Mass.: Harvard University Press, 1965).

[43] The rigid, totalitarian and monolithic representation of the communist era in Hungary has been widely utilised in political discourse since the 1990s. One of the most striking examples of this view is the House of Terror museum in Budapest, which presents an undifferentiated image of the forty years and merges the Stalinist government of the early 1950s with Kádár's Hungary in the 1980s. See Zsolt K. Horváth and Zsófia Frazon, 'A Megsértett Magyarország. A Terror Háza Mint Tárgybemutatás, Emlékmű és Politikai Rítus', *Regio*, no. 4 (2002): 303–47; Péter Apor, 'Eurocommunism: Commemorating Communism in Contemporary Eastern Europe', in *European Memory? Contested Histories and Politics of Remembrance*, ed. Malgorzata Pakier and Bo Strath (New York and Oxford: Berghahn Books, 2010), 233–47.

referred to, and often perceived, the complex system of governance as one unit. As the structure of the state and party were entwined in a complicated web of responsibilities and functions,[44] the two words were often used interchangeably in the vernacular. Moreover, the government also invested significantly in appearing homogeneous, organised and efficient in its communication. Therefore, in a study of perceived and performed roles and responsibilities of state and society it remains a useful unit of analysis.

The research specifically focuses on epidemics in Hungary between the years 1952 and 1963. During these years, the country saw a rapid growth in the rate of incidence of polio, the arrival of a vaccine from the West, followed by one from the East, and the challenge of long-term care for disabled children. Meanwhile, this troubled decade of Hungarian history witnessed drastic changes in the number and composition of its population, the transformation of its industrial and agricultural production, and the greatest political upheaval of the century. The year 1952 marked the first major epidemic of the century, which initiated a significant political and medical response, while 1963 brought the end of involvement on the part of the state with the successful elimination of the disease and the closing down of the specialised treatment centre.

The periodisation of this study might be somewhat surprising for those whose eyes are trained to see Eastern European history of the early communist era divided into clear and distinct eras: in Hungary's case the communist takeover between 1945 and 1948; the Stalinist era from 1948 to 1956; the 1956 revolution and its aftermath until 1963; and the consolidation of the Kádár-era (with the introduction of the New Economic Mechanism, a major economic reform in 1968) that lasted until the late 1980s.[45]

Polio challenges this periodisation of history.[46] The disease was very much present in the Stalinist era, in the days of the revolution and in the early years of the Kádár regime and, in accordingly, so was political and social concern about it. Polio's history thus in many ways disregards the watersheds that are traditionally held as dividing the early history of communist regimes in Eastern Europe, and more visibly it overrides decisive moments in Hungarian history. I do not wish to claim that such periodisations are superfluous. One cannot minimise the effect of the 1956 revolution on the lives of those who were also touched by epidemic diseases, and, of course, a clear difference can be traced

---

[44] Csanádi, 'Honnan Tovább? A Pártállam és az Átalakulás'.
[45] See for instance the periodization of Romsics, *Hungary in the Twentieth Century*; Pittaway, *Eastern Europe 1939–2000*.
[46] Similarly, Zsuzsa Gille has contested conventional periodisation of the socialist era in Hungary through a conceptual lens different from economy or political institutions, namely waste regimes. Zsuzsa Gille, *From the Cult of Waste to the Trash Heap of History: The Politics of Waste in Socialist and Postsocialist Hungary* (Bloomington and Indianapolis: Indiana University Press, 2007).

between political and social life in the Stalinist era and the later years. The way polio does affect our view of the history of the 1950s and early 1960s is that it directs attention to continuities and consistencies where traditionally we expect ruptures. The virus spread among children regardless of the current political stance on collectivisation or counter-revolutionary actions, and continuously initiated responses from society and government. Moreover, the particularities of the disease often gave opportunities to individuals and governing bodies to look for cooperation where the usual course of action was animosity, or to go against their own proclaimed policies and ideologies if the need for disease prevention and treatment dictated.

Looking at the personal experiences of polio in Hungary, the book turns to the interaction of medical staff, parents and children in the prevention and treatment of the disease. On the one hand, I explore the particular social and political context of Hungary in the 1950s, in which patients, parents and physicians operated. My analysis is influenced by studies on the relationship of the party-state and factory workers.[47] As historian Mark Pittaway has pointed out, 'working-class Eastern Europeans were not simply acted upon by the operation of dictatorial state power, but played a role in state formation'; he describes the complicated relationship of communist states and societies as 'characterized by consent, accommodation and conflict that varied from locality to locality, state to state, period to period'.[48] My aim is to probe this relationship through other segments of society, ones that were not the pro-claimed centre of the regime's rhetoric and policies. This level of analysis also makes it possible to explore continuities and ruptures in medical professions,[49] processes that greatly influenced access to knowledge and treatment options for many children.

On the other hand, through the personal experiences of polio treatment in Hungary I investigate post-war concepts of production and the able body. The ideal of the worker-citizen glaring at the everyday onlooker from murals, statues, magazines and posters had a significant effect on setting goals for

---

[47] László Kürti, '"Red Csepel": Working Youth in a Socialist Firm', *East European Quarterly* 23, no. 4 (1990); Mária Schadt, *'Feltörekvő, Dolgozó Nő'. Nők az Ötvenes Években* (Budapest: Pannónia, 2005); Mark Pittaway, 'The Reproduction of Hierarchy: Skill, Working-Class Culture and the State in Early Socialist Hungary', *Journal of Modern History* 74, no. 4 (2002): 737–69; Eszter Zsófia Tóth, 'The Memory of the State Award in the Narratives of Women Workers' in *Regimes and Transformations: Hungary in the Twentieth Century*, ed. István Feitl and Balázs Sipos (Budapest: Napvilág, 2005); Sándor Horváth, ed. *Mindennapok Rákosi És Kádár Korában: Új Utak a Szocialista Korszak Kutatásában* (Budapest: Nyitott Könyvműhely, 2008).

[48] Mark Pittaway, 'Introduction: Workers and Socialist States in Postwar Central and Eastern Europe', *International Labor and Working-Class History* 68, Fall (2005): 1–8, 1.

[49] Mária Kovács, *Liberal Professions and Illiberal Politics: Hungary from the Habsburgs to the Holocaust* (Washington: Woodrow Wilson Center Press, 1994); Hoffman, 'Professional Autonomy Reconsidered', 1997.

rehabilitation treatment, on choosing educational options for polio patients and on the way children, later grown up to be disabled adults, thought about their place in society. Disability historians like Catherine Kudlick have argued for the use of disability 'as a key defining social category on a par with race, class and gender',[50] and I use this lens to analyse the meaning of production and how it was paired with the relegation of disabled bodies to seclusion both physically and socially. Furthermore, I look at the way in which the obsession with production affected the changing meaning of polio itself. In this I draw upon the work of a wide array of scholars, such as Susan Sontag, Charles Rosenberg, Emily Martin and Daniel Wilson, who have shown how the metaphors, names and meanings used in conceptualising illness and its effect on the body shape medical treatment, the experience of disease and the place of the patient in society.[51]

Scientists, parents and children worked within and challenged the political, social and medical systems in which their lives were integrated. Virologists and physicians drew on their transnational relations and personal network to be participants in international conferences and study trips and to gain knowledge of cutting-edge research and technology. Parents smuggled vaccines, if necessary; children openly resisted medical procedures; and both crossed the Iron Curtain in hope of a better treatment option. Patients obtained skills in operating intricate respiratory machines and reinterpreted childhood games to include all levels of mobility. When the state lost interest in polio, they became depositories of medical knowledge.

Polio shaped and overrode Cold War policies and forged unlikely alliances. Doctors and politicians watched the rising numbers of epidemic cases with growing concern, while parents feared the summer lest it should bring polio. Even today, over two decades after the end of the Cold War, the memory of the fear that children might contract the disease in swimming pools and other summertime activities is still very much alive, as it has been handed down to generations with no immediate experience of polio.

With its focus on polio in 1950s Hungary, this book shifts attention from the two superpowers to focus on the circulation of medical knowledge and technology in global contexts. It uncovers cooperation where animosity would be expected, and finds continuities in the place of traditional watersheds in Cold

---

[50] Catherine J. Kudlick, 'Disability History: Why We Need Another "Other"', *American Historical Review* 108, no. 3 (2003).
[51] Susan Sontag, *Illness as Metaphor and AIDS and Its Metaphors* (New York: Picador, 1990); Emily Martin, *Flexible Bodies: Tracking Immunity in American Culture-from the Days of Polio to the Age of AIDS* (Boston: Beacon Press, 1994); Daniel J. Wilson, *Living with Polio: The Epidemic and Its Survivors* (Chicago: University of Chicago Press, 2005); Charles Rosenberg and Janet Golden, eds., *Framing Disease: Studies in Cultural History*, 2nd edn (New Brunswick: Rutgers University Press, 1997).

War history. Thus, the book aims to enrich our understanding of what the Cold War was, among whom it was 'fought', and in what ways it did and did not affect public health policies, research and medical treatment. It asks if it was possible to operate outside the framework of the Cold War in countries fully involved in the political and military conflict.

The history of polio in Hungary matters. It presents another face of the global Cold War, a new perspective on our view of communist societies and an important moment in the history of medicine and global public health, all of which have repercussions for the present. More importantly, this history links the personal, national and institutional stories of an effort to meet a global epidemic challenge in an increasingly divided world all too familiar to today's reader.

1   The Power of Polio

The year 1952 was a tumultuous one. It saw the Cold War gain full speed: the United States detonated its first hydrogen bomb, while Britain announced that it was now in the possession of an atomic bomb. East Germany started forming the National People's Army and the B-52 aircraft flew for the first time. As the division of the world between East and West deepened, another crisis was unfolding as the summer of 1952 arrived: a severe polio epidemic wave swept over the world, leaving tens of thousands of children disabled and thousands dead. The worst epidemic outbreak in the history of the United States and Denmark, polio in 1952 marked a turning point in the history of the disease. The severe epidemic boosted vaccine research in the former country, and prompted innovation in respiratory technology in the latter, making it the European centre of polio research.

The epidemic wave also hit Hungary, a small Eastern European country whose society was still struggling with the aftermath of a destructive war and whose communist government was grappling with the task of laying down the foundations of a new era. The epidemic started with an outbreak in North-Eastern Hungary,[1] a region that continued to show the highest incident rates of polio throughout the decade. Cases of poliomyelitis started rising in June and peaked in August and September, paralysing nearly 500 patients and leaving 29 dead[2] out of a total population of roughly 9.5 million.[3] This was the first major epidemic since 1948. At first glance, the numbers do not seem to be particularly high, especially compared to the over 21,000 paralytic cases in the United States[4]

---

[1] Gábor Debrődi, 'A Mesterséges Lélegeztetés és az Újraélesztési Eljárások Története Magyarországon a Felvilágosult Abszolutizmus Korától az 1960-as Évekig, a Hazai Modern Mentéstudomány (Oxyologia) Megszületéséig', *Kharón* 7, no. 4 (2003): 52–76.

[2] Károly Nagy, *Medical Microbiology* (Budapest: Institute of Medical Microbiology, Semmelweis University, 2008).

[3] The population of Hungary in 1952 was 9,453,000 according to the figures of the Hungarian Central Statistical Office. Központi Statisztikai Hivatal, 'Népesség, Népmozgalom (1949–)' (Budapest: Központi Statisztikai Hivatal, 2012).

[4] *Poliomyelitis*, vol. 74, Health Information Series (Washington, D.C.: U.S. Department of Health, Education and Welfare. Public Health Service, 1963).

or the 3,000 cases in Copenhagen alone.[5] However, this was the first instance in which the healthcare system of the new People's Republic of Hungary was faced with such an epidemic crisis.

Following general guidelines of contagious diseases, polio patients needed to be quarantined for four weeks, preferably in one of the six infectious disease wards in the country, but if the paralysis was not too severe home care was also possible. There were two iron lungs operating in Hungary at the time, both in the László hospital in Budapest, therefore all respiratory cases needed to be directed to the capital.[6]

It soon became clear that an epidemic of this volume challenged the meagre resources of post-war Hungary. In a meeting prompted by the epidemic, the leading epidemiologists and hospital directors of Budapest agreed that infectious disease and post-treatment facilities were badly needed for the rehabilitation of polio patients. The absence of 400 beds in the infectious disease hospital – they had been destroyed in a bombing in the war – was particularly felt and resulted in crowded conditions in time of epidemics.[7] As a report from the Health Ministry pointed out in 1953, 'In the war the [Hungarian] healthcare network collapsed'. An epidemiological network was put in place in 1951 and the number of doctors was constantly increasing, but hospital buildings had not been renovated since the 1930s and shortages in beds, medical equipment, food and heating were everyday concerns for most medical institutions.[8]

In these days Hungary, along with other Eastern European countries, was not only facing the challenges of recuperating from a devastating war, but also undergoing a major transformation that ranged from the political system to the social makeup. Eastern Europe was the hardest hit area of the Second World War: millions of its population killed in concentration camps and vigorous ethnic cleansing campaigns, its cities and bridges bombed, its infrastructure destroyed. Rebuilding the country coincided with the construction of a new political and social structure. The 'communist takeover' in 1949[9] marked the

---

[5] H. C. A. Lassen, 'The Epidemic of Poliomyelitis in Copenhagen, 1952', *Proceedings of the Royal Society of Medicine* 47 (1953): 67–71.

[6] 'Járványos Gyermekbénulás Elleni Védekezés.' Budapest: Budapest City Archives, Fővárosi Tanács Egészségügyi Osztálya, 10. doboz, B/8/2558/952.VIII.19, 1952.

[7] 'Jegyzőkönyv a Folyó Évi Október 24-Én Pénteken Délután 3 Órakkor Megtartott Járványügyi Ankéton Elhangzott Felszólalásokról.' Budapest: Budapest City Archives, Fővárosi Tanács Egészségügyi Osztálya, 10. doboz Tanácsi iratok gyűjteménye, B/8/3280/952, 1952.

[8] Antal Greiner. 'Magyarország Egészségügyi Helyzete 1953. Évi Adatok Alapján.' Budapest: National Archives of Hungary, Simonovits István iratai, Egészségügyi Minisztérium, XIX-C-2-s Box 20, 7/1953, 1953.

[9] On recent critical histories of the communist takeover that argue against the seeming inevitability, uniformity and strictly oppressive nature of the communist regime changes see Kenez, 'The Hungarian Communist Party and the Catholic Church 1945–1948'; Mark Pittaway, 'The

beginning of a new era, as the Cold War unfolded and the Hungarian Stalinist regime headed by Mátyás Rákosi set out to build the communist People's Republic. Forced collectivisation, show trials and empty shelves accompanied the construction of a classless society.

Polio might seem a trivial matter against this background, especially since, in terms of numbers, it was not a major health threat. Even at the climax of an epidemic, the increased incidence numbers were not particularly high when compared to the morbidity and mortality of other diseases. For example, in 1959, the year of the second largest epidemic in Hungary, ten times as many people were diagnosed with hepatitis and twice as many patients died as a result than with polio. In the same year, nearly four times as many people fell ill with influenza and its complications, with a death toll 140 times larger than that of polio[10]. Moreover, among the causes of death, infectious diseases on the whole ranked quite low: in 1960 they were responsible for 4.4 per cent of total deaths in the Hungarian population, while cancer claimed 17 per cent and 40.3 per cent died due to cardiovascular diseases.[11]

However, the Hungarian government invested significantly in the disease. While Hungary came to see much worse epidemics than the one it faced in 1952, the year marked the beginning of the state's intensive and growing interest in the prevention and treatment of the disease, which culminated in the latter half of the decade. The importance of polio overarched regime changes, revolutions and retributions. Moreover, by the end of the decade the Hungarian communist government would sidestep conventional domestic and foreign policies in order to curb the disease.

Hungarian involvement in the prevention and treatment of polio was part of a broader process in the epidemic management of polio that spanned the globe in its range. The disease had a tremendous effect not only on Hungarian politics, citizens and scientific communities, but also on societies from New Zealand to Brazil to the Netherlands. Polio created spaces of international collaboration in which Cold War politics played out in unexpected ways. Throughout the 1950s vaccines, iron lungs, people and practices crossed the Iron Curtain back and forth in a mutual effort to prevent and treat the disease.

Politics of Legitimacy and Hungary's Postwar Transition', *Contemporary European History* 13, no. 4 (2004): 453–75; Katherine Lebow, 'Public Works, Private Lives: Youth Brigades in Nowa Huta in the 1950s', ibid. 10, no. 2 (2001): 199–219; Benjamin Frommer, 'Retribution as Legitimation: The Uses of Political Justice in Postwar Czechoslovakia', ibid. 13, no. 477–492 (2004).

[10] Központi Statisztikai Hivatal, 'Egészségügyi Helyzet 1963', 86.

[11] András Klinger, 'Magyarország Népesedése az Elmúlt Negyven Évben', in *Magyarország Társadalomtörténete III. (1945–1989)*, ed. Nikosz Fokasz and Antal Örkény (Budapest: Új Mandátum, 1999), 65.

Where did the power of polio to meddle with Cold War politics, initiate international cooperation and jumble the tasks and responsibilities of family, medical staff and state come from? How did a disease whose effect was never great in numbers gain so much attention from the scientific community, governments and international organisations? What was so special about this particular disease?

The answer lies in the details of the important aspects of poliomyelitis: it was a relatively new disease; it was present across the globe; it affected children; and it caused disability. Polio epidemics received especially heightened attention in the 1950s from scientists to bureaucrats in Hungary and elsewhere because the particularities of the disease amalgamated with the particularities of the post-war era. Polio challenged demographic goals, ideas of modern production, medical theories and practice, and spoke to a post-war confidence in technological and scientific progress and a renewed obsession with children in propaganda and humanitarian work.

The four factors discussed below played equally important roles in forming the Hungarian and international response to polio. In order to understand the significance of the disease in the 1950s and early 1960s and its Cold War history, we need to take a broader look at the attributes of polio that created spaces of cooperation and brought together unlikely allies.

A Twentieth-Century Disease: New Challenges Unite

Poliomyelitis was a relatively new disease in the mid-twentieth century. Severe and widespread epidemic waves had started appearing quite recently, most notably in Sweden in the late nineteenth century and in the United States in the early twentieth century. The rising number of cases gave way to an increase in scientific interest, as virologists and physicians tried to understand the virus and to figure out efficient ways of preventing and treating the disease.

Although polio is usually considered a success story, with the disease eradicated from most countries in the world, this story unfolded rather slowly. As Naomi Rogers argues in her book *Dirt and Disease: Polio before FDR*, 'polio epidemics highlighted tensions between old and new medical theories and practices as physicians, scientists, and the lay public debated the increasing authority of scientific medicine'.[12]

For almost half a century, the virus's point of entry into the human body was debated. The treatment of paralysis caused by polio was not standardised until well into the 1950s and, even then, different schools of thought and concepts

---

[12] Naomi Rogers, *Dirt and Disease: Polio before FDR*, ed. Judith Walzer Leavitt and Morris Vogel, Health and Medicine in American Society (New Brunswick: Rutgers University Press, 1992), 3.

about what counted as an efficient cure clashed regularly. Debates about vaccine efficiency and safety – first with Salk's killed virus vaccine, followed by several live virus vaccines – flared, as did difference of opinions on the right dosage, method of injection and age groups to be vaccinated.

These continuous, ongoing conversations (some more heated than others), the constant uncertainty about the best way to prevent and treat this virus and the new high-tech equipment and specialised knowledge needed by polio research and treatment all played a part in creating a space of intensive scientific interaction. As the following chapters of the dissertation show, this space was perceived as standing above Cold War divisions, and moreover it was a space that was, to certain extent, open to actors outside the medical profession as well.

Scientific Uncertainties

Marking two crucial turning points in the identification of the disease, the name Heine-Medin's disease became commonly used through the first half of the twentieth century; in some parts of the world, like Hungary, the term is still widely used today. In the late eighteenth and early nineteenth centuries, British physicians described the paralysis of the lower extremities in children as a separate disease.[13] One of the groundbreaking works in polio's history was published in 1840 by German orthopaedist Jakob von Heine,[14] who identified this particular type of paralysis as a disease entity and termed it spinal infantile paralysis (*Spinale Kinderlähmung*).[15]

Polio first appeared as an infectious disease in a presentation given by Karl-Oskar Medin, a Swedish physician at an international conference in Berlin in 1890. Provincial doctor Nils August Bergenholtz identified the first epidemics of infantile paralysis in Sweden in 1881, and the Scandinavian country experienced several epidemic waves before the turn of the century. Medin based his findings on an epidemic in 1887 and concluded that polio was an acute infectious disease, but not a contagious one. At the time concepts of contagious and non-contagious diseases were not clear-cut categories, therefore while considering it to be an epidemic disease, 'Medin thought of polio as caused by miasmatic conditions.'[16]

[13] J. M. S. Pearce, 'Poliomyelitis (Heine-Medin Disease)', *Journal of Neurology Neurosurgery and Psychiatry*, no. 76 (2005): 128.
[14] Jakob von Heine, *Beobachtungen über Lähmungszustände der untern Extremitäten und deren Behandlung: Mit 7 Steindrucktafeln* (Stuttgart: Köhler, 1840).
[15] Jakob von Heine, *Spinale Kinderlähmung: Monographie* (Stuttgart: J. G. Cottascher Verlag, 1860).
[16] Per Axelsson, '"Do Not Eat Those Apples; They've Been on the Ground!": Polio Epidemics and Preventive Measures, Sweden 1880s–1940s', *Asclepio. Revista de Historia de la Medicina y la Ciencia* 61, no. 1 (2009): 23–38, at 30.

It was in 1908 that Austrian physicians Karl Landsteiner and Erwin Popper identified the poliovirus as the cause of poliomyelitis.[17] Acting upon the news of the virus isolation, Simon Flexner, director of the Rockefeller Institute for Medical Research, took on experimental poliomyelitis; in 1908 he inoculated monkeys with human tissue containing poliovirus, and was able to pass polio from monkey to monkey as well.[18] Moving the study of the disease to the laboratory and the problem of applying findings to epidemics that played out in various populations was a characteristic of polio research throughout the next fifty to sixty years.

In the early twentieth century, polio epidemics became particularly severe in the United States. In 1916, Americans were faced with the world's then worst outbreak, counting 27,000 cases, with 8,900 in New York City alone.[19] This severe epidemic marked the beginning of the American history of polio, which soon became connected with the figure of Franklin D. Roosevelt, whose person determined the image of polio victims in pre-Second World War United States.[20] While hiding his disability in his public appearances, Roosevelt played an important part in the formation of American polio research and treatment, with the foundation of Warm Springs, a major treatment centre in Georgia, and the National Foundation for Infantile Paralysis, which provided the financial means for vaccine research and treatment through the March of Dimes.[21] Moreover, the national myth of Roosevelt's success in conquering polio was so pervasive that it greatly influenced polio patients' thinking of their own disease and disability, either by aligning with the president's myth, or challenging it.[22]

In this sense, polio in the United States was peculiar when seen in an international comparison. The personal involvement of a highly esteemed political leader was unique, and in some ways the funding of scientific research and medical treatment as well. In societies where free healthcare provided by the state was an organisational cornerstone and where discussions about the health of children were framed through paternalism, fundraising and individual donation were entirely missing from the steps taken against polio epidemics. This does not mean, of course, that citizens outside the United States were not called upon in one way or another to participate in the effort to curb the

---

[17] John R. Paul, *A History of Poliomyelitis*, Yale Studies in the History of Science and Medicine (New Haven: Yale University Press, 1971), 98.

[18] Saul Benison, 'Speculation and Experimentation in Early Poliomyelitis Research', *Clio Medica* 10, no. 1 (1975): 1–22.

[19] Rogers, *Dirt and Disease*, 10–11.

[20] Daniel J. Wilson, 'A Crippling Fear: Experiencing Polio in the Era of Fdr', *Bulletin of the History of Medicine* 72, no. 3 (1998): 464–95.

[21] See chapters 2 and 3 in Oshinsky, *Polio: An American Story*.

[22] Amy L. Fairchild, 'The Polio Narratives: Dialogues with FDR', *The Bulletin of the History of Medicine* 75 (2001): 488–534.

disease. Rather, the differences and similarities between the various experiences of the disease comprised overlapping and constantly moving maps of what polio meant and how it was approached by politics, society and science. Polio cases had been recorded in Hungary from the end of the nineteenth century and epidemics had been observed from 1911 onwards. From the following year, polio became a reportable disease in the country and the Health Minister ordered patients diagnosed with polio to be quarantined for three weeks, along with children in the patient's household. After the three weeks of seclusion, the patient's immediate environment was to be disinfected.[23] The regulation shows that polio was already perceived in Hungary as a public health threat in the early twentieth century and that the attempts at prevention followed the usual protocol of contagious diseases. The exact way the virus spread, however, would not be agreed upon until quite a while after the introduction of these early prophylaxis strategies.

The virus's entry point into the body was debated for over half a century. Flexner was an early proponent of the theory that the disease infected through the nasal mucus.[24] Coming from a microbiological approach, Flexner based his theory on the animal model. He succeeded in infecting monkeys by wiping their nasal passages with infected material in 1910.[25] The conclusion, that this was the mode of infection among humans as well, prompted a field trial in Alabama in 1936 where a nose spray designed to chemically block the nasal mucosa was tested – the trial closed as inconclusive in 1937. Meanwhile, in the same year, with pressure from the public due to an unfolding epidemic, the Ontario government in Canada conducted yet another trial to test the nasal spray that was already in use by many private physicians, with similar results.[26] The enthusiasm that initially surrounded this prevention technique did not spread further and the method was not tested or used elsewhere again. Following the unsuccessful trials and the lack of evidence for the nasal route infection, the theory was highly contested in the late 1930s and abandoned by the early 1940s.[27]

Other theories were more persistent. Armed with the relatively new germ theory of disease and the obsession with cleanliness it brought to the everyday

[23] Rezső Hargitai and Kiss, *A Gyermekbénulás Elleni Küzdelem: Beszámoló egy Ma Már Múlttá Váló Rettegett Betegség Ellen Folytatott Hősies Küzdelemről és Felszámolásának Lehetőségéről: A Szent László Kórház Centenáriumára Készült Összeállítás* (Budapest: Literatura Medica, 1994).

[24] Margaret L. Grimshaw, 'Scientific Specialization and the Poliovirus Controversy in the Years before World War II', *Bulletin of the History of Medicine* 69, no. 1 (1995): 44–65, at pp. 46–47.

[25] Paul, *A History of Poliomyelitis*, 243.

[26] Christopher J. Rutty, 'The Middle Class Plague: Epidemic Polio and the Canadian State, 1936–37', *Canadian Bulletin of Medical History* 13, no. 2 (1996): 277–314, at pp. 291–95.

[27] Grimshaw, 'Scientific Specialization and the Poliovirus Controversy in the Years before World War II'.

perception of diseases and health,[28] researchers as well as the lay public looked to that profound connection between filth and disease. As early as the 1916 New York epidemic, evidence suggested that polio preferred healthy, well-nourished children in affluent homes with good sanitation to impoverished households and filthy neighbourhoods.[29] Even as experience seemed to contradict the theory and new epidemiological thinking gained momentum, ridding households of flies, washing fruit and emphasising the cleanliness of the home continued to be a major part of prevention efforts well into the 1950s in many parts of the world.

Early twentieth century researchers were puzzled by the fact that polio can spread in a relatively wide geographical area with considerable speed while not producing a particularly high incidence rate. The conclusion was that there had to be 'abortive cases' of polio, meaning that the disease did not cause paralysis in everyone who contracted it. Based on observations of the 1905 Scandinavian epidemic, Ivar Wickman (a student of Medin) claimed that there were far more non-paralytic cases than paralytic ones and that these 'abortive' cases played a key part in spreading the disease.[30]

Equally puzzling was the seasonal nature of the epidemics. Polio usually arrived recurrently at a particular time of year, which also affected the cause that was attributed to the spread of polio. This attribute added to the unknown or debated aspects of the disease. An analysis of the 1939 epidemic in the Eastern Hungarian city of Debrecen[31] published in a public health journal in 1941 gives an overview of possible reasons, none of which, it concludes, can serve as a sole explanation for the pattern. Infection by insects, gastro-intestinal infection, the presence of dust in the dry summer weather, the amount of precipitation and dampness and even the general direction of wind were all raised and discarded, leaving the author with the conclusion that there was definitely an observable pattern in climate regarding polio epidemics, but no sufficient explanation to account for it. Moreover, the author felt the need to remark that 'the practice of meteoropathology is tiresome and the results obtained do not reflect the amount of work invested in the process'.[32] While finding a plausible explanation could be useful in developing adequate prevention measures, the results acquired in this kind of research were simply not worth the effort.

[28] Nancy Tomes, *The Gospel of Germs: Men, Women, and the Microbe in American Life* (Cambridge, Mass.: Harvard University Press, 1998).
[29] Rogers, *Dirt and Disease*, 161–63.
[30] Tony Gould, *A Summer Plague: Polio and its Survivors* (New Haven: Yale University Press, 1995), 112–13.
[31] László Mecseky, 'Meteorológiai Vonatkozások a Heine-Medin-Kór Epidemiológiájában', *Népegészségügy*, no. 14 (1941).
[32] Ibid. 9.

In the meantime, the scientific uncertainty that surrounded the recurrent spread of the disease trickled down to the public perception of environmental threats that could cause polio. Children were warned against over-exhaustion when playing outside, public swimming pools were to be avoided in the heat, fruit was to be thoroughly washed and homes were to be kept particularly clean. A theory in New Zealand blamed the inefficient clothing of children during the summer – the sudden changes in temperature taxed children's bodies, which were clad in short socks and short trousers or skirts, leaving their legs exposed to the elements.[33] Polio did not arrive in the summer months in every corner of the world, though. In Sweden, it was the autumn months that suffered the peak of epidemics, thus giving polio its popular name, 'the Autumn Ghost',[34] and prompting people to avoid falling leaves and rotting fruit in order to prevent polio.[35]

Vaccine Development

The scientific uncertainties surrounding polio continued well into the post-war era. Whenever one issue seemed to be resolved and a unison in scientific explanation achieved, three others jumped into its place. Even the development and spread of vaccines in the 1950s did not really help to stabilise the knowledge about polio. One of the key remaining questions to be answered was about how many strains of poliovirus there were. Australian and American researchers identified two strains of the virus and concluded, with animal experiments, that surviving polio of one strain did not provide immunity to the other. Confirming and identifying the number of strains was crucial, therefore, in developing an effective vaccine. This tedious and repetitive work was conducted in individual American laboratories in 1948 with funds from the National Foundation for Infantile Paralysis (NFIP).[36]

Another important step in providing the conditions for vaccine research in the 1950s was the breakthrough of virus culturing. In 1949, John Enders and his colleagues at Harvard University succeeded in culturing poliovirus *in vitro*, that is, in a test tube. Growing poliovirus under laboratory conditions had been possible for decades, though only in the nervous tissue of monkeys, which is dangerous to life when injected into humans and therefore was not an option to use in vaccine production. The intervention of Enders and his colleagues was to use tissues, among them kidney, in culturing that were safe for human use.

---

[33] Ross, 'A History of Poliomyelitis in New Zealand'.
[34] Per Axelsson, *Höstens Spöke. De Svenska Polioepidemiernas Historia* (Stockholm: Carlssons, 2004).
[35] '"Do Not Eat Those Apples; They've Been on the Ground!": Polio Epidemics and Preventive Measures, Sweden 1880s–1940s', 37.
[36] Daniel J. Wilson, *Polio* (Portsmouth: Greenwood Publishing Group, 2009).

This feat earned them a Nobel Prize in Physiology or Medicine in 1954 'for their discovery of the ability of poliomyelitis viruses to grow in cultures of various types of tissue'.[37]

As polio epidemics appeared with more frequency and with higher and higher incidence rates around the world, vaccine development became especially pressing and therefore had priority in securing funds. In the United States, where both the killed virus vaccine (by Jonas Salk) and the three live virus vaccines (by Hilary Koprowsky, Albert Sabin and H. R. Cox) were developed, the majority of the funding came from the NFIP. The first vaccine to be widely produced and distributed was the Salk vaccine, which induced immunity to the disease with the help of inactivated or killed poliovirus.

Developing the vaccine was one important step. Establishing its efficiency was quite another. American authorities moved quite fast when it came to approving and licensing the Salk vaccine;[38] it took them a mere two hours after Thomas Francis, director of the University of Michigan Poliomyelitis Vaccine Evaluation Centre, officially announced the results of the field trial involving 1.8 million schoolchildren on 12 April 1954.[39] However, in the following years, based on varying experience of the Salk vaccine around the world, its efficacy would be debated in the pages of medical journals well into the 1960s.

Live poliovirus vaccines fared even worse in creating consensus in vaccine efficiency and, more importantly, safety. Fears that vaccines made with attenuated live viruses could cause or spread polio instead of curbing the disease were persistent throughout the development of the live vaccines in the 1950s and early 1960s by Albert Sabin, Hilary Koprowski and H. R. Cox. The vaccine trials of the three vaccines, spanning five continents, aimed to soothe reservations about safety and efficiency, but, as Chapter 5 shows, were far from successful in bringing about consensus in the scientific community.

Questions about vaccine evaluation kept appearing with every trial and after every outbreak of polio. New answers to a new disease created yet another set of uncertainties. How would one translate laboratory results into effects on whole populations of a disease that came haphazardly and with varying force? How could one establish the length of the vaccines' protective power when such a short time had elapsed between the development, trial and widespread

---

[37] The Nobel Foundation, 'The Nobel Prize in Physiology or Medicine 1954. John F. Enders, Thomas H. Weller, Fredeick C. Robbins', www.nobelprize.org/nobel_prizes/medicine/laureates/1954/.

[38] The Secretary of Health, Education and Welfare was responsible for giving licence, acting on the recommendation of the Surgeon General. The latter was advised by the National Institute of Health and the Division of Biological Standards. Subcommittee on Health and Safety of the Committee on Interstate and Foreign Commerce, *Polio Vaccines*, First session on developments with respect to the manufacture of live virus polio vaccine and results of utilization of killed virus polio vaccine, 16 March 1961, 3–4.

[39] Oshinsky, *Polio: An American Story*, 203.

use of the serum? In the pages of medical journals, at international polio conferences and at personal laboratory visits, virologists, paediatricians and public health officials exchanged experiences, crunched numbers and debated results to establish proper prophylactic and treatment strategies for their respective countries and ultimately to aim for a consensus in curbing the disease worldwide.

The increasing preoccupation with polio prompted the application of new scientific methods, such as Wickman's statistical analysis and Flexner's use of the animal model in constructing knowledge about the virus. The conflicting theories and the scientific uncertainty that enveloped the disease opened yet new arenas of cooperation between virologists, therapists and physicians in a world already densely interwoven with an international scientific network,[40] and kept them in place during an unfolding Cold War.

In order to plan and execute prevention methods, develop vaccines and provide state of the art treatment for a new epidemiological phenomenon, scientific communities needed to be constantly in touch with each other, share new experiences and knowledge and cooperate in figuring out the next step. The lack of widely accepted standard procedures and the presence of intense debates in the fields of virology, medicine and public health ensured that a space for exchange and cooperation existed continuously, disregarding the barriers erected after the Second World War between East and West.

While scientific uncertainties were, in some ways, continuously present throughout the first half of the century, the meaning of polio changed over time. From its existence as a rhapsodically appearing and puzzling disease in the early twentieth century, it became a major threat to future populations by the early 1950s. In the early 1960s the disease changed meaning yet again and became synonymous with scientific triumph over nature and a symbol for international cooperation.

A Global Issue

Polio epidemics not only increased in their severity over time in the first half of the twentieth century, but also in their geographical scope. Outside Europe and North America, where polio outbreaks began to be registered in the late

---

[40] See for instance Anne Marie Moulin, 'The Pasteur Institute's International Network: Scientific Innovations and French Tropisms', in *Transnational Intellectual Networks. Forms of Academic Knowledge and the Search for Cultural Identities*, ed. Christophe Charle et al. (Frankfurt: Campus, 2004), 134–64; Clifford Rosenberg, 'The International Politics of Vaccine Testing in Interwar Algiers', *American Historical Review* 117, no. 3 (2012): 671–97; Joao Rangel de Almeida, 'The 1851 International Sanitary Conference and the Construction of an International Sphere of Public Health' (PhD thesis, University of Edinburgh, 2012).

nineteenth and early twentieth centuries, the disease made its appearance on a large scale in Africa, Asia, Latin America and Oceania in the 1920s.[41]

Research Cooperation

While global cooperation in polio research, prevention and treatment reached its climax in the 1950s, an international exchange of knowledge and specimens had existed from the outset. For instance, when asked for poliovirus samples to facilitate European research, Flexner sent specimens to Dr Arnold Netter, a French clinician, through personal contacts.[42] Interwar Hungarian publications on polio demonstrate an extensive knowledge of contemporary epidemiological research, and place their findings in the context of the up-to-date data and theories published by German, French, Romanian, Swedish, American and British colleagues.[43]

With the creation of the United Nations and the World Health Organisation (WHO), international scientific cooperation received new impetus. The WHO expressed interest in international research on polio from the very beginning of its existence. At the suggestion of the French delegation, who emphasised that polio should be studied by an international group of virologists, epidemiologists and clinical experts, the First World Health Assembly passed a resolution to investigate the disease and to base its report on international conferences.[44]

In the same year that the WHO held its founding meeting, virologists and public health delegates from 28 countries came together to discuss the crippling disease. The 1948 First International Poliomyelitis Conference in New York was funded by the National Foundation for Infantile Paralysis (NFIP), which was celebrating its tenth anniversary.[45] The conference covered a wide range of subjects related to polio, among them polio's global issues. The papers and discussions emphasised the presence of polio across the continents and the severe problems it raised in medical care, economy and social stability. Some papers followed arguments much along the ideas articulated a century before at the 1851 International Sanitary Conferences, the first international public health meetings: the economic reverberations of an epidemic; the feasibility of quarantine from the perspective of cost and its effect on trade;

---

[41] Matthew Smallman-Raynor, *Poliomyelitis: Emergence to Eradication*, Oxford Geographical and Environmental Studies (Oxford and New York: Oxford University Press, 2006), 192.

[42] Benison, 'Speculation and Experimentation in Early Poliomyelitis Research', 4.

[43] Jenő Barla-Szabó, 'A Heine-Medin-Kór Kezelése Lyssa Ellenes Oltásokkal', *Orvosi Hetilap*, no. 22 (1933): 465–66; Elemér Hainiss, 'A Heine-Medin-Betegség Kóreredete és Kezdeti Szakaszának Jelentősége', *Orvosképzés*, no. 2 (1936), 109–13; Ferenc Székely, 'A Poliomyelitis Anterior Acuta (Heine-Medin) Serumtherapiájáról', *Gyógyászat* 82, no. 32 (1942), 1–8.

[44] María Isabel Porras, María José Báguena, and Rosa Ballester, 'Spain and the International Scientific Conferences on Polio', *Dynamis* 30 (2010): 91–118.

[45] Ibid. 102.

and the question of submitting political independence to epidemic control in the name of efficiency.[46] Soon, a specifically European organisation followed in the footsteps of the International Congress and the European Association against Poliomyelitis was formed in 1951. Its first symposium was held in 1953 in Copenhagen,[47] a year after one of the most severe polio epidemics in the world, which had pushed Denmark to the forefront of European polio research and treatment.

Both the International Conferences and the Symposia of the European Association for Poliomyelitis became regularly occurring events. The former met every three years until 1960 and all of its meetings were funded by the NFIP. It would seem, then, that polio occupied a similar space in the Cold War politics of the United States to malaria control, in line with Marcos Cueto's argument. From the analysis of malaria eradication efforts in the 1950s in Latin America, Cueto argues that malaria prevention turned into a political tool of the Cold War in the hands of international agencies, the Rockefeller Foundation and the United States government, both on the rhetorical and the practical level.[48] However, polio did not follow the same pattern.

While it is clear that the NFIP did not fund a string of gigantic international events without a possibly political agenda, the Cold War rhetoric of polio worked in the opposite way to that of malaria. Emphasis was continuously on international cooperation and on standing above the Cold War itself. Moreover, the conferences gave an opportunity for intensive cooperation between researchers across the globe and for the exchange of information and experience of a disease whose laboratory research was hardly affordable for countries with weaker economies. This marked difference in the way these two diseases were handled during the Cold War politics of medicine and public health was at least partly due to the global presence of polio. While malaria affected areas of the world with a particular climate (and which coincided with the geopolitical interest of both East and West), polio was present on both sides of the Iron Curtain and thus acted as an equaliser in scientific exchange and international public health interventions.

Still, national agendas and local politics of science and economy intertwined with transnational goals of disease control: the severe post-war epidemics caught many countries in transformative moments. For instance, the location chosen for the 1954 meeting of the International Poliomyelitis Congress in Rome represented the opening of Italy's medical and professional community

---

[46] Rangel de Almeida, 'The 1851 International Sanitary Conference and the Construction of an International Sphere of Public Health'.

[47] Ballester and Porras, 'La Lucha Europea Contra la Presencia Epidémica de la Poliomielitis: una Reflexión Histórica'.

[48] Cueto, *Cold War, Deadly Fevers*.

after the fascist era and aimed to display the country's economic recuperation through the Marshall Plan.[49] Spain, not being a member of the WHO until 1958, used its participation in the European Symposium from 1954 onwards to promote its unpopular dictatorship in the European public health scene.[50]

It would be a mistake to over-evaluate the universality of the WHO's and Poliomyelitis Conferences' proclaimed goals as neutral and interest-free. The WHO was itself a venue where the Cold War was fought,[51] and decisions of aid and public health assistance were infused with geopolitical and economic interests.[52] It would equally be a mistake to under-value the opportunities that the global presence of the disease created. Individual scientists, who were in many ways hindered by the foreign policies of their governments, could connect or keep existing networks alive in international meetings. Delegates from countries of little geopolitical influence could voice concerns and contribute to a discussion that affected all parties in a roughly equal manner. Based on fresh statistics and detailed information presented at the conferences, as we see in the following chapter, iron lungs flew across the globe as they grouped and regrouped in epidemic areas, undoubtedly saving many lives.

A critical assessment of these spaces of cooperation can show us a more nuanced, and perhaps different, side of Cold War interactions and the role that polio played in forming them. The global presence of the disease, together with the lack of clear answers to it, created room in international public health for an elaborate dance of national agendas and scientific cooperation.

Epidemic Reporting

The World Health Organisation played a central role in epidemiological data collection and management. This task was one of the most powerful tools of the WHO: it encompassed a classification system that would have an effect on trade, travel regulations, aid distribution, markers of progress, national agendas and medical practices. The WHO was not the first to exercise the power of collecting, producing and analysing public health data: international health organisations prior to the founding of the WHO had long-standing involvement with international statistics organisations. The International Statistical Institute compiled the International List of Causes of Death in 1891, which

---

[49] Fantini, 'Polio in Italy'.

[50] Porras et al., 'Spain and the International Scientific Conferences on Polio'.

[51] Theodore M. Brown, Marcos Cueto, and Elizabeth Fee, 'The World Health Organization and the Transition from "International" to "Global" Health', in *Medicine at the Border: Disease, Globalization and Security, 1850 to the Present*, ed. Alison Bashford (Basingstoke: Palgrave Macmillan, 2006), 76–94.

[52] Randall Packard, '"No Other Logical Choice": Global Malaria Eradication and the Politics of International Health in the Post-War Era', *Parassitologia* 40, no. 1–2 (1998): 217–29.

was revised every ten years. In the interwar era the League of Nations developed the lists further (in cooperation with the Statistical Institute). The devastating effects on populations of the First World War and the forced and voluntary migrations in its wake, along with their traditional travelling companions, typhus and cholera, prompted the nascent Health Committee of the League of Nations to organise a more effective method of epidemic data exchange. To this end the *Annual Epidemiological Report and Corrected Statistics of Notifiable Diseases* was founded, with polio among the regularly reported morbidity and mortality rates.[53]

Epidemic reporting and statistical data management really took off after the Second World War, when the list of causes of diseases and death became one of the top priorities of the nascent WHO, which formally adopted the *International Statistical Classification of Diseases, Injuries and Causes of Death* at the First World Health Assembly in 1948.[54] The WHO not only worked out the system in which diseases and causes of death should be viewed, but also intervened directly in the data collection process. Regulations No. 1 of the WHO (also ratified in the First Assembly) set requirements for individual countries for the death certification process, and from 1952, WHO consultants travelled to member states to give 'advice on the institution or improvement of local statistical systems'.[55] From the information gathered by member states and national public health offices, the WHO published a monthly and annual *Epidemic and Vital Statistics Report* in which they included articles,[56] statistical tables on communicable diseases[57] and, later, vaccination statistics.[58]

The way epidemiological reporting worked in reality was a different question. WHO data relied on the collection and management system of national statistics, which could operate with various levels of rigour. Moreover, collecting data on polio was a tricky issue, as the case of Hungary shows. Although polio was considered a significant problem in the 1950s, the analysis of data compilation of polio incidences in Hungary shows a puzzling picture. Currently we cannot be sure about the exact number of people who fell ill with polio in the 1950s, partly because of the peculiarities of polio, partly because of organisational problems. Polio diagnosis remained problematic throughout the decade. Do these numbers then only refer to the children who needed to be

[53] Smallman-Raynor, *Poliomyelitis: Emergence to Eradication*, 194.
[54] *The First Ten Years of the World Health Organization* (Geneva: World Health Organization, 1958), 278.
[55] Ibid. 280.
[56] M. J. Freyche, 'The Incidence of Poliomyelitis in the World, 1947–1949', *Epidemiological and Vital Statistics Report* 4, no. 1 (1951): 3–18.
[57] 'Morbidity Statistics Acute Poliomyelitis', ibid. 14 (1961): 91–117.
[58] 'Number of Persons Immunized against Poliomyelitis', ibid. 11 (1958): 330–31.

hospitalised? Were the registered cases all paralytic? Were all paralytic cases registered? The novelty of the disease, the lack of standards in the diagnostic process and the costly and time-consuming method of virological identification all contributed to uncertainty in reporting. As historian Saul Benison argues, 'physicians at the time, like physicians everywhere, . . . from the point of view of reporting, paid no attention to non-paralytic cases'.[59] The problem persisted in countries like the United States, where, since 1951, epidemic reporting separated paralytic and non-paralytic cases. Some patients did not seek medical care, while others could be underdiagnosed, or simply not reported.[60]

The problem of polio reporting as a widespread phenomenon is also addressed in the WHO report 'Poliomyelitis' from 1955. In relation to polio data compilation in general, the report remarks that:

in certain countries, only cases of the acute paralytic form of the complaint are registered under the heading of 'poliomyelitis'; in addition, even in the most carefully compiled series, diagnostic errors of the order of 14% have been found. Elsewhere, notifications also cover a varying proportion of febrile states with signs of meningeal irritation, without symptoms of spinal or bulbar paralysis, and perhaps abortive forms without manifestations, which can be ascribed to involvement of the central nervous system. In such cases, a clinical diagnosis can only be one of probability, even when it refers to patients who have been in close contact with a confirmed case of poliomyelitis and the possibility of error is very large.[61]

Inaccurate registration and belated reporting further complicated the compilation of statistics in Hungary. Epidemic reporting on polio began in Hungary in 1926, when an outbreak prompted János Bókay, the renowned paediatrician, to persuade the Minister for Welfare and Labour to classify polio as a reportable disease.[62] This reporting, however, was not always up to expectations, and was a cause for frustration as epidemics turned more frequent and more severe. Ottó Rudnai of the National Public Health Institution pointed out the deficiencies in the reporting process in 1952.[63]

The problems, mainly concerning the lack of thoroughness of local physicians in their paperwork, their responsibility to overlap with hospitals and the lack of follow-up from the Health Ministry, seemed persistent throughout the decade. As late as 1959, records indicate the burning necessity of

[59] Saul Benison, 'International Medical Cooperation: Dr. Albert Sabin, Live Poliovirus Vaccine and the Soviets', *Bulletin of the History of Medicine* 56, no. 4 (1982): 460–83, at 461.
[60] Richard L. Bruno, 'Paralytic Versus "Non-Paralytic" Polio: A Distinction without a Difference?', *American Journal of Physical Medicine and Rehabilitation* 79 (2000): 1–9.
[61] Matthieu-Jean Freyche and Johannes Nielsen, 'Incidence of Poliomyelitis since 1920', in *Poliomyelitis*, ed. Robert Debré (Geneva: World Health Organization, 1955), 59–109, at 59.
[62] János Bókay, *Az 1926. évi Heine-Medin-Járvány Csonka-Magyarországban* (Budapest: Pest könyvnyomda részvénytársaság, 1927).
[63] Ottó Rudnai, 'Járványügyi Munkánk Néhány Hiányosságáról', *Népegészségügy*, no. 33 (1952): 343–47.

revising the questionnaire about the incidence of polio.[64] As a result of diagnosing difficulties and lack of rigour in reporting, the political system, which appeared to be efficient at organising and enforcing regular reports on individuals for its secret service, spent a whole decade unable to overcome the chaotic and disorderly reporting practice of a recurring epidemic that threatened the whole population.

In whatever way public health officials interpreted epidemiological data, and regardless of the problems with numbers that we may raise today, polio epidemics were definitely gaining momentum up until the 1960s in Europe, and in many other parts of the world even after that. Whether the numbers can be considered accurate or imprecise, they were consistently growing, and more importantly, the threat of polio was perceived to be growing by parents, the scientific community and the state.

Access to epidemic data across the globe made an expansion of scope in polio research possible. The analysis of incidence rate from Cairo to Tokyo to Greenland provided an opportunity to corroborate theories that were based on the study of a limited geographical area. The observation that paralytic polio was at its worst in social groups that were relatively well off, rather than the expected poor and crammed neighbourhoods where most epidemic diseases flourished, could now be extended on a global scale. Middle class families became first world countries, while slums became equivalent to post-colonial and 'backward' societies.

One of the conclusions drawn about the rapid emergence of polio and the difference in the ways in which it attacked various populations across the globe was that polio went from being endemic with low paralytic rates to epidemic and highly paralytic because of changes in sanitation and lifestyle. Increasing sanitary conditions and personal hygiene reduced the fecal-oral route of infection and thereby reduced the exposure of the population in early infancy. This meant that a latent immunisation could not develop in the majority of society, leaving children and adults unprotected against the disease.[65]

By mid-century, polio became a disease of civilisation. As Albert Sabin put it: 'The poorer the population, its standard of living and sanitation, the more extensively is poliomyelitis virus disseminated among them and the lower is the incidence of paralytic poliomyelitis when virulent strains of virus come their way.'[66] If a country had epidemic polio, it was one of the civilised nations. This

---

[64] Bakács, 'Poliomyelitis Betegek Védőoltására Vonatkozó Adatgyűjtés.' Budapest: National Archives of Hungary, 1959.

[65] M. R. Smallman-Raynor et al., *Poliomyelitis. A World Geography: Emergence to Eradication* (New York: Oxford University Press, 2006), 127.

[66] Albert B. Sabin, 'Paralytic Consequences of Poliomyelitis Infection in Different Parts of the World and in Different Population Groups', *American Journal of Public Health* 41, no. 10 (1951): 1215–30, at 1229.

marker of civilisation and progress later lost its force, and a complete lack of polio became the new signifier as vaccination became widely used.

Infantile Paralysis: Children as Catalysts for Cold War Cooperation

While scientific uncertainties and the global scale of the disease can serve as sufficient explanation for why polio could create international cooperation and exchange by the early Cold War era, it is important to consider that the incidence rate and the death toll of polio was far from reaching the scale of many other infectious diseases of the time, such as influenza or tuberculosis. The fact that it was a relatively rare disease demands a look into the other attributes of polio. One of the most important explanations for the exceptional status of polio in the Cold War era was that it attacked children.

'Is there a greater joy for the parent than his child, and is there a greater worry?' begins a popular Hungarian handbook from 1957 titled *The Healthy and the Sick Child*.[67] Indeed, concern over the health of children lay at the heart of many parents' fear of the summer months, and they found a partner for their concern in the state – whether that be the self-proclaimed champion of freedom, or the pioneer of international communism.

One of the severe diseases threatening the Healthy Child was polio: in many parts of the world it remained perceived as infantile paralysis, as the virus mostly attacked the bodies of children. While in some countries, like the United States, the age distribution of the disease changed over time to higher and higher age groups[68] (and thus changed the widespread use of its name from infantile paralysis to polio), in many other states the childhood nature of the disease remained. In Hungary, for instance, between 1952 and 1957, the age group most affected by polio comprised those between 1 and 2 years old. In 1959, the largest group to fall ill with the disease was under one year of age.[69]

While polio's status as a new disease opened spaces for knowledge exchange, equally important, if not even more important, in this process was the widely held view that it was most prevalent among children. In an era of post-war recuperation, at a time when ideologies that claimed to have the exclusive answer to a bright future clashed, the fledglings of a new generation received heightened attention. Seen as key subjects of national security and

---

[67] Alfréd Berndorfer et al., *Egészséges és Beteg Gyermek* (Budapest: Gondolat Kiadó, 1957).
[68] Albert Sabin, 'Epidemiologic Patterns of Poliomyelitis in Different Parts of the World', in *Poliomyelitis: Papers and Discussions Presented at the First International Poliomyelitis Conference* (Philadelphia: Lippincott, 1949), 3–33.
[69] Ottó Rudnai and Gyula Barsy, *The Results of Salk Vaccination in Hungary as Measured on the 1959 Poliomyelitis Epidemic*, Acta Microbiologica (Budapest: Akadémiai Kiadó, 1961).

economy, children of the 1950s were considered particularly precious to states on both sides of the Iron Curtain.

Cold War concepts of the role of children in the new world order were paired with long-standing ideas of children as symbols of innocence. The figure of the universal and untainted child could be used concurrently to opposing ends: Cold War cooperation and the reinforcement of nationalist and antagonist agendas.

One of the most striking features of polio as a disease was that it threatened those who were perceived as the most vulnerable segment of society: children. Moreover, the victims of the disease were mostly considered to be faultless in contracting the debilitating virus. This is not to say that polio was without powerful metaphors. Cold War interactions over polio utilised the military metaphor extensively, and polio treatment was imbued with military and industrial metaphors in the 1950s.[70] Moral considerations, however, played little or no part in the understanding of the disease, which, together with the fact that polio did not affect the face or skin, led Susan Sontag to consider polio 'unmetaphorical'.[71] However, upon closer inspection, Sontag's conclusion does not hold up, as Marc Shell's work, *Polio and Its Aftermath*, also demonstrates.[72] Polio was laden with ideas of production and masculinity, and its prevention and treatment more often than not operated with a militaristic language.

However, the lack of moral issues that so much permeated sexually transmitted diseases and contagious diseases connected to a particular social class or poverty was a crucial feature of polio. It opened an apparently neutral space by putting forth an image that could be universally appropriated: a disease unfairly attacking the symbols of innocence. The innocence of children, by no means a new perception,[73] gained new momentum in the post-war era. Ideas of childhood that had become prevalent a few centuries previously resurfaced in new ways after the Second World War. The preoccupation with innocence, parent–child relations and the rights of children significantly formed the way in which polio was talked about and acted upon in the 1950s.

Most historians agree that as far as the visual representation of innocent childhood is concerned, it is a modern phenomenon. It first appeared in the works of eighteenth-century British portrait painters, which diffused into

---

[70] David Serlin, 'The Other Arms Race', in *The Disability Studies Reader*, ed. Lennard J. Davis (New York: Routledge, 2006), 49–65; Basil O'Connor, 'The Setting for Scientific Research in the Last Half of the Twentieth Century', in *Fifth International Poliomyelitis Conference*, ed. International Poliomyelitis Congress (Copenhagen, 1960); József Vető, 'A Sabin-Cseppek', *Népszabadság* 1960, 1.

[71] Sontag, *Illness as Metaphor and AIDS and Its Metaphors*, 127.

[72] Marc Shell, *Polio and Its Aftermath: The Paralysis of Culture* (Cambridge, Mass.: Harvard University Press, 2005), 186–89.

[73] Albrecht Classen, ed. *Childhood in the Middle Ages and the Renaissance* (Berlin: Walter de Gruyter, 2005), 3–8.

popular consciousness during the nineteenth century. Anne Higonnet explains the pervasiveness of these images: 'childhood innocence was considered an attribute of the child's body, both because the child's body was supposed to be naturally innocent of adult sexuality, and because the child's mind was supposed to begin blank'.[74]

The idea of children's innocence played a large part in forming children as universal and politically neutral citizens in the early twentieth century. During and following the First World War, children were the primary publicity tool and main recipients of relief efforts, since their innocence protected them from being seen as enemies. Moreover, representing children as universal played an essential part in establishing the neutrality of humanitarian aid in the early years of the war.[75]

International medical relief for children became an important component in foreign diplomacy from the First World War onwards, with the participation of international organisations such as the Red Cross[76] and the Save the Children Fund.[77] The Declaration of the Rights of the Child, adopted by the League of Nations in 1924 – a document not binding by international law, but rather perceived as guidelines – proclaimed rights specific for children for the first time and established adults' responsibility towards children.[78] The first, legally binding legislation to secure the rights of children transnationally was the document of the same name, adopted by the General Assembly of the United Nations in 1959, which proclaimed the rights of children to medical care and to special education and treatment if they were handicapped.[79] Concerns over the physical, mental and social development of children at once became a unifying pursuit, but also created a battleground for ideological clashes in the Cold War era. Both of the Declarations worked with a fluid concept of what a child was, as neither set any limit of age or otherwise to define where childhood began and ended.

The abstract idea of the child, a flexible term that can be added to give weight to a multitude of arguments, has become so naturalised over the course

---

[74] Anne Higonnet, *Pictures of Innocence: A History and Crisis of Ideal Childhood* (London: Thames and Hudson, 1998).

[75] Dominique Marhall, 'Children's Rights and Children's Action in International Relief and Domestic Welfare: The Work of Herbert Hoover between 1914 and 1950', *The Journal of the History of Childhood and Youth* 1, no. 3 (2008): 351–88, at 362.

[76] Julia Irwin, 'Sauvons Les Bébés: Child Health and U.S. Humanitarian Aid in the First World War Era', *Bulletin of the History of Medicine* 86, no. 1 (2012): 37–65.

[77] Friederike Kind-Kovacs, 'Child Transports across and beyond the Empire: World War I and the Relocation of Needy Children from Central Europe', *Revue d'histoire de l'enfance 'irréguliere'* 15, no. Enfances déplacées. (II) en temps de guerre (2013): 75–109.

[78] 'Geneva Declaration of the Rights of the Child of 1924', in *O.J. Spec.Supp. 21*, ed. League of Nations (Geneva, 1924).

[79] United Nations General Assembly, 'Declaration of the Rights of the Child', in *Resolution 1386 (XIV)* (Geneva, 1959).

of two centuries that it has become a concept that is rarely problematised or questioned. Moreover, this perceived universality and flexibility has provided space for the justification of various, often opposing political positions since the nineteenth century, as Robin Bernstein argues in her analysis of American dynamic 'racial innocence'.[80] In scientific and political reasoning, on national and international levels, the image of the innocent child was called upon to rationalise policies, voice concerns or promote cooperation. The innocent child, a universal concept, was used on both sides of the global divide, often with opposing ends: either fighting against or reinforcing Cold War antagonisms.

The Imagery of the Child in 1950s Eastern Europe

Children were extensively used as symbols of the communist and democratic future and as innocent victims of the opposing political system throughout the Cold War. Images of children were especially used in the Vietnam War in order to justify the political and military aims of all sides.[81] As Karen Dubinsky remarked in a recent piece: 'While children rarely achieve political citizenship, the world's political posters provide an extensive visual argument that children are political subjects.'[82]

In the case of polio, the idea of innocent children was utilised to place the scientific, economic and political effort to curb the disease above the global conflict. The innocence of children turned scientific work into a noble enterprise. The pursuit of a vaccine, development of treatment options and provision of access to medical technology was furthered by the concept of protecting the universal child on both sides of the Iron Curtain. Meanwhile, this set of imagery was highly politicised and, as the following two sections show, connected to the physical reality of children and their place in society in the post-war era.

In her book *The Lost Children: Reconstructing Europe's Families after World War II*, Tara Zahra argues that the post-war era was a time when 'basic ideals of family and childhood were reinvented'.[83] Children were increasingly seen as a form of national property, as the European population was reshuffled

---

[80] Robin Bernstein, *Racial Innocence: Performing American Childhood from Slavery to Civil Rights* (New York: New York University Press, 2011).

[81] Margaret Peacock, 'Broadcasting Benevolence: Images of the Child in American, Soviet and Nfl Propaganda in Vietnam 1964–1973', *Journal of the History of Childhood and Youth* 3, no. 1 (2010): 15–38.

[82] Karen Dubinsky, 'Children, Ideology and Iconography: How Babies Rule the World', ibid. 5 (2012): 5–13, at 6.

[83] Tara Zahra, *The Lost Children: Reconstructing Europe's Families after World War II* (Cambridge, Mass.: Harvard University Press, 2011), x.

through DP camps, forced resettlement and mass migration. Exhibiting universally perceived values (and at the same time following an East–West divide, as discussed in the section below), the figure of the child and its importance in the biological and political future of the nation became a central issue in reconstruction policies and emerging state systems. After a world war that permeated all areas of life and left almost the whole European civilian population compromised in one way or another, children seemed to have remained the only innocent victims of the destruction.[84] It was this innocence from which communist propaganda drew its powerful images.

On a national level, the representation of the child in communist societies was part of a complicated perception of family. The patriarchal state, which acted as a parent to the child-citizens, formed one family. In this superstructure nested the domestic family. The resources, tasks and responsibilities were shared among the members. The state – at least on a rhetorical level, much less in reality – provided healthcare, childcare and mass dining for the workers, who in return were expected to pay with their loyalty, their production and, most importantly, their reproduction.[85]

On the one hand, the figure of the child was used as a model for adults and children alike. In Russia, visual and literary depictions of children in the Stalinist era showed children as 'the ultimate model citizens of the Soviet state, more perfectly grateful than any adult could be' and their portrayal indicated expectations of citizenship as well.[86] We can see this strategy at work in Hungarian imagery as well, which looked to the Soviet example in much of its propaganda.[87]

On the other hand, the child, happy and healthy, represented the bright future of the nation. Communist propaganda was one of promise: there might be hard times now, but we are all striving to build the ideal world in which our children will be living. 'The chiming laughter of our children is carried far by the wind . . . the people's struggle is not in vain, they want to see their children laughing' captured the message of a poem published in the Hungarian women's magazine *Nők Lapja* in 1952.[88]

[84] Ibid. 241–42.
[85] Joanna Goven, 'Gender and Modernism in a Stalinist State', *Social Politics* 9, no. 1 (2002): 3–28.
[86] Kelly, *Children's World*, 110–11.
[87] Csilla Halász, 'Agitáció és Propaganda a Népművelésben a Rákosi-Rendszer Idején' (PhD thesis, Eötvös Loránd Tudományegyetem, 2011).
[88] Uj Rezső, 'Kacagjanak a gyermekek' *Nők Lapja*, 10 April 1952. Cited in Katalin Kéri, 'Gyermekképünk Az Ötvenes Évek Első Felében ' *Iskolakultúra*, no. 3 (2002): 47–59. *Nők Lapja* was the most important women's magazine of the whole socialist era, focusing mainly on working women, women's career choices, social issues, and giving advice on everyday life. Attila Horváth, *A Magyar Sajtó Története a Szovjet Típusú Diktatúra Idején*, ed. András Koltay and Levente Nyakas, Médiatudományi Könyvtár (Budapest: Médiatudományi intézet, 2013).

Children as the future of Hungary – based on Soviet practice – were often contrasted with children of the past or children suffering in imperialist countries.[89] Contrasting the social benefits of childcare and support of communism with the poverty and high infant mortality of the interwar era was a powerful way to communicate the superiority of the new regime. Furthermore, depictions of children who had fallen victim to racism and imperialist exploitation invariably portrayed unwashed, uncombed, ragged and emaciated children as opposed to the round, pink, healthy and well-groomed young pioneers of the Eastern Bloc.[90]

While the innocence and malleability of children was used to reinforce Cold War divides in the national rhetoric, the universal child served as a symbol of cooperation and key to world peace on the international scene. This symbol was, to a large extent, thoroughly politicised in Cold War interactions. Catriona Kelly argues that

in the peculiar circumstances of the Cold War, children's rights, like other areas of international diplomacy, became an arena in which key points of political difference – the extent to which state control over the family was ideologically desirable, the importance or otherwise of explicit political indoctrination – could be brandished, and where set positions of hostility or rapprochement could be adopted. Significantly, it was not until the Cold War was coming to an end that a broader agreement about international standards of children's welfare began to emerge.[91]

However, if we look at polio from the Hungarian angle, another story unfolds. In scientific and political exchanges over the disease, the fact that the virus attacked children created a common ground, a cause to unite efforts and disregard Cold War politics. The argument that 'the Russians love their children, too', as captured by the well-known song by Sting in 1985,[92] was drawn upon when dismantling Cold War stereotypes in the evaluation of the scientific results of vaccine testing.[93] Furthermore, as the following chapters show, governments on both sides of the Iron Curtain were ready to step over the boundaries of their own international and domestic politics in the name of children. In short, the rhetoric of protecting innocent children from polio

[89] Dina Fainberg, 'The Heirs of the Future: Foreign Correspondents Meeting Youth on the Other Side of the Iron Curtain', in Winter Kept Us Warm Cold War Interactions Reconsidered, ed. Sari Autio-Sarasmo, Brendan Humphreys and Katalin Miklóssy (Helsinki: Aleksanteri Institute, 2010), 126–36.
[90] Kéri, 'Gyermekképünk az Ötvenes Évek Első Felében'.
[91] Catriona Kelly, 'Defending Children's Rights, "in Defense of Peace": Children and Soviet Cultural Policy', Kritika: Explorations in Russian and Eurasian History 9, no. 4 (2008): 711–46.
[92] Sting and Sergei Prokofjev, Russians: The Dream of the Blue Turtles (Santa Monica: A&M, 1985), Single.
[93] See Chapter 4.

played an important part in creating a safe haven in the troubled sea of Cold War politics.

The role of childhood and the importance of the child in Cold War rhetoric often did not match everyday experiences in the 1950s. The ways in which the rhetoric used by the Hungarian communist state in social issues played out in governmental actions and in the experiences of women, families and children have been explored by feminist scholars,[94] and some aspects are covered in this book. The distance between representation and experience does not mean, however, that they did not significantly influence policies. Professional organisations, governments and individuals drew on rhetorical elements to justify their policies and aims, or support their claims and needs. Children played such a role in creating a neutral place in the international and national politics of polio. The image of the innocent child and the role of scientists, governments and international organisations to protect them from the harm of the debilitating disease provided an opportunity to transcend boundaries and political limitations.

Demographic Context and Pro-Natalism in Hungary

Children became the focus of the Hungarian government not only from a propagandistic view, but also from a demographic one. Between the years 1949 and 1960, 24.9–25.4 per cent of Hungary's population was aged under 15 years.[95] This means that in the 1950s, the age group most endangered by polio constituted a quarter of the country's inhabitants. Following the demographic shock of the Second World War, the spectre of such destruction elevated the significance of the disease and placed it at the centre of the state's attention as polio epidemics became more frequent and more powerful throughout the decade.

As in many post-war societies, population politics became increasingly important in the wake of long years of devastating and bloody battles, deportations, genocide and starvation. In the course of the war, Hungary lost 40 per cent of its national wealth and over 10 per cent of its population, around 1 million people.[96] A severely damaged infrastructure and housing shortage brought challenges for post-war governments, and demographic problems

---

[94] See Éva Bicskei, "'Our Greatest Treasure, the Child'': The Politics of Child Care in Hungary, 1945–1956', *Social Politics* 13, no. 2 (2006): 151–88; Joanna Goven, 'Gender and Modernism in a Stalinist State', ibid. 9, no. 1 (2002): 3–28.
[95] Gyula Benda, 'Budapest Társadalma 1945–1970', in *Magyarország Társadalomtörténete III. (1945–1989)*, ed. Nikosz Fokasz and Antal Örkény (Budapest: Új Mandátum, 1999), 8–31, at 22.
[96] Ignác Romsics, *Magyarország Története a XX. Században* (Budapest: Osiris Kiadó, 2001).

were further exacerbated by the reorganisation of industry and labour in the early years of the communist takeover. While the number of live births increased in the years following the war, and between 1947 and 1950 population increase stabilised at a rate higher than preceding the war (2.1 per cent),[97] a more significant growth in the future labour force was needed to make up for the lack of resources and to fulfil the industrial goals of the new communist state. To further boost population increase, in 1952 the Hungarian government enforced a strict pro-natalist policy. The Hungarian government was not alone in introducing the policy; other Eastern European Peoples'Democracies also decided to ban the termination of pregnancies at this time.[98] While Hungary's method was nowhere near as extreme as the infamous abortion ban of Ceaucescu's Romania over a decade later, the general idea and goal undergirding such pro-natalist policies was a shared attribute in the Eastern Bloc. As historian Gail Kligman put it,

mobilization and control of the population were of critical strategic importance for the maximization of development potential, and attention to demographic phenomena was essential to securing long-term interests. In order to meet the relatively high labor needs of such economies, reproduction of the labor force became a priority planning item.[99]

The *Decree on the Further Development of Mother and Child Protection* was a short lived regulation, with significant effects – in the years between 1953 and 1955, the population increase more than doubled to 5.1 per cent.[100] This jump was achieved by limiting access to contraceptive methods, financial incentives and propaganda. Women were severely punished for undergoing abortions, as were doctors who performed them. Public show trials of abortionist doctors and midwives began in the autumn of 1952 and concluded with exceptionally severe sentences.[101] All pregnant women were required to register at state offices, and the state imposed a special tax on childless citizens over 20 years of age. If they had no children, women between 20 and 45 and men between 20 and 50 had to pay a tax equalling 4 per cent of their salary. Both women and men were exempt from the tax until the age of 24 if they were students.[102] Propaganda efforts went as far as to urge childbearing both among

---

[97] Kéri, 'Gyermekképünk az Ötvenes Évek Első Felében'.
[98] Andrea Pető, 'Women's Rights in Stalinist Hungary: The Abortion Trials of 1952–1953', *Hungarian Studies Review* 29, no. 1–2 (2002): 49–76.
[99] Kligman, *The Politics of Duplicity*, 19.
[100] Kéri, 'Gyermekképünk az Ötvenes Évek Első Felében'.
[101] Pető, 'Women's Rights in Stalinist Hungary: The Abortion Trials of 1952–1953', 53.
[102] 'Határozat Az Anya– és Gyermekvédelem Továbbfejlesztéséről. 1004/1953. (II.8.) M.T.', in *A Családjogi Törvény*, ed. Jenő Bacsó, Géza Rády and Viktor Szigligeti (Budapest: Közgazdasági és Jogi Könyvkiadó, 1955), 365–74.

married couples and out of wedlock, emphasised by the slogan of the movement: 'To give birth is a duty for wives, and glory for maidens.'[103]

The pro-natalist policy was connected to the name of Anna Ratkó, Welfare Minister and later Health Minister, and the only female member of government of her time. The population policies of the early 1950s were soon termed 'Ratkó-era', and the members of the baby boomer generation, born between 1952 and 1956, are even today called 'Ratkó children'. However, according to archivist Piroska Kocsis, the welfare minister had little to do with the development and implementation of the policy herself.[104] A textile worker with a long history of activism in the communist movement, Ratkó, in her own words, 'had nothing to do with health issues … Comrade Rákosi told me that I could not choose what I wanted to do, I had to do what the Party wished.'[105] Her career as a government member ended in April 1953, but her name forever became one with this exceptional period in the Hungarian history of population policy.

The harsh anti-abortion decree met significant resistance from citizens, as well as from the state administration itself, from the beginning. Historian Andrea Pető has shown that those who did not want to have children found a way to have abortions independent of regulations.[106] The decree was enacted on 8 February 1953, and less than a month later, Josip Stalin died on 5 March. The new Imre Nagy government was not keen on enforcing the criminalisation aspect of the decree, and certain parts of the regulation began to be revoked in the autumn of the same year. From 1 January 1954 the government permitted abortions due to social considerations. The decree was finally fully revoked under Soviet pressure in 1956.[107]

The short increase in live births was soon followed by a sharp decrease after abortions became available and the childless tax was withdrawn. Statistics show that families simply rescheduled having children – there was no major increase in the number of children per families; instead, parents had the same amount of children they would have had anyway, crammed into the few years when the decree was effective.[108] This did result in a high peak in the number of young children by the mid to late 1950s, however. Incidentally, this was also the time when polio epidemics began claiming more and more lives and affected the health of more and more children.

---

[103] Piroska Kocsis, 'A Szövőszéktől a Miniszteri Bársonyszékig', *Archívnet* 6, no. 4 (2006).
[104] Ibid.
[105] Gyuláné Králl: Ratkó Anna visszaemlékezése életútjáról. (Interjú, 1979 január. Politikatörténeti és Szakszervezeti Levéltár). Cited ibid.
[106] Pető, 'Women's Rights in Stalinist Hungary: The Abortion Trials of 1952–1953', 52.
[107] Kocsis, 'A Szövőszéktől a Miniszteri Bársonyszékig'.
[108] Klinger, 'Magyarország Népesedése az Elmúlt Negyven Évben', 47.

Moreover, the state's concern with population growth was renewed by the lives lost in the 1956 revolution, coupled with a massive emigration of dissidents. Over 200,000 out of a total population of 9 million citizens left when the revolution was suppressed, about 40 per cent of them industrial workers. According to Austrian official sources, between late October 1956 and the end of April 1957, over 180,288 people crossed the border from Hungary, most of them in November 1956. A further 34,000 exited the country through Yugoslavia, after the Austro-Hungarian border was closed down. Around 8,000–10,000 emigrants returned during this time frame.[109] Approximately 25 per cent of emigrants returned in early summer 1957, after the post-revolutionary Kádár government offered amnesty to emigrants who were not affiliated with revolutionary actions.[110]

The modernist communist state showed great interest in demography. Its goals in industrial production rested on having an adequate workforce available, and for that it needed healthy and physically able children who would grow up to be productive miners and steel workers.

Disabled Bodies and Post-War Production

With an insight into the significance of the disease both for the scientific community and in the eyes of the state and the public, one more important aspect needs to be investigated in order to understand the particular space that polio created and which is explored in more detail in the next five chapters. Polio was a debilitating disease that worked against modern ideas of production based on able bodies. The economic and political challenges of the post-war era and the changes in economic structure and production in the nineteenth and twentieth centuries placed physically disabled children in a new position. As part of their family units and living in relatively small communities, disabled children were often integrated into the family economy. However, an emerging market economy, the spread of wage labour and industrialisation made it more and more difficult for disabled people to find employment.[111] Their disability became increasingly divided from the productive capacity of their able-bodied peers, and many became marginalised, especially in urban areas.

In parallel with physically disabled work falling out of the concept of production, philanthropic organisations became more and more involved in care for the disabled, especially for children. Institutions for crippled children

---

[109] Ernő Deák, 'Adatok az 1956-os Menekülthullámról', in *Magyarország Társadalomtörténete III. (1945–1989)*, ed. Nikosz Fokasz and Antal Örkény (Budapest: Új Mandátum, 1999), 72.
[110] Romsics, *Magyarország Története a XX. Században*.
[111] Brad Byrom, 'The Progressive Movement and the Child with Physical Disabilities', in *Children with Disabilities in America: A Historical Handbook and Guide*, ed. Philip L. Safford and Elizabeth J. Safford (London: Greenwood Press, 2006), 49–64.

started cropping up in the late nineteenth and early twentieth centuries, often functioning as homes, vocational schools and sites of medical treatment.[112]

The first such institution in Hungary, the Home for Crippled Children (Nyomorék Gyermekek Otthona), was established in 1903 by the Ferenc Deák Masonry Lodge. As was typical for charitable organisations of the time, the leadership included barons and counts among its ranks.[113] The association, established to raise funds and manage the institution, set a goal

to establish asylums in Hungary for physically crippled (with the exception of blind, deaf-mute, moron) children and in these institutions to train crippled children of both sexes, without regard to religion or ethnicity in body and in mind, and provide them with medical treatment and education, and perhaps vocational training.[114]

The goal of the institution was primarily to train future adults to care for themselves; medical care took a backseat.

The concept of children in policymaking as future workers has been present for centuries. In the nineteenth century, 'campaigners against child labour in the factories liked to appeal to the self-interest of manufacturers, by suggesting that abuses risked compromising the future quality of the industrial workforce', and on a more patriotic note also sought to protect them as future soldiers.[115] Modern ideas of production soon became entwined with modern warfare, which on the one hand required the physical ability of a previously unseen amount of citizens, and on the other hand turned out disabled bodies by the thousands. War disability in such large proportions presented the medical profession with new challenges (e.g. the production and design of prosthetic devices) and highlighted concerns about welfare systems from the mid-nineteenth century onwards.[116] War veterans' disability often became entwined with children's disability – either by forming each other's perception and treatment,[117] or by playing a part in making disability invisible.

Disability caused by war was especially problematic in the Socialist Bloc. The Second World War had a devastating effect on the population as

---

[112] Seth Koven, 'Remembering Dismemberment: Crippled Children, Wounded Soldiers, and the Great War in Great Britain', *American Historical Review* 99, no. 4 (1994): 1167–1202.

[113] Béla Kun, *A Fiatalkorúak Támogatására Hivatott Jótékonycélú Intézmények Magyarországon* (Budapest: Wodianer F. és fiai könyvnyomdai műintézete, 1911), 146.

[114] In the 1950s many children with polio ended up in this institution as wards of state. Nyomorék Gyermekek Menhelye Alapszabálya 1903. 20, cited in Éva Bán et al., eds., *Száz Esztendő a Mozgáskorlátozott Gyermekek Szolgálatában* (Budapest: Nádas Pál, 2003), 14. Nóra Schweitzer, *Polio 2.0* (Budapest: Magyar Polio Alapítvány, 2016), 93.

[115] Colin Heywood, *A History of Childhood* (Cambridge: Polity Press, 2001), 145.

[116] Beth Linker, *War's Waste: Rehabilitation in World War I America* (Chicago: University of Chicago Press, 2011).

[117] Koven, 'Remembering Dismemberment: Crippled Children, Wounded Soldiers, and the Great War in Great Britain'.

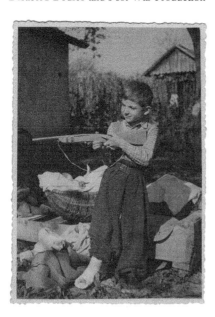

Figure 1.1 *György, age 10, after his last, sixth operation due to polio. Kisvárda, 1961. From the personal collection of Dr. György Vargha.* **This image is protected by copyright and cannot be used without further permissions clearance.**

destructive fronts moved back and forth for years. The bloodshed left nearly 3 million people disabled in the Soviet Union alone, in whose war effort manpower was a central element on the battlefront and home front alike.[118] Yet the social and political status of disabled veterans, as well as their representation and provision, was complicated at best. Second World War veterans' sacrifice in defending the country and contributing to the victory of the army was acknowledged through iconographic imagery in newspapers, films and plays, and some veterans, such as the developer of a prosthetic arm, were hailed as celebrities. At the same time, bodily disability was often invisible in this representation and was always 'cured' either by physicians or through technology.[119]

[118] Frances L. Bernstein, 'Rehabilitation Staged: How Soviet Doctors "Cured" Disability in the Second World War', in *Disability Histories*, ed. Susan Burch and Michael Rembis (Urbana: University of Illinois Press, 2014), 218–36.

[119] 'Prosthetic Promise in Late-Stalinist Russia', in *Disability in Eastern Europe and the Former Soviet Union: History, Policy and Everyday Life*, ed. Michael Rasell and Elena Iarskaia-Smirnova (London: Routledge, 2013), 42–64.

The invisibility of disabled war veterans was even greater in Hungary. Veterans whose bodies had been permanently distorted or mutilated on the battleground had been fighting for a bad cause. In fact, they were the enemy themselves: the new Hungarian state was under the Soviet Union's political and military control, while its citizens a few years before had been involved in armed conflict against that power on the side of Nazi Germany. The disability of war veterans thus raised an uncomfortable issue – the implication of the Hungarian population and their relationship with the Soviet Union. Silencing and erasure was the answer to this vexing problem, as veteran disability associations were discouraged and then forbidden outright, and disabled adults were pushed to the peripheries of the paternalistic state care.[120]

Innocent children were quite another matter. They were not tainted with the history of their forefathers and therefore were 'safe' to address openly. Moreover, since their disability threatened the progress for which the communist government had promised and strived, the prevention and treatment of polio became highly important in the 1950s. This does not mean, however, that disabled children were visible. Concepts of production and the individual's role in society did not permit a visual contrast to the ideal that bodies ridden with polio represented.

Industrial production and the productive body became a focus of attention in the post-war era in many countries, albeit for different reasons and with different attributes. David Serlin has shown that 'with the excitement of industrial production from a military economy still fresh, using one's body remained one of the primary ways that citizens … forged identities and affiliations with industrial economies'.[121] The Soviet Union also worked with a functional model of disability from revolutionary times onwards, privileging work capacity as the primary norm for citizens throughout the twentieth century. This framework resulted in a hierarchy of disabilities where children did not always fare well.[122]

Key issues forming the prevention and treatment policies of the communist state were ideological conceptions of the body and particular visions of the role of the individual in society. In this sense, the state expected and supported the construction of perfect productive bodies capable of performing physical labour – the base of the idealized worker-citizen. The muscular and healthy socialist body became a reference point, which in the case of children meant rosy cheeks and a plump figure. One hardly needed to look for signs of the

---

[120] Monika Baár, 'Disability and Civil Courage under State Socialism: The Scandal over the Hungarian Guide-Dog School', *Past and Present* 227, no. 1 (2015): 179–203.

[121] Serlin, 'The Other Arms Race', in *The Disability Studies Reader*, 49.

[122] Sarah D. Phillips, '"There Are No Invalids in the USSR!": A Missing Soviet Chapter in the New Disability History', *Disability Studies Quarterly* 29, no. 3 (2009), www.dsq-sds.org/article/view/936/1111 (last accessed 11 June 2018).

healthy socialist body, as it was ever-present in public statues, book illustrations, murals and propaganda imagery. The pages of Nők Lapja, for instance, were filled with pictures of mothers and children bursting with health and happiness. This women's magazine was controlled by the Party management and was an established medium to communicate the Party's ideals to worker and peasant women. The editors made a point of presenting success stories about ideal socialist, productive women on a regular basis, in order to give the impression that the number of ideal women was constantly growing in reality, and thereby to convince their readers to follow the example.[123] Since the magazine was illustrated with photographs as well as sketches, it gave an opportunity to the editors to display the ideal bodies to accompany the texts. Children were often represented on these photographs, for another task assigned by Party ideology to the socialist woman was to maintain the ideological and bodily health of her children. Even if the theme was healthcare or women in the medical profession, the photos showed smiling young women examining healthy-looking round babies.

The bodies of children with polio deviated from these idealised forms. Spines distorted by muscle spasms, disfigured arms and immobile legs failed to meet the requirements of production and health demanded by communist ideology. Therefore, it became a central issue in polio care to change the diseased bodies of children back to normal and productive. Restoring children's bodies so as to make them capable of becoming a productive member of socialist society was not particular to Hungary at the time.

Children whose bodies did not conform to the ideal and whose appearance threatened the early Hungarian communist project were often hidden from view. Magazines, newspaper articles and propaganda films showed healthy-looking, completely recovered, cheerful children,[124] while the disability of polio patients was secluded in polio hospitals and wards. Paradoxically, the same reasons – preoccupation with ideal images of the socialist, productive body – that brought polio to the centre of attention also made its reality invisible. This ambivalent perception of polio, its publicly acknowledged importance and its simultaneous invisibility and marginality created a unique space in the society and politics of communist Hungary: polio hospitals and wards became the terrain of contesting bodies of production and disability.

In a report about the Heine-Medin Hospital, the largest daily newspaper, Népszabadság, wrote in a bright and affectionate tone, 'The community of the little patients lives in total isolation. They are not broken in soul like those who

---

[123] Mária Schadt, 'Feltörekvő, Dolgozó Nő'. Nők az Ötvenes Években (Budapest: Pannónia, 2005), 98.
[124] 'A Heine-Medines Mozgászavarok Utókezeléséről', Hungary, 1957. Gábor Vajda, 'Visszaadják Őket az Életnek', Népszava, 26 March 1961.

are teased by their healthy peers because they are temporarily crippled.'[125] The obvious solution was thought to be removing disabled children from society. Polio did not fit with the ideal socialist body; therefore the distorted and disabled bodies of the victims were undesirable to public sight. The reminders of the disease could have compromised the image of the hard but successful struggle against polio that would eventually lead to victory.

Discussion about children with polio rarely appeared on the pages of newspapers and their images even less so.[126] Whenever they were depicted, their disability was invisible; a little boy standing still, a girl reading on a bed: they could have been any child from the neighbourhood. Disabled children were rarely talked about, let alone pictured. This was even true in the case of Heine-Medin Hospital's own internal magazine. In an article reporting on orphan and state ward polio patients being patronised by two factories, a sketch shows two industrial buildings with open arms and perfectly healthy, round little babies in nappies hurrying to them on their hands and knees.[127]

When stories did appear about children with polio, they always told of success and the children presented in them had always made an almost full recovery; disabled children remained invisible in spite of the visibility of polio: '[treatments and surgeries] give more and more paralytic patients their health back, who can grow up to be productive adults'.[128] Children with polio appeared only as future healthy children, rendering their disability invisible. One of the articles from 1957, describing the Heine-Medin Hospital as a beautiful wonderland for children, quite bluntly gives an explanation of why the work of the institution is so important: 'A large number of the children are totally or partially recovered and are not a burden on society.'[129] The function of the Heine-Medin Hospital therefore was not perceived as an institution for disabled children, but one whose goal was to rehabilitate them into useful members of society by making their bodies productive, thereby making them un-disabled.

This invisibility had profound effects on the experience of the disease, and, ultimately, on national and international policies. There were no poster children for the effort against polio, as disabled children did not fit into the representational or physical landscape of communist Hungary. Not when the

[125] András Faludi, 'Az Élet Nevében. Látogatás a Heine-Medin Utókezelő Kórházban', *Népszabadság*, 7 March 1958.
[126] Photographs and illustrations often appeared in medical literature; however, in this section I focus exclusively on representations of the socialist body and polio children in the popular press.
[127] 'Heine Medin Híradó' (Budapest: Heine Medin Utókezelő Kórház, 1959–63).
[128] Rózsa Fehér, 'A Gyógyító Torna', *Magyar Nemzet*, 24 January 1956.
[129] 'Ötszáznyolcvan Újabb Ágy a Heine-Medin-Kórban Megbetegedettek Utókezelésére', *Magyar Nemzet*, 10 September 1957.

state focused its efforts on demonstrating power over an epidemic disease that was spiralling out of its control, and even less so when Hungary's encounter with polio ultimately became a global success story in itself.

The overall scientific and political discourse on polio in Hungary fitted into a larger Cold War strategy: evasion. Severe public health problems concerning adults and the issue of war disability could be pushed to the background or even made invisible by concentrating on the health of children. Questions of inequalities in access to medical technologies (partly because of Cold War embargoes) could be escaped by the celebration of scientific cooperation. Finally, the common fight against polio rechannelled conversations on hostility: participation in a war on disease, instead of a Cold War on each other.

Yet these mostly rhetorical evasions did create concrete opportunities for cooperation. The universal concept of the innocent child paved the way for international conferences and budding international organisations to provide actual knowledge transfer and transnational assistance in times of polio epidemics. Scientific cooperation did lead to the development and trial of a vaccine that is still used today in global polio eradication efforts.

All of the crucial attributes of polio discussed above played an important part in shaping Cold War interactions between scientists, governments and citizens, with far-reaching ramifications. Medical communities, patients and public health regimes grappling with scientific uncertainties crossed international political divides in the name of children. The global nature of the disease facilitated research and kept the stakes of the disease high. The constant reminder of disability caused by polio contributed to the priority of the disease in comparison to other ailments and public health challenges.

The significance of the disease was fixed in time and place. The era of post-Second World War reconstruction and development made polio a priority, a disease that was not great in numbers, but attacked and debilitated children. It also mattered on which side of the Iron Curtain one contracted the disease, as communist ideals of the body made polio-ridden ones invisible. However, the characteristics of polio were in constant flux. Some uncertainties became established facts, causing other uncertainties in the process. The meanings of the disease changed in space and time, reacting to and interacting with social, political and cultural changes on both sides of the Iron Curtain. The following chapters explore moments in the Hungarian history of polio in which the constantly changing and flexible disease mapped onto an equally fluctuating and shifting Cold War. In these flashpoints, the various attributes of polio come to the foreground to highlight underlying problems or to be used by actors to achieve political or professional goals.

2   Iron Curtain, Iron Lungs

On the late autumn day of 2 November 1956, Russian commander-in-chief Marshal Ivan Konev established the Hungarian headquarters of the Soviet army in Szolnok. Two days later he would give orders to attack and put an end to the Hungarian uprising against the communist regime. Ten days had passed since the mass demonstration initiated by university students took a revolutionary turn on 23 October. The Hungarian revolution, this key moment of the Cold War, would be crushed in little over a week.

On the same day, Imre Nagy, the revolutionary prime minister, also gave orders in Budapest. However, the nature of the Hungarian leader's orders could hardly have been more different from that of his Soviet counterpart: amidst the turbulent events of the revolution, he took the time to establish a polio hospital.[1] Even though the revolution would come to an end in a matter of weeks, the Heine-Medin Post Treatment Hospital would survive and continue to operate for seven more years treating children with polio, a cause that seemed to override political ideologies and regimes.

The revolution of 1956 was a key event in the history of the Cold War. Millions of people worldwide followed the unfolding of the October events. International efforts were aimed at accommodating – and protecting – hundreds of thousands of refugees who left the conflict-torn country. The Hungarian Revolutionary became man of the year on the cover of *TIME* magazine. The events of the revolution have been widely discussed in Cold War historiography,[2] and the uprising overshadows the Hungarian historical narrative of the era.

---

[1] Lukács, 'Feljegyzés a Fővárosi Heine-Medin Kórház és Rendelőintézet Alapításáról, Működéséről, Eredményeiről és ezzel Kapcsolatos Tevékenységéről'. Budapest: Personal archives of Dr. Prof. Ferenc Péter, 1993, and Budai Gyermekkórház és Rendelőintézet, 'A Kórház Története', www.budaigyk.hu/site.php?inc=0&menuId=5.

[2] M. János Rainer and Katalin Somlai, *The 1956 Hungarian Revolution and the Soviet Bloc Countries: Reactions and Repercussions* (Budapest: The Institute for the History of the 1956 Hungarian Revolution, 2007); Johanna C. Granville and Raymond L. Garthoff, *The First Domino: International Decision Making during the Hungarian Crisis of 1956*, 1st edn, Eastern European Studies (College Station: Texas A&M University Press, 2004); Charles Gati, *Failed*

It is less well known that there was a polio outbreak during the revolution in the eastern part of the country. It was an unexpected, autumn epidemic that could not have come at a worse time. As infrastructure and state services collapsed with the turmoil of the revolution, those affected by the disease had difficulties in getting help. The country was already in a dire situation in terms of basic medical services, especially in the conflict-stricken areas, and was badly in need of aid; an epidemic on top of the battles only exacerbated the public health emergency. Yet the breakdown of transportation systems and the lack of safety on the roads might have contributed to the relatively contained nature of the outbreak: other than fleeing to the West, not many travelled in late October that year.

Cold War relations, with their thaws and frosts, affected polio in Hungary in various ways. Some watershed events of the Cold War, like the 1956 revolution in Hungary, had unexpected effects on the epidemic management of polio. The political and social upheaval of revolution propelled Hungarian polio treatment forward with the establishment of a specialised hospital, plans for which had already started in the early 1950s. Access to technologies and knowledge ebbed and flowed in ways that did not necessarily map onto the usual Cold War narratives. In this sense, the preoccupation with polio presents us with more continuity than is allowed for by Cold War history.

The politics of polio in the 1956 revolution also point to the importance of considering individual actors on the ground when examining international humanitarian and medical interventions. Putting polio at the centre of this well-known event in the history of the Cold War sheds light on the important and life-saving role that international organisations such as the Red Cross played at a time of political and epidemic crisis. However, the actions of these organisations were put into motion and often executed by individuals who had no official connection to international organisations. They were physicians, amateur radio users, virologists, nurses and religious scholars, who utilised their professional and political connections and resources to tackle the tasks of preventing and treating polio in a time of turmoil.

The humanitarian crisis in the wake of the uprising not only facilitated the influx of hospital equipment, but also highlighted international and local responses to scarcity through an emerging network of iron lungs that criss-crossed the Iron Curtain. This scarcity was partly due to the destruction caused by past and current armed conflict in Hungary and the result of national and

Illusions: Moscow, Washington, Budapest, and the 1956 Hungarian Revolt, Cold War International History Project Series (Washington, D.C., Stanford, Calif.: Woodrow Wilson Center Press; Stanford University Press, 2006); Csaba Békés, Malcolm Byrne, and M. János Rainer, *The 1956 Hungarian Revolution: A History in Documents*, National Security Archive Cold War Readers (Budapest and New York: Central European University Press, 2002).

global Cold War politics. At the same time it was also a universal problem, caused by the insufficient supply of a costly technology that had trouble meeting the huge demand of severe outbreaks not just in Eastern Europe but all over the world.

The 1956 Revolution and International Aid

On 23 October 1956, university students, joined by workers, intellectuals and even the communist youth organisation Union of Worker Youth, flooded the streets of Budapest demanding reforms. Crowds assembled at the Radio and tried to have their demands broadcast, while some assembled in front of the parliament and others joined forces to knock down a great statue of Stalin. By the late evening, shooting had started at the Radio, where the demonstrators, armed with the help of workers from ammunition warehouses and factories, besieged the studios and took over the building by dawn.

The roots of the revolution lay in the changes in Soviet policy towards the Eastern Bloc triggered by Stalin's death in 1953. This did not necessarily mean that the status of satellite states was up for negotiation: in the same year, the states of the Eastern Bloc and the Soviet Union signed the military alliance Warsaw Treaty Organisation, signalling a tightening of Soviet control over Eastern Europe.[3] However, after Nikita Khrushchev announced 'peaceful coexistence' with Western nations and condemned Stalinism in 1955, debates cropped up across the region on fundamental political issues, most of all in Poland and in Hungary.

By 1953, the Hungarian economy was on the brink of collapse, and the Soviet leadership initiated changes in policy and personnel. Imre Nagy became prime minister and initiated several reforms, but he and his reforms soon became caught up in power struggles and Moscow became increasingly dissatisfied. The Hungarian economy had not improved as they had hoped, and Nagy's effort to democratise the party resulted in Mátyás Rákosi, a devout Stalinist, making a comeback in 1955 and having Nagy removed from his seat. By the end of the year, Rákosi had expelled him from the party. There was no going back to the pre-1953 era, however. Nagy's reforms opened a Pandora's box of dissatisfaction and opposition within Hungarian society, which was experiencing new economic and political pressure; the masses lived in extreme poverty, but now had a sense of an alternative. Through Soviet intervention, Rákosi was removed, but it was too little too late.[4]

In October 1956 it all came to a head. In Poland, Wladyslaw Gomulka's reformist faction rose to power, prompting university students in Hungary to

---

[3] Békés et al., *The 1956 Hungarian Revolution: A History in Documents.*   [4] Ibid.

formulate their own demands for reforms and organise a march of sympathy with Poland for 23 October 1956. It was from this demonstration that the revolution erupted. The next few days saw fierce street battles among protesters, the Soviet army, the Hungarian secret police and occasionally the Hungarian army, which was joining the ranks of the rebels in increasing numbers. The revolutionaries erected street barricades, tore down Stalinist statues, occupied public buildings and even captured tanks. The revolution was occasionally peaceful, and sometimes extremely violent on both sides. A massacre in front of the Parliament took the lives of over 300 civilians, and in the turmoil of the revolution demonstrators lynched several members of the secret police and strung them up on lampposts as gruesome reminders. The country, Budapest first and foremost, suffered great damage as fighting between armed rebels and the military took place on crooked streets, in squares and on bridges.

Imre Nagy took the seat of prime minister once more and in an effort towards consolidation promised significant reforms. On 30 October he announced the end of the one-party system and the formation of a coalition government. A few days later Hungary declared itself neutral and withdrew from the Warsaw Pact. Ultimately, however, Soviet tanks rolled into Hungary and Budapest came under artillery fire on 4 November 1956.[5] By 11 November, the Soviet military had broken armed resistance, Nagy had sought refuge at the Yugoslavian embassy and János Kádár had taken the oath of office; meanwhile, sporadic demonstrations continued well into mid-December.

The crisis and revolution of 1956 opened up discussions about the failings of the communist healthcare system. It was a rare instance when fundamental critiques and the admission of failure on several fronts were openly verbalised and gained publicity. The double-speak that permeates the archival materials of the time lifts for a brief moment in the professional meetings and newspaper reports of the days preceding the revolution.[6] In a meeting with leaders of health institutes on 19 October 1956, Health Minister József Román admitted that contrary to the goals of the first five-year plan, no new hospitals had been

---

[5] Head of the General Department of the Central Committee, Vladimir Nikiforovich Malin had taken notes during the discussions of the Soviet Presidium on the Hungarian situation between 23 October and 4 November. The so-called Malin notes have revealed that the Soviet invasion and military suppression of the revolution was uncertain for a while and several scenarios were in play. János M. Rainer, 'The Road to Budapest, 1956. New Documentation on the Kremlin's Decision to Intervene', *Hungarian Quarterly*, no. Summer (1996): 24–41; Timothy Garton Ash, 'Introductory Essay: Forty Years On', in *The 1956 Hungarian Revolution: A History in Documents*, ed. Csaba Békés, Malcolm Byrne and János M. Rainer (Budapest: Central European University Press, 2002), xix–xxvii.

[6] One report written by the executive party committee of Budapest heavily criticised the Health Ministry for its excessive bureaucratisation, its centralisation and ineffective management of healthcare on over thirty pages. 'Beszámoló.' Budapest: National Archives of Hungary, Vilmon Gyula iratai, Egészségügyi Minisztérium, XIX-C-2-o 1956–1957, 1956.

built. He pointed out that the growing demand for health services had been met by the further overcrowding of extant facilities or the appropriation of buildings that were not originally intended for healthcare use.[7] The minister also conceded that the areas of public health and epidemiology had been particularly neglected in recent years.[8] The simultaneous outbreak of a revolution and a polio epidemic further exacerbated these conditions. Some hospitals and clinics were badly damaged during street battles, especially in Budapest.[9] By December, even basic hygiene supplies such as soap were hard to find.[10] During and after the revolution, Hungary was decidedly in need of foreign aid.

Humanitarian aid and the intervention of the Red Cross in the Hungarian Revolution became symbolic acts in the Cold War, albeit ones with very important consequences on the ground. Donations of food, clothes and medicine from Western countries became powerful expressions of support for the cause of the revolution,[11] while the Soviet army and the post-revolutionary Hungarian regime saw the humanitarian intervention as a political and military scheme.[12]

In fact, the International Committee of the Red Cross (ICRC) was the only international organisation that was granted access to Hungary during and immediately after the revolution. The Hungarian Red Cross contacted the ICRC on 27 October to request aid and the first shipment arrived two days later. In the meantime, the ICRC requested that twenty-six national Red Cross societies send blood, medical equipment and medicine to Vienna, where the shipments were assembled. The humanitarian intervention was not uncontested by the Soviet army. In one case, the aircraft carrying medical supplies and food had to turn back due to Russian tanks having blockaded the airport, and convoys were suspended between 4 and 11 November because the border between Hungary and Austria was closed off.[13] The Soviet occupying forces

---

[7] 'Román József Egészségügyi Miniszter Egészségügyünk Problémáiról', *Népszava*, 21 October 1956.

[8] 'Az Egészségügy Legégetőbb Problémái és az Egészségügyi Dolgozók Rehabilitációja', *Népszava*, 23 October 1956.

[9] The teaching hospitals, which served as main healthcare providers were particularly hard hit in Budapest – Dermatology, Internal Medicine, Surgery, Ophthamology, Gynaecology. The Bókay children's Hospital was also injured in a fire. 'Van Építőanyag a Kórházak Helyreállításához, Vöröskereszt Táborikonyhák Létesülnek, Szappant, Mosóport, DDT-t Kapnak a Kerületek', *Népakarat*, 21 November 1956.

[10] 'Lesz Szappan', *Népakarat*, 7 December 1956.

[11] Françoise Perret, 'L'Action du CICR en Hongrie en 1956', *International Review of the Red Cross*, 78, no. 820 (1996): 449–63.

[12] A good example of this narrative can be found in the only monograph to date on the history of the Hungarian Red Cross from 1981: János Hantos, *A Magyar Vöröskereszt 100 Éve. Emberiesség Háborúban és Békében* (Budapest: Akadémiai Kiadó, 1981). 149–51.

[13] Isabelle Voneche Cardia, *Magyar Október Vörös Zászló És Vörös Kereszt Között [L'octobre Hongrois: Entre Croix Rouge Et Drapeau Rouge]* (Budapest: Socio-typo, 1998).

were very suspicious of the aid workers during and after the revolution. Evidence suggests that several ICRC workers were arrested and held by the KGB for ten days, during which they were questioned about their actions and movements.[14]

Despite these difficulties, the ICRC continued to send convoys and aeroplanes to provide aid throughout the revolution.[15] Clothing, infant milk, food and medical supplies were in great need, especially in Budapest, a city that had barely had time to recover from the destruction of the Second World War, only to be torn apart by tanks, machine guns and Molotov cocktails once again. Aid continued to flow into the country – with the subsequent approval of the new Hungarian government backed by the Soviet Union – until the summer of 1957.[16] Industrial production stopped as strikes continued well into the winter, and infrastructure was badly damaged.

Red Cross aid was tolerated and even welcomed by the post-revolutionary government. Moreover, the need for food, clothes and medical supplies created a space for cooperation with the Hungarian branch of Actio Catholica, the Catholic international movement, which had been established in 1932.[17] On 11 December 1956 the ICRC, the Hungarian Red Cross society and Actio Catholica signed a trilateral agreement stating that all aid received should be distributed by the Hungarian Red Cross. However, the Catholic group did distribute 150 train wagons of aid, for which it was heavily criticised in 1957; it was accused of using resources unfairly, for instance giving out tinned whale to rich Catholics.[18] Shortly after, the religious organisation was co-opted by the Hungarian post-revolutionary government. The Hungarian Red Cross faced a similar fate.[19]

---

[14] György Lupkovics, 'A Nemzetközi Vöröskereszt Aktivistái a Magyar Forradalomban és a KGB Fogságában', *Betekintő*, no. 3 (2009).

[15] Cardia, *Magyar Október*.

[16] David P. Forsythe, *The Humanitarians: The International Committee of the Red Cross* (Cambridge: Cambridge University Press, 2005).

[17] For more on the history of Actio Catholica in Hungary, see Paul A. Hanebrink, *In Defense of Christian Hungary: Religion, Nationalism, and Antisemitism, 1890–1944* (Ithaca, NY: Cornell University Press, 2006) and András Gianone, 'Az Actio Catholica Története Magyarországon 1932–1948' (PhD thesis, Eötvös Loránd Tudományegyetem, 2006).

[18] 'A MVK Átszervezése és az ezzel Kapcsolatos Hatósági és Belső Vizsgálatok.' P 2130 MVK: National Archives of Hungary, The papers of the Hungarian Red Cross, 1957; György Tamás. 'Élelmezésügyi Minisztérium Vizsgálatáról Készült Jelentés.' ibid.

[19] There is little written on the takeover of the Hungarian Red Cross in the late 1950s. The only Hungarian monograph available dates from 1981 and delivers the very clear political agenda of the new, coopted organization. Hantos, *A Magyar Vöröskereszt 100 Éve*. Cardia's work on the ICRC in the 1956 revolution is based exclusively on the archives of the ICRC in Geneva, and therefore reveals little about the relationship between the ICRC and the Hungarian Red Cross. Cardia, *Magyar Október*.

In the early days of the 1956 revolution, Imre Nagy appointed a commissioner to head the Red Cross, along with a committee of university professors to take over the leadership of the organisation. In the months following the failure of the uprising, the new government had no time or energy to deal with the internal structure of the Red Cross, whose services were needed to distribute the still incoming shipments of aid. In June 1957, the new government commissioner and committee were dismissed and a new leadership appointed: the rector of the Budapest Medical University and Academy member, Dr Pál Gegesi Kiss, became president, while József Kárpáti, a former ambassador, became secretary. The takeover involved an inspection of the organisation's actions in 1956–57, its stocks and membership. All activists who had been involved in providing aid to revolutionaries were expelled from the society. In 1959 the Hungarian Red Cross was still struggling with its heritage, as the presidential committee strove to communicate a marked difference between 'pseudo-civil humanism and the current, socialist Red Cross'.[20]

As the Hungarian Red Cross society saw a complete changing of the guard, the relationship with the ICRC slowly began to deteriorate. A report on the takeover of the Hungarian Red Cross and its status in 1957 lambasted the ICRC for 'not keeping control over the distribution of aid during and following the revolution. Instead, they were caught up in their own and their supporters' propaganda and took great care not to be inspected by Hungarian governmental authorities, saying it would be political intrusion.'[21] In his inauguration speech, Győző Kárász, the new vice-secretary of the Hungarian Red Cross, went as far as to accuse the ICRC of abusing the Red Cross emblem and smuggling guns and ammunition into the country during the revolution.[22] The ties between the international and national organisation were further strained by a struggle over the attempts at the 'repatriation' of youths and children after the revolution. The ICRC blocked any attempts by the Hungarian Red Cross and the government to send out the names of underage refugees in order to bring them back to Hungary.

The impact of Red Cross activities in Hungary during and after the revolution had global significance. The actions of the ICRC during and immediately after the revolution became one of the major success stories that served to re-establish the organisation's battered reputation after 1945. In the 1950s, the

---

[20] 'Jegyzőkönyv 1959. Március 27-én Megtartott Elnökségi Ülésről.' Budapest: National Archives of Hungary, Vezető testületek, Elnökség ülésjegyzőkönyvek 1957–1962, P2130 MVK, 1959, 11.
[21] Tamás, 'Élelmezésügyi Minisztérium Vizsgálatáról Készült Jelentés.' Budapest: National Archives of Hungary, 1957.
[22] 'Jegyzőkönyv Felvéve Az 1957 Június 25-Én Megtartott Országos Vezetőségválasztó Értekezletről.' Budapest: National Archives of Hungary, The papers of the Hungarian Red Cross, XXVIII-C-1, 1957.

ICRC was battling against a damaged reputation from its controversial role in the Second World War, especially with regard to the Holocaust. The ICRC had not acted when the German Red Cross went against the fundamental ideas of the movement, such as the universality of the Red Cross, as Jews were forced out of the society.[23] Despite their knowledge of the genocide in Nazi Germany from 1942 onwards, the ICRC had decided to remain silent on the issue, and had shied away from issuing even a mild and vague public statement reminding belligerent states of humanitarian principles.[24] Following the war, the ICRC needed to prove that it was a viable organisation.

Moreover, the humanitarian intervention in the Hungarian revolution became a reference point for the armed conflicts that followed, among them the Algerian liberation movement in 1956. The National Liberation Front (FNL) and the newly established Algerian Red Crescent (not acknowledged by the League of Red Cross societies) both contrasted the indifference of Western powers to the Algerian struggle and the accompanying lack of humanitarian assistance with the aid provided to Hungarian freedom fighters and refugees, in order to highlight the difference in standards applied to European and Third World countries.[25]

Revolutionary Skies: Iron Lungs on and in the Air

Strikingly left out of the story of Red Cross intervention in the Hungarian revolution was the organisation's role in supporting polio treatment during and immediately after the uprising. While supplying aid for long-term treatment was not among the declared priorities in providing assistance to conflict-torn countries, the geopolitical significance of this particular conflict made possible the inclusion of diverse needs. The revolution thus provided windows of opportunity for physicians invested in polio treatment to obtain medical technology and hospital equipment from abroad to which they otherwise would not have had access. This aspect of humanitarian intervention in the 1956 revolution is entirely missing from the historical narratives of the uprising itself or of the Red Cross. The reason might be that, as we will see, these transactions did not involve governments; in some cases, they hardly involved international organisations at all. As such, most of the international aid and collaboration in preventing and treating polio was initiated – and carried out – on the ground, and its history remains invisible when studied from above.

---

[23] Jean_Claude Favez, *The Red Cross and the Holocaust* (Cambridge: Cambridge University Press, 1999).
[24] Forsythe, *The Humanitarians,* 44–50.
[25] Young-sun Hong, *Cold War Germany, the Third World and the Global Humanitarian Regime* (New York: Cambridge University Press, 2015), 135–36.

As the revolution was unfolding in Hungary, a polio epidemic erupted in the north-eastern part of the country, leaving parents and doctors in a desperate situation. The country's infrastructure came to a full stop, and administrative services and communication ran into severe problems. For many cities, the only means of establishing contact with the outside world was radio. Broadcasts were used not only to inform people of the events and goals of the revolution, but also as channels for family members to look for each other or notify each other of their safety, to reach over borders for aid and to coordinate processes that would have otherwise fallen under the tasks of the state. Occasionally, doctors would send each other messages about incoming aid or transporting blood to the wounded.[26]

On 29 October the radio stations of Miskolc and Nyíregyháza broadcast an appeal for an iron lung for the hospital of Debrecen, since its only iron lung was broken.[27] Iron lungs were life-saving devices that essentially breathed for polio patients suffering from respiratory paralysis. By the 1950s the machines came to symbolise the horrors of polio epidemics in the imaginations of parents all over the world. Iron lungs and other respiratory machines, such as swing beds (rocking beds), were crucial in the treatment of the acute phase of the disease.

Iron lungs, no longer in use today, were large, tubular metal machines that operated with negative pressure. The patient lay on her back, her whole body inside the machine, with only her head on the outside. The machine created a vacuum inside the tank, which made the patient's chest rise, resulting in inhalation. The pressure then changed in the tank, letting the chest fall and creating exhalation.[28] This device could only work for patients without complications, since any infection or mucus would cause significant problems – patients with respiratory paralysis cannot cough. Another important respiratory method, developed in Denmark in the early 1950s, was called intratracheal positive-pressure respiration. A portable machine applied positive pressure into the lung of the patient directly through the trachea. This meant that a tracheotomy was necessary; however, getting rid of mucus also became easier, and the less mucus, the lower the risk of infection. The least invasive respiratory device was the rocking bed. This bed, swinging back and forth like a

---

[26] György Vámos, ed. *A Szabad Európa Rádió és a Magyar Forradalom. Műsortükör 1956. Október 23–November 5*, vol. 7, História Könyvtár Okmánytárak (Budapest: MTA Történettudományi Intézete, 2010).

[27] Rádió Miskolc, '1956 Október 29: A Debreceni Kórház Felhívása!', in *A Forradalom Hangja. Magyarországi Rádióadások 1956. Október 23–November 9*, ed. Gyurgyák János (Budapest: Századvég kiadó és Nyilvánosság Klub, 1989), 216.

[28] Ákosné Dr Kiss, 'Tartós Gépi Lélegeztetéssel Életben Tartott Postpoliós Légzésbénultak Sorsa' (Candidate thesis [kandidátusi értekezés], Semmelweis University, 1989), 9.

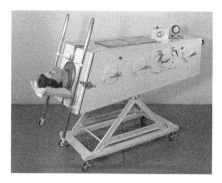

Figure 2.1 *Both-type iron lung, London, England, 1950–55. By Science Museum, London. Credit: Science Museum, London. CC BY.* **This image is protected by copyright and cannot be used without further permissions clearance.**

seesaw, used gravity to help breathing. Internal organs pushed and pulled the diaphragm as the body swayed up and down in a lying position.

The first iron lung arrived in Hungary in 1948, with the cooperation of the American embassy and Andor Bossányi, director of the László Hospital of Infectious Diseases.[29] This machine became the basis of the respiratory ward of the infectious disease hospital organised by Dr Domokos Boda under the direction of Pál Ferenc.[30] Nevertheless, for a long time, access to the treasured respiratory device was difficult.

In the first half of the 1950s, iron lungs began to be produced in Czechoslovakia and the GDR.[31] By 1959, over 100 Hungarian iron lungs were in use in the country.[32] Most of the iron lungs arrived in Hungary during the 1957 epidemic, the worst year for polio in the country's history. However, the arrival of a much-needed iron lung during the 1956 revolution tells perhaps one of the most dramatic stories of international cooperation during the Cold War.

The hospital's request for help found its way to Munich through Radio Free Europe (RFE), which was monitoring and documenting radio transmissions in

---

[29] 'Megérkezett Hazánkba az Első Vastüdő', Hungary, 1948.
[30] 'Tartós Gépi Lélegeztetéssel Életben Tartott Postpoliós Légzésbénultak Sorsa', 1989; Rezső Hargitai and Kiss, *A Gyermekbénulás Elleni Küzdelem: Beszámoló egy Ma Már Múlttá Váló Rettegett Betegség Ellen Folytatott Hősies Küzdelemről és Felszámolásának Lehetőségéről: A Szent László Kórház Centenáriumára Készült Összeállítás*, 2.
[31] Boda, *Sorsfordulók*, 60.
[32] Dr Kiss, 'Tartós Gépi Lélegeztetéssel Életben Tartott Postpoliós Légzésbénultak Sorsa'.

Hungary and had its headquarters in the German city.[33] Requests for help through radio waves were not uncommon during the revolution, especially requests for medical aid. In contrast to requests for political and military intervention, guns and ammunition from the West, which mostly went unanswered,[34] appeals for public health intervention made through domestic radio broadcasts travelled a long way with the help of RFE. In a telegraph to Geneva, RFE notified the Red Cross about a call 'to all international helping organisations' about the polio epidemic in the North-Eastern region, stating that thirty people had already died and asking for 'a serum against this malady'.[35]

In reply to the appeal for an iron lung, the RFE station sent back a message through its broadcast that same afternoon:

We have important news for the hospital of Debrecen. We have heard your urgent appeal regarding the iron lung. We will immediately help and we have done everything for the desired iron lung to leave today for Debrecen. The only reason for delay is that there is no iron lung for sale in Munich at the moment. Keep listening to our broadcast; we will let you know immediately when the iron lung begins its journey.[36]

Apparently, the shortage of respiratory devices was not unique to Hungary. In their next message, RFE let the Hungarian hospital know that there were no available iron lungs for sale on the whole continent, due to the epidemic outbreak in the Netherlands.[37]

It is uncertain how the RFE managed to secure a device in the end. Only 20 minutes after stating that they were not able to obtain an iron lung, the presenter suddenly interrupted his account of the events in Hungary to announce once again that they would do everything in their power to send

---

[33] Much of the history of Radio Free Europe is written by journalists or former directors of the radio. See Sig Michelson, *America's Other Voice: The Story of Radio Free Europe and Radio Liberty* (New York: Praeger, 1983); Richard H. Cummings, *Cold War Radio: The Dangerous History of American Broadcasting in Europe, 1950–1989* (Jefferson, NC: McFarland, 2009); George R. Urban, *Radio Free Europe and the Pursuit of Democracy* (New Haven: Yale University Press, 1997). A. Ross Johnson, *Radio Free Europe and Radio Liberty: The Cia Years and Beyond* (Washington and Stanford: Woodrow Wilson Center Press; Stanford University Press, 2010); Gyula Borbándi, *Magyarok Az Angol Kertben* (Budapest: Mundus, 2004). A critical history of the radio in the early 1950s is provided by historian Irén Simándi, *Magyarország a Szabad Európa Hullámhosszán*, ed. Ferenc Kégli and István Monok, Nemzeti Téka (Budapest: Gondolat Kiadó, 2005).

[34] Csaba Békés, *Az 1956-os Magyar Forradalom a Világpolitikában* (Budapest: 1956-os Intézet, 2006), 44–45.

[35] Fischer, 'Telegraph Message to Mr. Ammann International Red Cross Geneva.' Geneva: International Committee of the Red Cross Archives, Demandes d'aide pour secours en Hongrie, B AG 280 094–031.01, 280 (65), 1956.

[36] '14:00 Hírszolgálat. October 29, 1956. Vámos', *A Szabad Európa Rádió és a Magyar Forradalom. Műsortükör 1956. Október 23–November 5.* 566.

[37] '18:09 Figyelem, figyelem!', ibid.

the life-saving machine that day. A few hours later, on the evening of 29 October 1956, an iron lung onboard a German aeroplane arrived in the skies above Hungary. The was almost certainly organised by the West German Red Cross, but the origin of the device at this point remains a mystery. What we do know, however, is that landing the aircraft was more than challenging: in the midst of the revolution, airports were not functioning and there was no one to control the aeroplane from the ground.

At 10:10 p.m., the radio station of Miskolc broadcast an urgent message for Hajdúszoboszló, the town neighbouring Debrecen, to illuminate their airport for the arrival of the iron lung. All they needed to do then was to direct the aeroplane there. Four minutes later, the radio broadcast the following message: 'Attention, attention! We ask all amateur [radio transmitters] to help with landing the plane! Seek connection with [the aeroplane] and direct it to Hajdúszoboszló, where a lit-up airport will receive it.'[38] A few minutes later, the radio revealed that the plane was flying above Debrecen, close to the target airport. However, something must have gone wrong; the plane had to be redirected to yet another city through public radio: 'Attention, attention, radio stations of [Budapest], Debrecen and all Hungarian airports, and radio control of the German aircraft! Direct the aeroplane to Miskolc! We are waiting for it. It will be able to land at the airport there. We will transport the iron lung to its destination!'[39] There is no way of knowing how many amateurs took part in this community effort, using low-tech, amateur devices and knowledge to navigate the plane and ensure the safe arrival of the iron lung. From the initial appeal for help through radio, in a time of upheaval and during the breakdown of infrastructure and services, the life-saving equipment reached its destination with efficiency that would put a communist dictatorship to shame.

This iron lung did not follow the usual route of aid flowing into the country at the time. Other donations from various locations were mostly collected in Vienna and transported from there via aeroplane or convoy to Budapest, where the resources were distributed,[40] and were not flown individually to specific locations. The arrival of the iron lung in the autumn of 1956 was, it seems, an exceptional event under the exceptional circumstances of the revolution.

What makes this feat particularly interesting is that it was accomplished with the help of a technology that was right in the centre of ideological and political contestation: radio. Since radio waves crossed borders with ease and were a relatively simple and cheap way of reaching a theoretically unlimited number

---

[38] Rádió Miskolc, '1956 Október 29. 22.14 H: Halló, Halló, Figyelem!', in *A Forradalom Hangja. Magyarországi Rádióadások 1956. Október 23–November 9*, ed. Gyurgyák János (Budapest: Századvég kiadó és Nyilvánosság Klub, 1989).

[39] '1956 Október 29, 23.54 H: Figyelem!', ibid.

[40] Judit Gyurcsán, 'The ICRC's Operations in Hungary between 1956 and the 1960s', *Miskolc Journal of International Law* 3, no. 3 (2006): 28–40.

of people on the other side, radios were considered to be crucial weapons in waging the media war of the 1950s.[41] Hungary was also an active participant on this front: the state vigorously communicated the achievements of peoples' republics to a potential audience ranging from East Asia to Latin America, while Hungarian language programmes from the West attempted to reach behind the Iron Curtain. 'The enemy works against us on 110–120 different frequencies, in an accumulated 210–220 hours per day', stated a report prepared for the Hungarian Workers' Party's Political Committee in 1954.[42] The Hungarian government attempted to curb access to these transmissions by issuing radios that were technically unable to receive anything except the two official stations. Later, in an international project with neighbouring countries, they built transmitters designed to jam the radio signals of Radio Free Europe and Voice of America.[43] Radio Free Europe was naturally very much under the watch of the Hungarian secret police (ÁVH), who had installed regularly reporting agents in the Munich headquarters from at least 1955 onwards.[44] Even listening to the programme was punishable by law.

There is little information about radio amateurs of this era. Amateur radio clubs were permitted in limited numbers and the Association of Hungarian Shortwave Radio Amateurs was re-established in 1948 after having been banned in 1944. By 1954 there were fifteen clubs active in the country, three of which were in Budapest, and by December 1955, 101 amateur radio users were registered nationwide.[45] While we do not know their exact relationship with the communist regime, at least some of them were clearly critical and took part in the 1956 uprising in their own way. One amateur radio user recounts having 'fixed' a high number of radio receivers in 1956, enabling them to receive all frequencies instead of only the state-sanctioned ones.[46]

While the dramatic story of the iron lung flying over the country in revolution is an exceptional one, the speedy transport of a respiratory device over political borders during an epidemic crisis was not entirely unusual at the time.

---

[41] For more on radio in the Cold War, see Michael A. Krysko, *American Radio in China: International Encounters with Technology and Communications, 1919–41* ed. Bill Bell, et al., Palgrave Studies in the History of the Media (Basingstoke: Palgrave Macmillan, 2011); A. Ross Johnson and R. Eugene Parta, eds., *Cold War Broadcasting: Impact on the Soviet Union and Eastern Europe* (Budapest-New York: Central European University Press, 2010); Alban Webb, *London Calling: Britain, the BBC World Service and the Cold War* (London: Bloomsbury Academic, 2014).

[42] Cited in Béla Révész, 'Manipulációs Technikák a Hidegháború Korai Időszakában', *Acta Juridica et Politica* 10 (1996): 3–90, at 4.

[43] Ibid.

[44] László Kasza, 'A Magyar Állambiztonsági Szervezet és a Szabad Európa Rádió', in *Közelítések a Kádárizmushoz*, ed. Pál Germuska and János Rainer M. (Budapest: 1956-os Intézet, 2008), 144–89.

[45] Zoltán Papp to Régi rádiók és egyebek, 22 July 2011.

[46] Ferenc Kósa, 'Az Amatőr Rádiózás Gyulai Emlékei', *Gyulai Hírlap*, 2 July 2010.

In a country strained by the effects of the Second World War, forced industrialisation and collectivisation and a bloody revolution, medical supplies were
often scarce and facilities were not readily available to accommodate the long-
term care of polio patients. Moreover, polio was a disease that required highly
specialised equipment – most importantly life-saving respiratory machines
such as iron lungs.

The devices were expensive and hard to come by, especially on the eastern
side of the Iron Curtain. This lack of resources triggered innovation, with new
ways of using existing devices or developing new machines. However,
Hungary was not alone in its difficulties in accessing high-tech machinery.
In the midst of the Cold War, in a network spearheaded by the International
Committee of the Red Cross, iron lungs criss-crossed Europe (and, in fact, the
globe) to assist polio patients wherever an epidemic crisis was unfolding.

The idea of mutual assistance in polio epidemics and the establishment of a
global network of respiratory devices first came up in May 1948 at the
European Regional Conference on Poliomyelitis in Brussels. Among other
recommendations for procedures during epidemics and questions of recuperation and treatment centres, the conference identified access to respiratory
devices as a crucial problem in tackling polio. The attendees expressed the
wish that various countries undertake the mass production of respiratory
devices with the aim of reducing the cost of the expensive machines. Secondly,
each country should keep a stock of iron lungs in proportion to its population,
and, in case of an epidemic emergency,

> if local resources are insufficient, to provide for, to study and to determine the ways and
> means for a rapid mobilisation of means of assistance. Such mobilisation should include
> not only iron lungs and necessary equipment, but expert medical advisors and trained
> helpers belonging to the regional areas or to neighbouring countries.

The Belgian delegation then put forward the conclusions of the conference
at the First World Health Assembly of the newly formed World Health
Organisation.[47]

The WHO sent out a circular letter to all European countries the following
year, to which fifteen countries had replied by 1950. Based on the replies, the
WHO took stock of the available respiratory devices across the continent; the
advantages and disadvantages of the various models; the way in which access
to respiratory devices was organised (i.e. national or regional level, whether
there was a central stock etc.); and the availability of specialised staff. The
questionnaire also gauged interest in the establishment of an international iron

---

[47] 'Poliomyelite Antérieure Aigue (Paralysie Infantile)'. Geneva: WHO Archives, European
Regional Conference on Poliomyelitis, Brussels, May 1948, WHO 1 484–1–2, A/Prog/
40, 1948.

lung loan system. The options on the table were an international loan network, loans based on bilateral agreements or, alternatively, the establishment of a European, central stock of respirators to be utilised in the case of epidemic emergency.[48]

Not all countries were enthusiastic about the proposal. Opinions were divided over whether a network or a centralised stock would be the best solution, and a significant number of countries decided against the whole scheme. Among them was Hungary.[49] It is important to note here that in 1950 countries like Hungary had yet to experience severe epidemic waves of polio. The acute problem of respiratory paralysis on a mass scale had not been a reality at that time and it is doubtful that anyone would have anticipated the escalation of epidemics in the 1950s across the globe. Finally, due to the varied responses as to how the international loan of respiratory devices should be organised, if indeed they should be organised at all, the Executive Board of the WHO decided to hold off on taking any steps unless the initiative garnered wider support.[50]

However, the lack of available respiratory devices remained a problem for most of the decade. In 1954, Austria identified the insufficient number of iron lungs available as one of its main challenges,[51] while polio experts from the Netherlands considered the issue of respiratory paralysis to be 'of extreme importance' and planned to organise training courses for specialised physicians and nurses.[52] Scandinavian polio experts formed a special respiratory committee to advise the North European states and give 'suggestions for acquiring a respirator emergency stock'.[53] The Scandinavian scheme for cooperation was soon put to the test when the Nordic countries were required to provide aid to Iceland during an epidemic in 1955.[54]

In the end, it was the Red Cross – not the WHO – that became the organising force behind the international network of iron lung loans. With polio epidemic outbreaks on the rise worldwide, the network of loaning respiratory devices reached far beyond the original European area. The League of Red Cross Societies became increasingly invested in providing aid during polio epidemics. In a report from 1957, the Red Cross considered polio epidemics to fit

---

[48] 'Use of Respirators in the Treatment of Poliomyelitis and Proposed Organization of a System of International Loan of These Apparatus', in *Report of the Executive Board. Fifth Session. Held in Geneva from 16 January to 2 February 1950*, ed. World Health Organization (Geneva: World Health Organization, 1950).
[49] Ibid.   [50] Ibid.
[51] Gerald Grinschgl, 'Austria', in *Third International Poliomyelitis Congress* (Rome: J. B. Lippincott Company, 1955), 31.
[52] G. D. Hemmes, 'Netherlands', in *Third International Poliomyelitis Conference* (Rome: J. B. Lippincott, 1955), 50–52.
[53] E. Juel Henningsen, 'Denmark', ibid.
[54] 'Denmark', in *Fourth International Poliomyelitis Conference* (Geneva: J.B. Lippincott, 1957).

perfectly with their main goals of 'diffusion among the population of humanitarian principles and, respectively, the application of these principles in the *prevention* and *relief* of human suffering'. Accordingly, the League advised all national societies to 'participate as actively as possible' in combating the disease.[55] The national societies took on the new challenge and carried out various tasks, from the sterilisation of syringes and needles for mass vaccination campaigns (in the United States) to supplying orthopaedic appliances (Ecuador) and increasing stocks in medical loan depots (Sweden).[56]

National Red Cross societies were not only involved in epidemic management in their own countries, but were active in transnational interventions as well. In 1957, a severe epidemic in Argentina prompted the West German, Italian and American Red Cross to send iron lungs and respiratory devices, while other countries, such as India and Czechoslovakia, contributed with specialists, hospital linen and vehicles to facilitate care for polio patients. In the same year, about seven months after the revolution was suppressed, Hungary became once again the focus of international aid when the Hungarian Red Cross asked the League to supply twenty respiratory devices as quickly as possible. Now there was peace, there was no need for radio.

The Hungarian case gives us an idea of what the use of the loaning network looked like in practice. In 1957 the International Committee of the Red Cross (ICRC) and the League of the Red Cross Societies coordinated an international effort to identify heavy-respiratory machinery all across Europe and send it to Hungary. The Hungarian delegate of the ICRC, who in early July found the epidemic severe but not catastrophic, deemed the insufficient number of respiratory devices as the most pressing problem.[57] Meanwhile, the ICRC headquarters was waiting for the reports of two Swedish polio specialists, Dr Lindhal and Dr Werneman, who were sent by the Swiss Red Cross to Hungary to determine the country's needs.[58] The international experts were seen by the Health Ministry as 'being able to provide significant assistance in getting aid from foreign organisations as soon as possible'[59] and thus were supported by the Hungarian government in their mission.

In the opinion of the Swedish doctors, the Hungarian hospital staff, including physicians, nurses and technicians, were sufficient in number and their treatment methods and expertise were 'modern'. The most urgent issue was,

---

[55] Z. S. Dr Hantchef, 'An Outline of Red Cross Activities in the Fight against Poliomyelitis', ibid.
[56] Ibid.
[57] F. Dr Züst. 'Note an Das I.K.R.K. Budapest, Z. Hd. Von Herrn Ch. Ammann: Poliomyelitis-Epidemie in Ungarn.' Geneva: International Committee of the Red Cross Archives, Epidémie de poliomyélite, B AG 280 094–031.02, 164, 1957.
[58] Dr Hantchef, 'An Outline of Red Cross Activities in the Fight against Poliomyelitis', 1957.
[59] Anna-Ma Toll and Bengt Aman, 'Letter to the Health Ministry.' Budapest: Magyar Nemzeti Levéltár, Drexler Miklós Egészségügyi Miniszterhelyettes iratai, XIX-C-2-p, 336/1957, 1957.

they concluded in accordance with the ICRC delegate, the lack of respiratory equipment. According to their findings, about 15–20 per cent of paralytic polio cases involved respiratory paralysis. Before the peak of the epidemic wave at the end of July, thirty-five patients needed artificial respiration. However, there were only twenty-four iron lungs in the country. The experts who visited treatment sites were apparently impressed by the innovation of Hungarian physicians and technicians born out of necessity and meagre resources. The report describes iron lungs transformed into devices that could serve three infants at a time instead of one and rocking beds accommodating up to six children.[60]

A detailed description of this latter technology in the Hungarian medical journal *Orvosi Hetilap* [trans. *Medical Weekly*] reveals that, in fact, even more children could be treated with a single respirator than in the cases encountered by the Swedish experts. Patients were connected to the tank of the iron lung through the side openings with rubber tubes and breathed through a humidifier receptacle.[61] This addition was important, keeping the patients' mucous membrane humid and thereby preventing infection.[62] With this technology, in an extreme situation in December 1956, Hungarian physicians were able to connect ten infants to one iron lung. Between June 1956 and July 1957, more than 100 patients were treated by the common use of a single iron lung.[63]

In response to the appeal from the League of Red Cross Societies, East Germany lent Hungary seven iron lungs,[64] which travelled to their destination by train.[65] The British Red Cross immediately sent two iron lungs by air and prepared three more for transportation.[66] West Germany dispatched five iron lungs, fifteen poliomats (smaller respiratory devices developed by the Dräger company, developer of the iron lung)[67] and four pieces of respiratory

---

[60] Bengt Aman, 'Epidemie de poliomyelite en Hongrie. Informations communiquées par le Bureau Médico-Social, Ligue des Sociétés de la Croix-Rouge.' Geneva: International Committee of the Red Cross Archives, Epidémie de poliomyélite, B AG 280 094–031.02, 7275, 1957.

[61] László Nagy, 'Vastüdő Felhasználása Intratracheális Szakaszos-Túlnyomásos Lélegeztetésre', *Orvosi Hetilap* 2, no. 7234 (1959): 86–7.

[62] Domokos Boda and László Murányi, *Respiratiós Therapia* (Budapest: Medicina Könyvkiadó, 1963). 113.

[63] Nagy, 'Vastüdő Felhasználása Intratracheális Szakaszos-Túlnyomásos Lélegeztetésre', 1959.

[64] Z. S. Dr. Hantchef, 'Rapport de Dr. Hantchef Directeur du Bureau Médico-Social, Ligue des Sociétés de la Croix-Rouge.' Geneva: International Committee of the Red Cross Archives, Epidémie de poliomyélite, B AG 280 094–031.02, 1957.

[65] Bengt Aman, 'Epidemie De Poliomyelite En Hongrie. Informations Communiquées Par Le Bureau Médico-Social, Ligue Des Sociétés De La Croix-Rouge', ibid., 7275.

[66] Evelyn Bark, 'Letter to Monsieur Amman, International Committee of the Red Cross.' ibid., 3096.

[67] Ernst Bahns, *It Began with the Pulmotor: One Hundred Years of Artificial Ventilation* (Lübeck: Dräger Medical AG & Co. KG, 2007).

equipment.[68] The Swedish Red Cross dispatched six respiratory devices and ten mucus aspirators,[69] key equipment in preventing infections in polio patients with respiratory paralysis. The iron lungs and devices arrived by air in Vienna and were transported by Malév Hungarian Airlines to Budapest with the coordination of the Austrian and Hungarian Red Cross societies.

Hungarian patients with respiratory paralysis were not exclusively dependent on loans and donations from international agencies and foreign governments. In fact, a locally developed and produced machine called the *Electrospirator* soon became the most widely used device. The result of a technology transfer from one medical speciality to another, from one side of the Iron Curtain to the other, the *Electrospirator* became a central element in the life of many patients.

During an especially severe polio epidemic in Copenhagen in 1952, Dr Alexander Lassen, chief physician at the Blegdam hospital, faced an influx of respiratory paralysis cases in unprecedented numbers and sought the help of anaesthesiologists to find a solution to the problem of the meagre number of respiratory machines.[70] A common procedure in anaesthesiology, applying positive pressure ventilation through the trachea, became an innovative method in polio treatment and went on to have a significant effect on the overall treatment of respiratory paralysis. The most important trait of this type of ventilation was that it was conducted through the trachea, which made getting rid of mucus easier, thereby lowering the risk of infection. However, the initial version was manually operated during the Copenhagen epidemic, mainly by medical students. This worked as an emergency measure, but required many staff to operate in the long run.

Using manpower in extreme ways in cases of emergency was not unusual in the history of polio, especially when it came to respiratory paralysis. An otherwise healthy-looking child or young adult suddenly unable to breathe was a shocking and powerful image that mobilised resources to exhaustion and shaped public health policies and medical practices. In his book *Beginnings Count*, David J. Rothman argues that the personal choices of doctors and the moral imperative of trying to help each and every case of respiratory paralysis with iron lungs, regardless of the efficiency of the technology or the prognosis of the particular patient, formed ideas about access to medical care.[71] While

---

[68] Deutsches Rotes Kreuz. 'Telegraph Message to M. Ammann International Committee of the Red Cross.' Geneva: International Committee of the Red Cross Archives, Epidémie de polio-myélite, B AG 280 094–031.02, 1118, 1957.

[69] Z. S. Dr. Hantchef. 'Rapport de Dr. Hantchef Directeur du Bureau Médico-Social, Ligue des Sociétés de la Croix-Rouge', ibid.

[70] Luise Reisner-Sénélar, 'The Birth of Intensive Care Medicine: Björn Ibsen's Records', *Intensive Care Med*, no. 37 (2011): 1084–86.

[71] David J. Rothman, *Beginnings Count: The Technological Imperative in American Health Care* (New York: Oxford University Press, 1997), 41–67.

Rothman analyses a 'democratisation' process of technology use and expectations and concludes that such ideas could be counterproductive from a medical perspective, the Hungarian case raises different issues. In an economy of shortage, the question of whether to use a certain medical technology, in this case the iron lung, never came up. The dilemma was, rather, how to make the best use of given resources and maximise access to the available technology.

Dr Kiss Ákosné, who later became head of the respiratory ward at the Heine-Medin Hospital, considered the dramatic story of a relative who contracted polio to have shaped her medical career. In 1946, two years before the first iron lung was to arrive in Hungary, the young doctor's distant relative fell ill on her sixteenth birthday and became paralysed first in the legs, then in the arms and finally in her respiratory muscles.

Since in these cases you could never tell if the respiratory paralysis would last five hours, three days, or a month ... Three of us, another doctor, a pianist cousin and I tried to help, like relay horses, with the Silvester method, the most efficient method available then.[72]

This way of artificial respiration, so often pictured in films, involved raising the patient's arm above her head to induce air into the lungs and pressing them down on her chest for exhalation.[73] It was a huge physical strain on both the givers and the receiver. The efforts of the doctors and friends lasted one and a half days, by which time the girl's skin on her forearms and chest was so damaged from the continuous friction that she could no longer stand the pain and begged them to stop. The young doctor could do nothing but arrange a morphine injection to ease the girl's struggle as she died.[74]

With such alternatives at hand, similarly to his Western colleagues, Boda started working on the mechanisation of the new Danish respiratory method in 1953. Iron lungs were scarce in Hungary and the epidemic of 1952, along with epidemic patterns all over Europe and beyond, made many physicians wary that epidemic crises were looming in the near future. Boda's first attempt was an 'inspirator', based on glass technology and completed the same year. He encountered a Swedish version, the Engström respirator, for the first time on his trip to Switzerland in 1954, which gave him new momentum for

---

[72] Interview with Dr. Kiss Ákosné by Ádám Csillag in Ádám Csillag, 'Gyermekbénulás I', Csillag és Ádám Film; Fórum Film, Hungary, 1995.

[73] The method was named after Henry Robert Sylvester, British physician who developed this technique in 1858. In the 1940s this method was still widely considered to be the most effective means of artificial respiration. See D. G. Cordier, 'Methods of Artificial Respiration', *British Medical Journal* 2, no. 4316 (1943): 381–83; Thomas F. Baskett, 'Silvester's Technique of Artificial Respiration', *Resuscitation* 74, no. 1 (2007): 8–10.

[74] Interview with Dr. Kiss Ákosné by Ádám Csillag in Csillag, 'Gyermekbénulás I', Csillag és Ádám Film; Fórum Film, Hungary, 1995.

developing his own device.[75] In cooperation with Pál Kerekes, an engineer at the Research Equipment Manufacturing Company of the Hungarian National Academy of Sciences, Boda built his final version and named it *Electrospirator*. The device was later patented and manufactured for export.[76] In the late 1950s, domestic iron lung production started, along with Electrospirators and rocking beds. By 1963 a wide variety of machines were in use in Hungary,[77] some of which, mostly Electrospirators and one iron lung, were continuously used until the early 2000s in the respiratory ward.[78]

The challenge that respiratory paralysis posed to public health systems was the same irrespective of ideological stance or political alignment. Both East and West struggled with the prospect of the sudden need for these costly and complicated machines in time of epidemic crises. Scientists and engineers on both sides of the Iron Curtain worked on similar projects at a parallel pace in order to solve the problem of providing breath to paralysed patients. As such, it would be too simplistic to see the arrival of iron lungs in Hungary as a story of technological transfer from West to East. Neither was it a story of Western countries providing aid to make up for Eastern insufficiencies. Instead, in this network of assistance, originally conceived in the West, all countries participated as potential givers and takers. It was easy to see that polio did not distinguish between capitalism and socialism when it came to outbreaks.

The Heine-Medin Hospital and the ICRC

It was the fact that polio outbreaks straddled the Iron Curtain and cut across political systems and regimes that contributed to the continued investment in the disease throughout the 1950s in Hungary. From the perspective of polio, the revolution was less of a watershed event than it is usually considered. This is the reason why the Heine-Medin Hospital, mentioned in the beginning of this chapter, was able to survive its founder and flourish in the years of political retribution following the revolution. At the same time, the revolution opened windows of opportunity in terms of pursuing public health agendas and access to aid; nevertheless this, too, appears different through the lens of polio. The various ways in which the hospital mobilised connections, initiated international donations and engaged with the ICRC sheds light on the agency of the actors involved, and thereby provides an excellent example of the way interventions by international organisations in political and social upheaval play out on the ground.

[75] Boda, *Sorsfordulók*, 56.   [76] Ibid. 62.
[77] Boda and Murányi, *Respiratiós Therapia*, 115–17.
[78] Csillag, 'Gyermekbénulás I', Csillag és Ádám Film; Fórum Film, Hungary, 1995.

One of the main sites of international aid in Hungary in 1956 was the Heine-Medin Hospital, established during the revolution. Although Imre Nagy signed off on the foundation of the hospital, the story of the institution that became a key player in polio treatment in Hungary began a few years earlier, in the Stalinist era. Dr László Lukács, an orthopaedic doctor and future director of the hospital, initiated the process in 1954, a year after poliomyelitis research began at the State Hygienic Institute (SHI) in cooperation with the epidemics department of the Health Ministry.[79]

Lukács handed in a petition to the Health Ministry, pointing out the necessity of a national polio hospital and emphasising the urgency of establishing such an institution.[80] Lukács made his case by pointing out the insufficient resources for treating the increasing number of polio patients.[81] At the time, polio patients were mainly treated in the László infectious disease hospital in the acute phase, and most polio patients received restorative treatment in the Heine-Medin Rehabilitation Institute, established in 1947 with fifty beds under the direction of Dr Annna Szívós, which became part of the National Institute of Rheumatology and Physiotherapy in the early 1950s.[82] The Under-Secretary of Health supported Lukács's proposal in a letter to the Health Minister,[83] and according to an internal document, the case of the future Heine-Medin Hospital was included in the second five-year plan to hold 150–200 beds.[84] However, for a while nothing happened: a year later, only twenty beds for polio patients were ordered to be issued to the Bókay János Children's Hospital, where Lukács worked at the time.[85]

The plans of Dr Lukács became a reality with the signature of Imre Nagy, and the hospital started working during the months of retribution. The institute, its acquired buildings and the appointment of Lukács as head of the hospital were reconfirmed on several occasions after the revolution was suppressed with the aid of the Soviet army.[86] The institute officially opened on

---

[79] Dr Bakács, *Az Országos Közegészségügyi Intézet Működése 1927–1957*, 82

[80] László Dr Lukács. 'Letter to the Health Minister.' Budapest: National Archives of Hungary, XIX-C-2-d-8113/L/1–1954, 1954.

[81] Lukács. 'Feljegyzés a Fővárosi Heine-Medin Kórház és Rendelőintézet Alapításáról, Működéséről, Eredményeiről és ezzel Kapcsolatos Tevékenységéről.' Budapest: Personal archives of Dr. Prof. Ferenc Péter, 1993.

[82] Schweitzer, *Polio 2.0*, 83–86.

[83] István Dr. Simonovits. 'Feljegyzés Zsoldos Elvtárs Részére Lukács László Dr. Javaslatáról.' XIX-C-2-d-8113/L/1–1954, 1954.

[84] Röthler. 'Házi Feljegyzés.' Budapest: National Archives of Hungary, XIX-C-2-d-8113/L/ 1, 1954.

[85] Ibid.

[86] József Dr. Karossa-Pfeiffer. 'Megbízás.' Budapest: Budapest City Archives, Budapest Főváros Tanácsa Végrehajtóbizottságának XII. Egészségügyi osztálya, 1956 and János Dr. Vikol, 'Határozat' (Budapest: Budapest Főváros Tanácsa Végrehajtóbizottságának XII. egészségügyi osztálya, 1956).

12 November 1956 with 160 beds, and was organised under the authority of the City of Budapest.[87]

Even though the importance of the fight against polio overrode political changes, this heritage put the hospital in a delicate situation. A brief manuscript, which became the basis of the chapter in a volume celebrating the hospital's fiftieth anniversary, gives insight into the political manoeuvring of its director, László Lukács, as he states:

> The Health Minister proposed that the institution belong directly to the Ministry, but I could also choose to put it under the authority of the City of Budapest instead. I chose the latter.... . The chief doctor of the city was Dr János Vikol, who had ... firmly supported the cause of the disabled. The other reason was that I didn't trust the leaders of the Health Ministry, I feared [undoing], a hope of the 200 leading party members with the intention of getting back the distinguished treatment of their children.[88]

Although maintaining the new institution and its buildings after the revolution clearly required political skills, the fact that the doctor-director could choose the authority to which the institution should belong implies the great importance assigned to the cause, granting Lukács a certain political independence. Meanwhile, he also had to deal with the hostility of the political elite, who felt that the establishment of the hospital would curb their privileges in childcare.

The reason for this was that the Heine-Medin Hospital used five buildings that had previously belonged to the Rákosi Mátyás[89] kindergarten, a childcare home for privileged party officials in the prestigious district of the Rózsadomb in the Buda hills. It is no coincidence that an institution founded during the 1956 revolution was established in buildings with such a history: this was a small, but obvious, attack on the hated political elite.

The houses were, for the most part, nationalised residences of the economic and political elite of another era. The villas were scattered in the most sought-after part of the city, among green lawns, small patches of woods and swimming pools. In many ways, they were ideal for the long-term care of disabled children, but they also threw up obstacles that were difficult to overcome.

First of all, the hospital's location posed problems: reaching the relatively remote location on the hilltop without proper public transportation on poor-quality roads[90] was often hard on staff and patients alike, neither of whom

[87] 'Új Gyermekbénulás-Utókezelő Intézetet Állítottak Fel', *Népszabadság* 1956, 3.

[88] Lukács. 'Feljegyzés a Fővárosi Heine-Medin Kórház és Rendelőintézet Alapításáról, Működéséről, Eredményeiről és ezzel Kapcsolatos Tevékenységéről.' Budapest: Personal archives of Dr. Prof. Ferenc Péter, 1993, 2.

[89] Hungarian Stalinist leader, head of the Hungarian Worker's Party and the most influential political figure from 1949 to 1956. The Stalinist era in Hungary is named after him.

[90] 'Polio Epidemic Feared', *Washington Post and Times Herald*, 5 June 1957, 8.

lived in the elegant neighbourhood. This was especially true in the early days. Public transportation came to a complete stop during the desperate street battles of the revolution, and it took months to reorganise trams and buses and to rebuild damage to the infrastructure. It could take nurses hours to reach their workplace on foot, even with the director giving them a ride as often as he could.[91]

Getting children to the hospital was equally hard. In the fights of the revolution, the hospital's only van was hit severely and had a gaping hole on the side and bottom. When transferring children from the infectious disease hospital to the Heine-Medin Hospital, nurses put infants into laundry baskets (along with the fresh laundry), which they tied to the inside of the van, and hoped for the best.[92] In later years, once in possession of more resources, the hospital organised a minibus to pick up children daily in the city centre for outpatient care – 4,500 on a monthly basis. Severely disabled outpatients were transported by two minivans door to door. Since the same vehicles were used to transport hospital patients between buildings (to X-ray, surgery, physical therapy, etc.), and were often under repair, these journeys often involved long waiting times.[93]

The buildings themselves were never intended to house a hospital, let alone a treatment centre for disabled children. Steep, curving stairways and slippery floors made each day in the hospital challenging for staff, parents and children as they made their way between bedrooms and spaces of treatment.[94] When the hospital opened, the buildings were partially damaged from the war and the revolution. After the fighting settled down in the winter of 1956–57, the Hungarian army contributed by repairing the buildings and heating them.[95]

The hospital was still in dire need of medical supplies. 'The bad conditions prevailing in Hungary are affecting and hindering the beginning of our work and are causing us great difficulties', wrote the director, Dr Lukács, in a letter to the Red Cross. 'It is quite impossible to obtain supplies of equipment, especially instruments, in Budapest.'[96] Even basic necessities like bed linens and beds were scarce. Katalin Parádi remembers her first weeks in the hospital, not long after it opened. She was a teenager when she contracted the disease, an exception to the rule in Hungary, where the overwhelming majority of polio

[91] Enyedi Judit Dr. Dékány Pálné, interview by Dora Vargha, 11 January 2008; Elvira Mészáros, interview by Dora Vargha, 11 January 2008.
[92] Dékány Pálné, interview by Vargha, 11 January 2008.
[93] 'Hungary Battle Polio', *Washington Post and Times Herald*, 2 July 1957.
[94] 'Salk Expects End of Polio Some Day', *New York Times*, 9 July 1957, 3.
[95] Péter Ferenc, ed. *Gyermekbeteg-ellátás a Rózsadombon 1956–2006* (Budapest: Tudomány Kiadó, 2006), 8.
[96] János Dr. Vikol. 'Heine-Medin Utókezelő-Intézet Szervezése.' Budapest: National Archives of Hungary, Egészségügyi Minisztérium XIX-C-2-d-40.318–1957 (16.d.), 1956.

patients were under 3 years old.[97] Since polio was truly an 'infantile paralysis' in Hungary, the hospital arranged its meagre resources accordingly – leaving exceptional patients like Katalin without a room of their own, or even a bed. 'They had only cots that they inherited from the childcare home, no proper beds for patients. I had to sleep in the same room with the little ones on a makeshift bed assembled of a couple of chairs.'[98]

Soon, help came from the International Red Cross. Both official and personal avenues were utilised to procure crucial donations. First, the Acting Minister for Foreign Affairs, István Sebes, sent a letter to the Secretary-General of the United Nations in reply to the UN's note 'requesting data on the Hungarian people's needs in medical supplies, foodstuffs and clothes from abroad'. In this, the minister gave a detailed list of urgent needs, including ambulances, insulin, gamma globulin, vitamins, surgical stitching materials, X-ray machines and iron lungs.[99] The request was forwarded to the Division of External Relations and Technical Assistance of the UN, which in turn forwarded it to the International Committee of the Red Cross (ICRC).

However, the general aid received from abroad was shared between all of the hospitals in the city and was mostly used to replenish stocks. It was not sufficient to equip a brand-new institution.[100] Thus, Lukács chose an unofficial, more targeted route to procure the necessary supplies that he needed for the treatment of the polio patients, now numbering more than 100, housed in the hospital: he mobilised his family.

An extensive exchange of letters between the American Red Cross, the ICRC and Hungarian physicians reveals the route of request for aid. On 28 December 1956, the American Red Cross contacted the ICRC with the following information:

Dr László Lukács, chief surgeon of the Metropolitan Heine-Medin Institute of Budapest ... has been in telephone communication with his wife, who is now in the United States on a visitor's visa, staying with her brother, a student at the Eastern Baptist Seminary in Philadelphia, Pennsylvania. In these telephone conversations, he spoke of the urgent need for Salk vaccine and essential operating room equipment for his hospital, equipment that had been lost when the hospital was moved from its previous location ... Since then, the brother-in-law has been trying to raise funds for the purchase of operating room equipment.[101]

[97] See Chapter 4.   [98] Parádi, interview by Vargha, 27 January 2010.
[99] Külügyminisztérium, 'A Külügyminisztérium Iii. Osztályának Feljegyzése a Magyar-Amerikai Viszonyról.' Budapest: National Archives of Hungary, XIX-J-1-j USA 4/bd, 99/1958, 11, doboz, 1958.
[100] Dr Vikol, 'Heine-Medin Utókezelő-Intézet Szervezése.' Budapest: National Archives of Hungary, 1956.
[101] 'Megérkezett Hazánkba Az Első Vastüdő', Hungary, 1948.

It is uncertain when and why Lukács's wife went to the United States, and if the trip took place before or during the revolution. It is certain that she was back in Hungary in 1959, as she was present as a member of the Women's Council at the annual school exams that were organised for the children staying and studying in the hospital.[102] This suggests that she was not considered to be an unwanted element of society by the communist government and could return safely to Hungary – perhaps thanks to the political connections of her husband.

The ICRC replied to the letter in mid-January with the promise of investigating it through their general delegate for relief in Hungary.[103] By the end of February 1957, a detailed report about the hospital and its needs was assembled by ICRC officials and was forwarded to the American Red Cross.[104] The report, containing an assessment by the head of medical services of the Hungarian Relief Action of the ICRC, highlighted: 'The poor and makeshift character of the therapeutic equipment stands out in sharp contrast to the modern fittings of the houses ... There is also a shortage of qualified staff.' The reason for urgency was the growing importance of the hospital in polio care in Hungary. Within mere months of its opening, without sufficient equipment or supplies, the patient load was growing fast. 'There are now 130 beds, all of them occupied. Except for two adults, this is purely a children's centre ... Besides the patients who live in, mostly children from the provinces, a further 200 children from Budapest visit the hospital every day for treatment.'[105]

This report, with detailed lists of requirements from different respiratory devices to surgical equipment, reached the American Red Cross too late. By the time the letter arrived, Lukács's brother-in-law had managed to secure some of the much-needed equipment and had sent it directly to the hospital.[106] However, the Red Cross was soon able to take a more active part in organising polio aid; when the 1957 epidemic rolled into Hungary, the ICRC, the League of the Red Cross Societies and national Red Cross societies coordinated their efforts in providing polio aid to the country.

Much of the equipment sent by Red Cross societies found its way to the Heine-Medin Hospital. The Swedish Red Cross and the Swedish Rädda Barnen society for child relief concentrated especial effort on this

---

[102] Ágnes Soós, interview by Dora Vargha, 7 April , 2010.
[103] 'Eljött a Nap...', Heine-Medin Híradó 1, July (1959), 2.
[104] Tamás Kertész and Tibor Szabó, interview by Dora Vargha, November 2010.
[105] Sándor Rádai, interview by Dora Vargha, 5 May 2010.
[106] Maria Roth, 'Child Protection in Communist Romania (1944–1989)', in Social Care under State Socialism (1945–1989): Ambitions, Ambiguities, and Mismanagement, ed. Sabine Hering (Opladen and Farmington Hills: Barbara Budrich Publishers, 2009), 201–11.

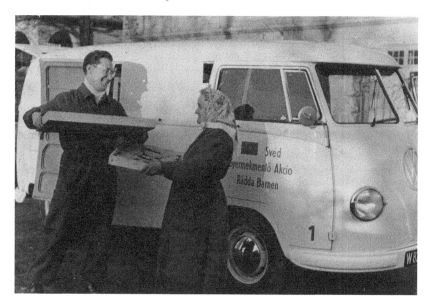

Figure 2.2 *Aid arriving from the Swedish Rädda Barnen. Hongrie
1956–57. Budapest. V-P-HU-N-00023–01 ICRC Archives (ARR).* **This
image is protected by copyright and cannot be used without further
permissions clearance.**

institution.[107] The hospital received important donations, such as rocking beds,
hospital beds, bed linen, blankets, surgical equipment and medicine. The
donations were vital and more than appreciated – hospital workers called the
high-quality blankets Swedish blankets for decades to come.[108] In this sense,
Swedish international aid achieved one of its central goals, as historian Ann
Nehlin has argued: exporting and promoting Swedish standards, values and
expertise on childcare.[109] The director of the hospital developed a personal
relationship with Anna Ma Toll, Rädda Barnen's representative in Hungary,

[107] Rädda Barnen's involvement in general Hungarian child relief dates back to December, 1956.
8. 'Agreement between the International Committee of the Red Cross, the Hungarian Red
Cross and Rädda Barnen.' Geneva: International Committee of the Red Cross Archives,
Accord conclu entre Rädda Barnen, le CICR et la Croix-Rouge hongroise au sujet des envois
non-Croix-Rouge acheminés par le CICR à Budapest. Signé le 3 décembre 1956, B AG 280
094–017.03, 1956.
[108] Dékány Pálné, interview with Vargha, 11 January 2008.
[109] Ann Nehlin, *Exporting Visions and Saving Children: The Swedish Save the Children Fund*,
Linköping Studies in Arts and Science (Linköping: The Department of Child Studies, Linköping University, 2009), 202.

and remained in contact even after the Swedish delegation had to leave the country following the fall of the revolution. The organisation continued to support the hospital with surgical equipment, bed linen and medicine well into the late 1950s.[110]

The Heine-Medin Hospital was the only institution in the country that exclusively provided specialised medical care for polio patients, and it quickly became the largest national centre for treatment by the end of the 1950s. Its establishment, from the foundational document to its physical location and the medical equipment it contained, was a profound product of the 1956 revolution. The same uprising that created chaos in politics, society and public health also created unique opportunities, of which a wide range of individuals took advantage in order to satisfy long-standing needs in polio treatment.

The capability of hospital directors, physicians and their family members to act quickly in the ensuing turmoil came from the realisation that they were part of a significant Cold War event. The procurement of life-saving devices and medical equipment was made possible by the international limelight thrown on this small Eastern European country in 1956. However, the arrival of iron lungs and the establishment of the Heine-Medin Hospital was not an intended and structural part of international aid to the country at the time. Rather, these Hungarian agents of internationalism tapped into the existing and emerging practices of international organisations dealing with political and humanitarian crises.

They also drew on transnational experiences that overarched Cold War barriers: the scarcity of specialised and high-tech medical equipment and the common understanding of a disease that did not halt at ideological and political dividing lines. It was the local poverty of a post-war Eastern European country that coincided with a global shortage and, in this cross-section, initiated innovation in respiration technology and in procuring essential medical equipment. In this sense, international aid during the revolution, with regard to epidemic management, was highly individualised and far from a one-way affair. Hungarian professionals actively utilised a particular political moment in the Cold War to address both acute and structural needs in public health and healthcare. Moreover, the networks they built proved to be invaluable as polio epidemic outbreaks erupted with renewed force in the following years.

---

[110] László Lukács, 'A Budai Gyermekkórház Történetének Periódusai. 1956. 12 November–1963. December 31', in *Gyermekbeteg-ellátás a Rózsadombon 1956–2006* , ed. Péter Ferenc (Budapest: Tudomány Kiadó, 2006).

3   Unlikely Allies

On the evening of 13 July 1957 a Swiss aeroplane, manned by a West German pilot, appeared above the skies of Budapest airport.[1] A prestigious group, including leading state officials and party members of the People's Republic of Hungary, greeted the tall, black-haired man as he descended from the cockpit. The Communist Party official shook his hand in the name of all Hungarian mothers, while experts from the Health Ministry and the State Hygienic Institute inspected the precious cargo: a long-awaited shipment of the Salk vaccine.[2]

Jonas Salk's inactivated vaccine was licensed two years before, in 1955 in the United States. This vaccine, administered as an injection, contained killed poliovirus strains that would provide immunity from paralytic poliomyelitis. The Salk vaccine became an important milestone in twentieth-century medicine. Its development within the March of Dimes movement, the role of the National Foundation for Infantile Paralysis in funding research and the orchestration of the exceptional field trial of the vaccine involving over 600,000 children have been the focus of many heroic and critical accounts.[3] Yet important stories about the Salk vaccine that reach beyond the 'American Story' are yet to be told. Polio represented a threat to societies all over the world and the news of an effective prevention spread fast. Just like the disease itself, the Salk vaccine transcended national and political boundaries with relative ease and soon became widely used on a global scale. As such, it made its way across the Iron Curtain as well.

---

[1] Part of the research and argument presented in chapters 3 and 5 was published in Vargha, Dora, 'Between East and West: Polio Vaccination Across the Iron Curtain in Cold War Hungary', Bulletin of the History of Medicine 88, no. 2 (2014): 319–342

[2] 'Szülők, Vigyázzatok!' (Hungary: Health Ministry, 1957); 'Július 18. És 19-én Megkezdődik a Gyermekbénulás Elleni Védőoltás. Az Egészségügyi Minisztérium Hivatalos Tájékoztatója', Népakarat, 14 July 1957.

[3] See for instance Paul, A History of Poliomyelitis; Jane S. Smith, Patenting the Sun: Polio and the Salk Vaccine (New York: Morrow, 1990); Nina Gilden Seavey, Jane S. Smith and Paul Wagner, A Paralyzing Fear: The Triumph over Polio in America, 1st ed. (New York: TV Books, 1998); Jeffrey Kluger, Splendid Solution: Jonas Salk and the Conquest of Polio (New York: G. P. Putnam's Sons, 2004); David M. Oshinsky, Polio: An American Story (Oxford and New York: Oxford University Press, 2005).

The Salk vaccine, whose first arrival was dramatically depicted in news broadcasts,[4] took a complicated route to Hungary. The vials of vaccine were developed in the United States and manufactured in and shipped from Canada; they then travelled to Amsterdam, where a West German pilot in a Swiss aeroplane picked it up and flew with it over the Iron Curtain, arriving in Budapest.

The West German pilot, who was immediately declared a national hero for volunteering for the job on his day off, had to return to Amsterdam soon after the boxes of Salk vaccine were unloaded and inspected by delegates from the Health Ministry. Had he been able to spend a few days in Hungary, he would have seen a country recuperating from one crisis and entering another one. Merely half a year had passed since Russian tanks had rolled along the streets of Budapest as the capital staged desperate battles in the revolution against the communist regime in the autumn of 1956. The new Kádár government had just started showing its teeth. The executions of those whom they had begun calling 'counter-revolutionaries' had started in early spring. Out of the total of 229 people executed as a retribution for the revolution between 1956 and 1961, 38 were killed by mid-1957.[5] Still, the country was slowly recovering from a complete standstill, restoring public transportation, removing rubble, moving on. The polio hospital founded by the revolutionary prime minister, Imre Nagy, who was soon to be imprisoned and executed, was up and running, if on meagre resources.

It was into this social and political environment that the most severe polio epidemic in Hungarian history made an entrance in the early summer of 1957. By October, nearly 2,300 children were paralysed by the disease, constituting a 23 per 100,000 incidence rate, one of the highest in Europe. The stakes were thus high: the new, post-revolutionary government was faced with a crisis of another kind and needed to show power and efficiency in providing an answer to the epidemic challenge.

Bringing the Salk Vaccine Home

As the stories of the polio hospital and flying iron lung show, the 1956 uprising opened up opportunities that revolutionised polio care itself. When it came to polio prevention, however, the chaos and destruction that the fighting left behind hindered efforts, rather than moving them forward. In the end, the revolution and the effect it had on the social and political

---

[4] 'Szülők, vigyázzatok!' (Hungary: Health Ministry, 1957).
[5] Attila Szakolcai, 'Az 1956-os Magyar Forradalmat Követő Politikai Megtorlás Áldozatainak Hivatalos Névsora', Beszélő 6, no. 24 (1994).

structure played an important part in the way subsequent polio vaccination strategies played out in Hungary.

Before mass vaccination became available, the use of gamma globulin was seen as the most effective, although imperfect, prophylactic technology. Gamma globulin is a part of the human blood that is rich in antibodies and therefore can be used to boost a person's immune system. In the 1950s, it was used in the form of injections derived from blood plasma, to build passive immunity against a number of diseases, like hepatitis and measles. In the early 1950s several trials explored the effectiveness of gamma globulin in polio control in the United States, although the trials proved to be inconclusive.[6] Since it was made from human blood, the serum was not readily available and its efficiency was debated in Hungary. The Health Ministry considered it to be an efficient way to curb both poliomyelitis and measles, and since 1954 had used the serum to provide protection in nurseries and kindergartens in which they registered polio.[7] In the early weeks of the outbreak of 1957, the International Committee of the Red Cross transferred 'a quantity of gamma globulin' to the Hungarian Red Cross to help curb the disease.[8]

A report by the Medical Research Council (*Egészségügyi Tudományos Tanács*)[9] in 1956, however, pointed out that according to its recommendation, gamma globulin was ineffective against polio and should be used only in measles and hepatitis prevention.[10] Indeed, contemporary international medical literature argued[11] that gamma globulin gave protection for a limited time only and was only effective if administered just days or weeks before exposure

---

[6] Stephen E. Mawdsley, *Selling Science: Polio and the Promise of Gamma Globulin*, ed. Rima D. Apple and Janet Golden, Critical Issues in Health and Medicine (New Brunswick, NJ: Rutgers University Press, 2016).

[7] Egészségügyi Minisztérium. 'Jelentés a Politikai Bizottsághoz Az Ország Közegészségügyi És Járványügyi Helyzetéről.' Budapest: Magyar Országos Levéltár, XIX-C-2-m, 115/1954, 1954, and Miklós Dr. Drexler. 'Gyermekbénulás Elleni Védekezés.' Budapest: National Archives of Hungary, Drexler Miklós egészségügyi miniszter iratai, XIX-C-2-n, 369/1956, 18 August 1956.

[8] 'Poliomyelitis. Papers Presented at the Fourth International Poliomyelitis Conference' (paper presented at the Fourth International Poliomyelitis Conference, Geneva, 1957), 6.

[9] The Medical Research Council was established in 1951 by the Ministerial Council, as a consulting body to the Health Ministry. Its task was to recommend or provide an opinion on issues of medical theory and practice. The Medical Research Council, comprised of twenty members, also directed medical research in Hungary (it shared this responsibility with the National Academy of Sciences). György Dr. Gál, László Dr. Medve, and Dr. Rák Kálmán, 'Az ETT Története', Egészségügyi Tudományos Tanács.

[10] 'Házi Feljegyzés.' Budapest: National Archives of Hungary, Zsoldos Sándor egészségügyi miniszter iratai, XIX-C-2-m, 821/v/1–16, 6 July 1956.

[11] Since scientists commissioned by the Health Ministry took part in international conferences regularly and had access to major international journals, they presumably had knowledge of major research findings on gamma globulin, such as W. McD. Hammon, L. L. Corlell, and P. F. Wehrle, 'Evaluation of Red Cross Gamma Globulin as a Prophylactic Agent for Poliomyelitis. IV. Final Report of Results Based on Clinical Diagnoses', *Journal of the American Medical Association* 151, no. 11 (1953): 1272–85.

to poliovirus. This was, given the difficulties in polio diagnosis, impossible to do on a large scale. In any case, the quantity of available gamma globulin was limited, since it was produced from human blood. For this reason, it was not seen as a viable solution, especially since it had to be divided for measles and hepatitis prevention.[12]

Prevention strategies involving technologies, such as the gamma globulin serum, reveal conflicting evaluations among the medical community and the political leadership. While the serum did not promise effective protection against polio, its risks were not considered substantial. However, the use of the serum could compromise prophylaxis against other diseases. This shows a prioritisation from the state: it considered the potential, limited effect of this particular technology in the prevention of polio to be more important than other, also common, childhood diseases. Thus, despite the conflicting views on efficiency and the limited availability of the serum, gamma globulin was officially considered to be one of several prophylactic tools that the state employed to protect its children from polio.[13]

However, it seems that the limited availability of the serum was sometimes paired with confused perceptions of its usage.

Soon after my son was diagnosed with polio in 1954, a big black car stopped in front of our house. Suddenly chills ran down my spine. The big black car usually meant that the political police was coming to take someone away. They knocked on our door and we opened it, trying to be as calm as possible. Two *ávós*[14] came in. They said that they heard that our son got polio, so they brought gamma globulin for him, hoping that it might help. This was very difficult to get at the time, but I guess they had special reserves. We thanked them and gave Gyuri the serum, but, of course, it was already too late for that. We wondered how they knew that our son was sick and why they wanted to help. My husband was a quite influential figure. He was the district vet in a rural area,

[12] To achieve protection against polio for 3 weeks, 0.3 ml per kg in bodyweight had to be administered – which would mean about 3–6 ml per child in a crèche (bölcsőde). According to a report from 1956, the widespread application of the serum is not possible because the total amount of available gamma globulin per month is 8,000 ml, and has to be divided among measles and hepatitis as well. József Román, 'Gyermekbénulás Elleni Védekezés' (Budapest: Egészségügyi Minisztérium, 1956). Even if the government spent all the available serum on polio immunization, it still would have been only enough to provide 1,300–2,600 children with it on a monthly basis, with each dose not even covering a full month.
[13] Passive immunisation practice in the United States was similar, after the gamma globulin field trials in 1951. See 'The Distribution and Use of Gamma Globulin: A Statement Issued April 20, 1953, by the Division of Medical Sciences of the National Research Council', *Public Health Reports* 68, no. 7 (1953): 659–65. Gamma globulin was used up to July 1957 in polio prevention, as new shipments were imported even in the days preceding vaccination with the Salk vaccine. 'A Minisztertanács Intézkedései a Gyermekparalízis Megelőzése és a Betegellátás Érdekében', *Népakarat*, 5 July 1957.
[14] Members of the political police. Although the political police was reorganised and renamed from Államvédelmi Osztály (ÁVO) to Államvédelmi Hatóság (ÁVH), the former name for its members continued to be used in the vernacular.

but he was by no means favoured by the system. They had already confiscated and nationalised his car by that time, for instance. Many years later he found out that his brother-in-law was an agent back then.[15]

While the confusion of treatment and prevention methods in this story highlight the uncertainties and lack of clear-cut ideas in the perception of the disease, the secret police's involvement is telling of the way access to goods, especially medical supplies and care, worked at the time. In a still recovering post-war Hungary, resources for the average citizen were quite scarce. 'I don't think there's a point in talking about poverty. After war displacement, the fronts moving about, we hardly had anything left, but as far as I remember, almost everyone was poor then', recalled one polio patient.[16] Political networks, connections and even key professions could facilitate access to certain goods or services, contributing to an informal economy of favours and exchange. On some occasions, it was these informal avenues of exchange and procurement that gained prevalence, with the blessing of authorities. These private and unofficial ways came forth and were supported by the state when the problem of fulfilling responsibilities, in this case toward the health of children, arose.

In the mid-1950s, a more efficient technology became available: an inactivated vaccine developed by Jonas Salk in the United States, released to the market in 1955. The vaccine contained dead viruses that helped the immune system of the body to develop a defence against the poliomyelitis virus. Salk finished work on the vaccine in 1952 at the University of Pittsburgh, but years of trials were needed before the vaccine could be marketed to the population.

On 25 April 1955, a child previously inoculated with the Salk vaccine was admitted to the hospital with signs of polio. The following day, five similar cases were reported. All of these patients received a vaccine produced by Cutter Laboratories, and on 27 April, the Surgeon General requested that Cutter recall all its vaccines. In the course of the next two months, 94 vaccinated patients, 126 family contacts and 40 community contacts were diagnosed with poliomyelitis[17] in what would be termed the *Cutter incident.* This situation had a tremendous impact: it shook public trust in the vaccine, changed vaccine regulation and control in the United States and ultimately affected the story of another, live, polio vaccine developed by Albert Sabin.[18]

---

[15] Irén Dr Vargha Jánosné Lázok, interview by Dora Vargha, 24 June 2008.
[16] Éva Paksáné Szentgyörgyi, interview by Dora Vargha, 12 November 2010.
[17] Nathanson and Langmuir, 'The Cutter Incident Poliomyelitis Following Formaldehyde-Inactivated Poliovirus Vaccination in the United States during the Spring of 1955'.
[18] Oshinsky, *Polio: An American Story*; Offit, *The Cutter Incident*; James Colgrove, *State of Immunity: The Politics of Vaccination in Twentieth-Century America* (Berkeley: University of California Press, 2006).

Hungarian newspapers could not let the opportunity of the Cutter incident go by without using it as yet another example of the West's disregard for the well-being and safety of its citizens. In May 1955, the newspaper *Szabad Nép* accused the United States of rushing into the vaccination process without proper testing due to negligence, thereby making children guinea pigs of the free market economy.[19] Incidentally, the Cutter fiasco had the opposite effect in the United States, sparking contradictory criticisms: the American Medical Association (AMA) viewed the mass trials as paving the way for mass vaccinations, which raised fear of the Red Menace in the form of socialised medicine.

Sentiments softened towards the Salk vaccine in Hungary (though not necessarily in the United States) when the renowned Russian virologist Mikhail Chumakov issued a favourable review of the serum, published in Hungary in April 1956.[20] In subsequent years, use of the Salk vaccination spread widely throughout Europe, with Denmark leading the way by immunising its entire endangered population through free vaccination by 1957.[21] The Netherlands started nationwide mass vaccination in 1957, along with Italy,[22] while Britain organised immunisation with the Salk vaccine a year later.[23] Of the Eastern European countries, in 1957, Czechoslovakia and Poland began using the Salk vaccination with a domestically produced vaccine.[24]

Plans to produce the Salk vaccine in Hungary started to form in June 1956, a year after it was introduced in the United States. In a report to the Ministerial Council, the Health Ministry deemed the production of the Salk vaccine 'extremely complicated and expensive'.[25] Among the problems, the report pointed out, were inadequate laboratories. The virus department of the State Hygienic Institute shared a building that had recently kept animals, and the Humán Vaccine Production and Research Institute was housed in a desolate space that did not permit expansion beyond the production of typhus and

[19] 'Halálos Áldozata Van az Amerikában Felfedezett Gyermekparalízis Elleni Védőoltásnak', *Szabad Nép*, 1 May 1955.
[20] Cited in Radio Free Europe. 'Polio in Hungary: Background Report.' Budapest: Open Society Archives, RFE News & Information Service – Evaluation & Research Section, 1957.
[21] Dr. E. Juel Henningsen, 'Poliovaccination in Denmark' (paper presented at the VIth Symposium of the European Association of Poliomyelitis, Munich, 7–9 September 1959).
[22] Crovari, 'History of Polio Vaccination in Italy'.
[23] Lindner and Blume, 'Vaccine Innovation and Adoption: Polio Vaccines in the UK, the Netherlands and West Germany, 1955–1965'.
[24] 'Poliomyelitis. Papers Presented at the Fourth International Poliomyelitis Conference', *Fourth International Poliomyelitis Conference* (1957).
[25] József Román. 'Gyermekbénulás Elleni Védekezés.' Budapest: National Archives of Hungary, Az Egészségügyi Minisztérium Iratai, XIX-C-n, 369/1956, 1956.

smallpox vaccines. Furthermore, a staff of 20 would have to be trained to handle such duties as caring for laboratory primates and to serve as lab technicians and scientists.[26]

A loan from the International Committee of the Red Cross was to be used for the developments needed for vaccine production, which included the establishment and building of a new institution in the SHI. The Health Ministry wished to speed up the decision-making process, given that even with the loan, it would take three years to build the required facilities.[27] In a newspaper interview in late summer 1956, however, the ministry unveiled plans to begin production as soon as the next year, pending the results of a study trip of experts to Western Europe.[28]

Before the Health Ministry would take a stand on the question of polio vaccine production, they stressed the urgent need for a study trip abroad to explore the details and to attain sufficient training in the process.[29] The destination would be Denmark, a European centre for polio research, where Polish colleagues also received their training in Salk vaccine production.[30] In addition to sending two virologists (Dr Elek Farkas and Dr Sándor Koch) to Copenhagen, the ministry also recommended sending the director of SHI to gain experience in organising the logistics of production and two directors from Humán to study the control procedures.

It is not clear why the Health Ministry assigned such importance to the research trip when it was already apparent from the outset that few of the necessary conditions for the production of the Salk vaccine could be fulfilled without significant investment. Of course, pushing for a larger scientific envoy could have originated from personal reasons – a chance to enjoy 'the West', and to build professional and personal connections. But there is also the possibility that the Health Ministry perceived that such a huge investment was indeed a realistic option for the government, in order to curb the crippling disease and dependency on the West all at once.

In the end, only one person joined the scientists: Dr Gábor Veres, director of the Humán Vaccine Production and Research Institute. The three delegates

[26] Ibid.
[27] Aladár Kátay. 'Polio-Vaccina Termelése,' Budapest: National Archives of Hungary, Dr. Vilmon Gyula Egészségügyi Miniszter Iratai, XIX-C-2-e, 50.654/1957, 1957.
[28] 'Nincs Gyermekbénulási Járvány: Hogyan Védekezzünk a Megbetegedések Ellen? Mikorra Várható a Hazai Oltóanyagok Termelése? Beszélgetés Az Egészségügyi Minisztérium Vezetőivel', Szabad Nép, 1956, 4.
[29] Román, 'Gyermekbénulás Elleni Védekezés', 1956.
[30] Arvid Wallgren. 'Some Observations Made during a Short Visit to Poland.' Geneva: World Health Organization, Reports on Maternal and Child Health (MCH) Conditions – Poland, M3–418-2POL JKT 1, 1957.

spent over a month in Denmark,[31] studying vaccine production and the process of vaccination. They also presented their own virus research work and reported intensive interest from Danish scientists, who requested written papers as well.[32]

The delegation decided to head back to Hungary earlier than originally planned, but were held up in Vienna for a week and arrived back in Budapest after the military victory of the Soviet Union on 14 November.[33] It is possible that they waited in Austria to see how the revolution would unfold before re-entering the country. Not surprisingly, the reasons for an almost fortnight-long trip back from Denmark were not detailed in the official documents submitted to the ministry.

The question, of course, arises: why did the scientists come back to Hungary at all? A significant number of medical professionals left the country during the revolution, creating an obvious deficiency in doctors. A year later, the Health Ministry publically called on them to return without any risk of retaliation and offered to help them find work again.[34] In an interview from 2006, Koch says that he thought a Hungarian's place was in Hungary.

The truth is that if you wanted to work, you could, even in that political system. Of course, there was not as much money and recognition as abroad. So I worked, I published a lot in journals abroad, I sometimes travelled and was okay ... I was at home ...[35]

This experience is similar to that of the paediatrician Domokos Boda. After a Swiss conference and study trip he took in 1954, he recounted feeling 'that there was a point to all the work. What's more, you could conduct successful

[31] It is not easy to see how the scientific innovation and travels of Hungarian doctors fits into an overall view of Eastern European Cold War interactions, for literature on Eastern European history of medicine and health is scarce. Lily M. Hoffman's article, Hoffman, 'Professional Autonomy Reconsidered: The Case of Czech Medicine under State Socialism', tells us that Czechoslovak doctors' opportunities were much more limited than their Hungarian colleagues in this respect, which may as well be, but at the same time, Czechoslovakia was one of the very first countries in the world to conduct mass polio vaccination with the Sabin vaccine in the late 1950s. Taking into account the Hungarian case, together with the much-debated cooperation of the USA and the USSR in polio prevention, it is safe to say that the debilitating child disease did create a space that sometimes overrode political rhetoric and action. The fight against polio, in a schizophrenic way, was also an avenue in which individual nationalist agendas and Cold War aspirations could be played out.

[32] Sándor Koch, Gábor Veres, and Elek Farkas. 'Jelentés a Koppenhágai Tanulmányútunkról.' Budapest: MOL Egészségügyi Minisztérium iratai, XIX-C-2-e, 50.911, 821/4/Virus/1957, 1957, 1.

[33] Ibid. 2.

[34] 'Két Érdekes Előadással Kezdődött Meg a Balatonfüredi Orvoskongresszus', Népakarat, 27 September 1957. There is another explanation, though, for this open call – this was a strategy of the state to lure home and incarcerate revolutionaries.

[35] Károly Mezei, '... Isten Van, Az Ember Történik.' Koch Sándor Virológussal Beszélget Mezei Károly, Miért Hiszek? (Budapest: Kairosz Kiadó, 2006).

research on an international level among the circumstances at home.'[36] Apart from the Danish trip, Koch had several occasions on which to revisit his commitment to staying in Hungary. Koch was thus not alone in remaining and working in Hungary out of a more or less free choice. In 1961, he spent a year working with Nobel Laureate André Lwoff in Paris at the Pasteur Institute.[37]

The revolution, as in so many areas of life, had effects on the polio epidemic in Hungary. In the middle of the fight, surprisingly, a window opened that facilitated polio treatment with the establishment of a polio hospital by Imre Nagy. At the same time, it significantly hindered polio prevention. Plans for Hungarian vaccine production stopped short in October 1956, only to regain some momentum in January 1957. However, the introduction of the Hungarian Salk vaccine would face one obstacle after another. A detailed look at the eventual failure of Salk vaccine production shows that while the revolution did indeed affect the way the history of polio unfolded in Hungary, there is something inherent in communist governmental practice that played a much larger role. The story of the Salk vaccine provides yet another example of the fragmented way in which the state operated in the communist era, the ways that ineffective ministries could not elicit action from multiple key actors in the process and the way that whole policies and important developments could be buried in bureaucratic labyrinths.

First of all, obtaining the report about the Copenhagen experiences ran into serious problems. What seemed to be a crucial element in the plan for vaccine production in June 1956 turned out to be a major hindrance in the spring of 1957. In February, the document was still not prepared.[38] Nearly four months had passed since the research and study trip and the Health Ministry was growing impatient. Following several requests, the report finally arrived at the ministry on 27 March 1957, signed by the three members of the delegation. The twenty-page document gave a brief account of the trip and detailed the steps necessary to start vaccine production. At the time of the report submission, there was disagreement among the three authors about the buildings needed to house the laboratories, and Veres promised a separate report due in April to detail his opinion. In May, the ministry was still waiting for the document,[39] unable to move forward, stranded in the planning process that had now spanned a whole year without any concrete results.

[36] Boda, *Sorsfordulók*, 57.
[37] Mezei, '... *Isten Van, Az Ember Történik.' Koch Sándor Virológussal Beszélget Mezei Károly.*
[38] Aladár Kátay, 'A Humán Intézet Vírus Osztályának Átköltözése Az Oki-Ba', Budapest: MOL, Egészségügyi Minisztérium iratai, XIX-C-2-e 1957, 50.189/1957, 821/1/Virus/1957. OKI, 1957.
[39] 'Koppenhágai Tanulmányútról Jelentés', Budapest: MOL, Egészségügyi Minisztérium iratai, XIX-C-2-e, 51406, 1957.

After nearly a year, plans for producing a polio vaccine were eventually lost in the attempt to fuse the virus department of SHI with Humán and centralise virus research and vaccine production. 'Domestic production of the Salk vaccine is not possible yet, since there are no facilities that would meet the requirements for production and testing', stated the Health Minister in a newspaper article in late June.[40] The Health Ministry's endeavour to merge the two institutions led to a tense power struggle, leaving a complicated paper trail of complaints infused with vitriolic comments.[41]

The struggle between the SHI, Humán and the Health Ministry points to the larger issue of a dispersed vaccine production and control, a structure that was inherited from the pre-war era and did not quite fit into the centralised notion of a communist healthcare organisation.[42] Humán was initially a department of a private pharmaceutical company, Phylaxia Serum Production Co. Ltd, established in 1924. The company was nationalised in 1948 and smaller vaccine and serum companies merged with it, creating Phylaxia National Serum Production Institute under the auspices of the Ministry of Agriculture. The State Hygienic Institute was established in 1927 with the support of the Rockefeller Foundation.[43] Vaccine production was divided between these two institutions after the war, with Humán producing diphtheria-tetanus-pertussis and smallpox vaccines and SHI producing BCG, rabies and influenza vaccines.[44] The production of this important new vaccine sparked a rivalry among the two, and the Health Ministry was caught in a power struggle that ultimately hindered the introduction of domestic polio vaccine production.

It would take two more years to achieve Salk vaccine production in Hungary. SHI finally won the battle, and the laboratory was completed in August 1958. The 250 litres of the first batch of vaccine produced would be used in July 1959 as the fourth, a booster shot for children who had received all compulsory injections before that time. The SHI planned to produce a maximum of 400 litres per year after that. However, Hungarian production would

[40] 'Az Egészségügyi Minisztérium Tájékoztatója a Gyermekbénulásos Megbetegedésekről és a Védekezés Módjairól', *Népakarat*, 27 June 1957.
[41] 'A Humán Intézet Vírus Osztályának Átköltözése az OKI-ba.' Budapest: MOL, 1957; Benyó, 'A Humán Vírus-Osztály Átvétele. Feljegyzés Dr. Vilmon Miniszterhelyettes Elvtárs Részére', ibid. National Archives of Hungary, XIX-C-2-e, 50.654.
[42] Sándor Koch, 'Present Status of Specific Poliomyelitis Prophylaxis in Hungary' (paper presented at the VIth Symposium of the European Association of Poliomyelitis, Munich, 7–9 September 1959).
[43] Gábor Palló, 'Rescue and Cordon Sanitaire: The Rockefeller Foundation in Hungarian Public Health', *Studies in History and Philosophy of Biological and Biomedical Sciences* 31, no. 3 (2000): 433–45.
[44] Lajos dr. Hegedűs, *The History of Human* (Budapest: HUMAN Pharmaceutical Works Co. Ltd., 2003).

still not be able to cover the whole population's needs, as yet another import from the Soviet Union was needed to complement the domestic stock.[45]

In early 1957 the state was still struggling to find an effective way of preventing polio in Hungary. Gamma globulin prevention was costly and its effectiveness was not convincing to the medical community and the public health administration. Domestic vaccine production was stalling, partly because of the long-term effects of October 1956 and partly because the structure of the public health system had not yet crystallised. As the country was recovering from the upheaval of the revolution, concerns about polio prevention remained in the background until a new and powerful epidemic brought about change in the summer of 1957.

The Unfolding of the 1957 Epidemic

The number of polio cases had been rising since the beginning of 1957. From January onwards, reported polio cases were mostly double – occasionally triple – that of the previous epidemic year, and were up to ten times that of other epidemic years' numbers.[46] Although the statistics of infectious diseases, among them polio, were routinely assembled by the Health Ministry and published in a public health journal every month, the high number of polio cases throughout the year did not stir concern earlier and failed to prompt the government and health authorities to act on disease prevention. The March epidemiology report reveals an explanation for this lack of concern: following the late autumn epidemic of 1956, the high numbers could have been an aftermath, rather than a forewarning.[47] A year later, Dr Otto Rudnai, an epidemiologist in the State Hygienic Institute (Országos Közegészségügyi Intézet, SHI), came to the same conclusion.[48] However, there might be another explanation as to why the government and public health authorities did not devote their full attention to the warning signs. This had to do rather with the aftermath of the 1956 revolution than the outbreak.

The revolution, like any armed conflict, had tremendous effects on public health issues. The consequences of destructive street battles and the absence of

---

[45] Aladár Kátay, 'Vaccination against Poliomyelitis in Hungary' (paper presented at the Eigthth European Symposium on Poliomyelitis, Prague, 23–26 September 1962), 45.

[46] For instance, according to data provided by the Health Ministry, while in March there were 4 reported cases in 1952, 6 in 1954 and 15 in 1956, 49 people were reported to have contracted polio in 1957. Egészségügyi Minisztérium, 'Az Egészségügyi Minisztérium Tájékoztatója Az Ország 1957. Évi Március Havi Járványügyi Helyzetéről', *Népegészségügy* 38, no. 4 (1957).

[47] Ibid.

[48] 'Tájékoztató a Gyermekbénulásos Megbetegedésekről', *Népszabadság*, 27 June 1957; Otto Rudnai, 'Az 1957. Évi Poliomyelitis Járvány. Közlemény Az Országos Közegészségügyi Intézet (Főigazgató: Bakács Tibor Dr.) Járványügyi Osztályáról (Osztályvezető: Petrilla Aladár Dr.)', *Népegészségügy* 39, no. 5–6 (1958): 121–27.

trade, production and transport for weeks, even months, manifested on several levels, from the mundane to the structural. Some hospitals and clinics were badly damaged during the battles in Budapest.[49] By December 1956, even basic hygienic supplies, such as soap, were hard to find.[50] As the country slowly recuperated from the shock of a failed revolution, with the people of Budapest standing in line for aid such as clothes and food and the new government beginning bloody retributions, starting up production and infrastructure and navigating hostile international waters, it seems understandable that the slowly rising numbers of polio cases did not ring alarm bells early on.

Beyond the material challenges to public health caused by the revolution, there is another important aspect of the way such an event could influence actions and concerns over epidemics among the medical community. The ways in which the new Kádár government – seen as traitors by many – publicly grappled with the traumatic shock of the previous year followed a pattern that led from solidarity with the revolutionaries through amnesia to an eventual vilification, labelling October 1956 as a counter-revolution.

The representation of the revolution and its changing political memory trickled down to everyday practices in the management of society, including public health practices and the interpretation of epidemic case numbers. While no records survive that reveal the internal debates about polio epidemic cases in the early months of 1957, the example of measles can give a general idea of the process in which current politics interacted with scientific observations of epidemics. While during and after the revolution polio cases rose to epidemic proportions, another strange thing happened: the number of measles cases plummeted. It was the lack of an epidemic, in this case, that caused concern for public health officials.

The infectious diseases report, intended to be published in the February 1957 edition of the public health journal *Népegészségügy*, addressed this unusual phenomenon and attempted to provide an explanation. The original report argued that schools and kindergartens were closed for a significant time in the autumn and early winter.[51] The school year was disrupted by the revolution, many buildings were damaged or destroyed in armed conflicts, and many, among them teachers and students, fled the country, while others

---

[49] The teaching hospitals, which served as main healthcare providers, were particularly hard hit in Budapest – Dermatology, Internal Medicine, Surgery, Ophthamology, Gynaecology. The Bókay children's Hospital was also injured in a fire. 'Van Építőanyag a Kórházak Helyreállításához, Vöröskereszt Táborikonyhák Létesülnek, Szappant, Mosóport, DDT-t Kapnak a Kerületek', Népakarat, 1956.

[50] 'Lesz Szappan', *Népakarat*, 1956.

[51] József Takó. 'Az Országos Közegészségügyi Intézet Járványügyi Tájékoztatója 1957. Február Haváról.' Budapest: National Archives of Hungary, Állami közegészségügyi felügyeleti és járványvédelmi főosztály, XIX-C-2-e, 50.189, 1957.

died in shootings or were incarcerated after the revolution was suppressed. This underlying knowledge was, however, deleted from the published version by order of the Health Minister.[52] So thorough was the silencing around the October events that even a seemingly harmless epidemiological observation could not be widely spread. This rare insight into the editing process of the journal suggests that political understandings of epidemics formed the way statistics and epidemic curves were interpreted and that certain scientific explanations of their anomalies could be dismissed based on politically unacceptable reasoning.

Silencing and the disregard of rising polio cases, for whatever reason, could not be long maintained. After the initial hesitation to declare a polio epidemic, by the end of June it was obvious to all that that summer would be different than in previous years. The health minister's polio report on the back page of the newspapers, planted among cinema listings, new inventions and accounts of enthusiastic workers, painted a bleaker and bleaker picture of the epidemic as the weeks passed. Polio had arrived with full force.

The initial response to the unfolding epidemic threat of 1957 reached back to broader and more traditional concepts of disease prevention that put the responsibility of families, in this case parents, at the centre. The effort of constraining the activities and movements of children was aided by guidelines issued by the Health Ministry, but was ultimately the task of parents, mostly mothers. Only when it became clear that the extent of this particular epidemic was unprecedented and that hitherto practised methods were no longer sufficient did responsibilities towards the health of children begin to shift and fluctuate.

Parents followed the unfolding epidemic through the radio and newspapers, from weekly reports that detailed the geographical spread of the disease and the number of people affected.[53] Mothers were called on to take care to wash fruit and vegetables thoroughly and to make sure that children washed their hands before eating.[54] Parents were also advised against letting children engage in excessive exercise like too much walking, intensive swimming or spending too much time in the sun.[55] Children under 3 years old would not be allowed to visit public baths and swimming pools,[56] a regulation that caused

[52] 'Note to the Editor of Népegészségügy', ibid.
[53] See for instance 'Az Egészségügyi Minisztérium Tájékoztatója a Gyermekbénulásos Megbetegedésekről És a Védekezés Módjairól', *Népakarat*, 1957. 'Az Egészségügyi Minisztérium Heti Tájékoztatója a Gyermekbénulásos Megbetegedésekről', *Népakarat*, 11 July 1957.
[54] 'Budapest Vezető Főorvosának Felhívása a Háziasszonyokhoz', *Népakarat*, no. 136, 13 June 1957, 1.
[55] 'Az Egészségügyi Minisztérium Tájékoztatója a Gyermekbénulásos Megbetegedésekről és a Védekezés Módjairól', *Népakarat*, no. 148, 27 June 1957, 3.
[56] 'Budapesten Nincsen Gyermekbénulási Járvány', *Népakarat*, no. 149, 28 June 1957, 1.

much suffering in the scorching summer heat. In order to preserve the cleanliness of baths and thereby curb the spread of infectious diseases, admittance into baths and open-air pools was limited. Moreover, not only the number of people but also the amount of time they spent at such facilities was capped through the issue of morning and afternoon instead of full-day tickets.[57]

At the onset of the epidemic, the Health Ministry released several films with imposing titles, which were shown in cinemas across the country. Since television broadcasting had started only a couple of months before[58] and its subscribers were scarce,[59] such propaganda films, shown in the news section in film houses, were one of the most effective ways for the government to reach the masses directly. The short film *Beware!* (*Vigyázz!*)[60] stressed the importance of personal hygiene and cleanliness of the home in polio prevention. Parents were advised not to let their children spend too much time in the sun, swim or exercise excessively. For instance, a bicycle tour could expose the tired body to contagion. The film also instructed parents what to do if they noticed that their child had a poor appetite or fever. A doctor had to be summoned immediately, and if it was polio, ambulances were to take the sick child to hospital no matter where they were in the country. The film also boasted that an aeroplane had recently been put into use to carry critical polio cases to hospital.

The state's preoccupation with cleanliness was not new. Silent propaganda films on contagious disease prevention from the interwar period operated with identical imagery and conveyed the same message as their 1950s counterparts.[61] Health and hygiene had long been considered fundamental in preserving political stability. Foucault argues that connecting physical and moral health with social order stemmed from the seventeenth century, as perception of death changed and power was increasingly 'situated and exercised at the level of life, the species, the race, and the large-scale phenomena of population'.[62] Public health practices and housing were (and are) tools through which populations were regulated. With the rise of germ theory and new directions in medicine developed in the 1870s and 1880s by scientists Louis Pasteur and

[57] 'Budapesten Nincsen Gyermekbénulási Járvány – Mondja a Tisztifőorvos. Egészségügyi Okokból Korlátozzák a Fővárosi Strandok Látogatását', ibid.
[58] Experimental broadcasting began on 23 February and broadcast available to the public began with the May Day celebrations on 1 May 1957. In: *A Magyar Televízió Története* (Szekszárd: Babits Kiadó, 1996–2000).
[59] According to 1958 figures, there were 16,038 television subscribers in the whole country a year after the broadcast started, while at the same time a total of 4,569 film theatres operated, reaching a much wider public for years to come. Ibid.
[60] 'Vigyázz!', Health Ministry, Hungary, 1957.
[61] 'Védekezzünk a Fertőző Betegségek Ellen', Hungary, n.d. [1920s].
[62] Michel Foucault, *The History of Sexuality: An Introduction*, 1st edn (New York: Vintage Books, 1980), 137.

Robert Koch, scientific approaches to power and population gained new momentum. Thus, by the twentieth century, a germ-free, clean and organised home became central, both as a reality and a metaphor, to a strong and successful state.

This new obsession with cleanliness in the everyday perception of diseases and health[63] prompted researchers as well as the lay public to make a profound connection between filth and disease. However, polio defied this association. As early as the 1916 New York epidemic, evidence suggested that polio tended to attack healthy, well-nourished children in affluent homes with good sanitation instead of impoverished households and filthy neighbourhoods.[64]

Since in epidemic proportions polio was a relatively new disease, scientific uncertainties regarding the mode of contagion lingered. One of these theories emerged in the transitional moment of reconciling the 'filth theory of disease', which sought to resolve epidemics with sanitary solutions, and the relatively new, but less visible, germ theory. The answer was that insects, as with malaria, transmitted polio. The main culprit became the housefly.[65] Dirt needed to be thoroughly purged in order to prevent germs from infecting the family.[66] Even as experience seemed to contradict the filth theory and new epidemiological thinking gained momentum, ridding households of flies, washing fruit and emphasising the cleanliness of the home continued to be a major part of prevention efforts well into the 1950s in many parts of the world.

Soviet ideals of hygiene followed the well-trodden path, arguing that clean living and working environments were crucial to preserving health. Tricia Starks argues,

Soviet hygienists associated mental acuity, political orthodoxy, and modernity with lives lived according to the concepts of balance and reason. These presumed benefits from a regulated, hygienic lifestyle informed medical inquiry, education and state programs. Soviet hygienists believed that ordered lives produced healthy bodies and politically enlightened, productive and happy populations; strong bodies generated balanced minds that, in turn, choose the most rational, equitable, and inevitable of political, social and economic structures, namely, socialism.[67]

These ideals were transferred to Eastern European public health perceptions,[68] giving a new incentive to essentially the same hygienic goals as in the era preceding the Second World War.

---

[63] Tomes, *The Gospel of Germs.*   [64] Rogers, *Dirt and Disease*, 161–63.   [65] Ibid., 16–19.
[66] Poverty and dirt were considered to be the hotbeds of the 1916 polio epidemic in New York City, which was blamed on the immigrant population living in tenements. See Oshinsky, *Polio: An American Story*; Offit, *The Cutter Incident.*
[67] Tricia Starks, *The Body Soviet: Propaganda, Hygiene and the Revolutionary State* (Madison: University of Wisconsin Press, 2008), 4.
[68] As an explanation for such a continuity, Bradley Matthys Moore argues that Czechoslovak public health officials and medical professionals were ready to take up the Soviet perception of hygiene without coercion, partly because celebrated Czech medical figures, such as Jan

94   Unlikely Allies

In both pre and post-Second World War Hungarian public health propaganda, maintaining a clean house, free of flies, and keeping an eye on the personal hygiene of children was the duty of mothers. The feminine tasks of controlling and maintaining the hygiene of spaces and people continued to be important in the preventive efforts of the 1957 polio epidemic. A newspaper article on polio prevention across the country attests to the assignment of hygienic practices and disease prevention, stating that 'women of the Red Cross are inspecting the baths and markets of Szolnok, and they are warning mothers to avoid busy areas with their children'.[69]

Children thus needed to be protected from polio outside the home as well as within it, and special attention was to be paid to children's communities. Summer was a time of organised holidays for children. City councils and the national and local organisations of trade unions offered mass holidaymaking for schoolchildren at Lake Balaton, various locations in hills, near thermal baths and even in the capital. The pioneer movement also organised summer camps. The subsidised or free vacations lasted two weeks, providing care for over 200,000 children per summer.[70] These holidays were not only an opportunity for families of lesser means to secure childcare and a summer experience for their children; they were also ideal grounds for any epidemic to spread quickly.

The same weekly newspaper reports that detailed the geographical spread of the disease and the number of people affected gave notification of bans on the public travel of children. The only way that children could take part in summer camps, organised hikes and group vacations was if they carried a medical document proving that there were no reported cases of polio among their family members or in their immediate environment.[71] As the disease spread, a complete ban on organised travel for children under 14 years old to and from certain areas and cities, such as the especially hard-hit Borsod, Abauj-Zemplén and Hajdu, as well as the cities of Miskolc and Nyíregyháza, was imposed.[72]

Purkyne, fit easily within a broad understanding of Pavlovian physiology. Bradley Matthys Moore, 'For the People's Health: Ideology, Medical Authority and Hygienic Science in Communist Czechoslovakia', *Social History of Medicine*, 27 no. 1 (2014): 122–43.

[69] 'Országszerte Hathatós Intézkedésekkel Küzdenek a Gyermekbénulás További Terjedésének Megakadályozásáért', *Népakarat*, 29 June 1957.

[70] V.M., 'Harmincezer Iskolásgyermeket Üdültet a SZOT, Kétszázezer Gyerek Megy Úttörőtáborba', *Népszava*, 4 June 1959.

[71] 'Az Ifjúság Csoportos Nyaraltatásának Egészségügyi Szabályai', *Népakarat*, 2 July 1957. Also see *A Magyar Forradalmi Munkás-Paraszt Kormány 1027/1958 (VIII. 3.) Számú Határozata a Gyermekbénulás Elleni Védekezésről* (1958).

[72] 'Az Egészségügyi Minisztérium Heti Tájékoztatója a Gyermekbénulásos Megbetegedésekről', *Népakarat*, no. 172, 25 July 1957, 1.

The geography of the banned areas kept changing over time, as it followed the disease.

Such regulations were not necessarily successful. Some children still travelled with their parents, which perhaps contributed to their contracting the disease,[73] while others remained in their isolated villages and were the only ones to come down with polio in their communities.[74] Many times the ban on travel was impossible to impose, and occasionally it was the ban itself that led to new cases when healthy children became trapped in epidemic centres. In late June 1957, Éva, then 6 years old, travelled from the westernmost part of the country to the East with her parents for her grandparents' 40th wedding anniversary. It was only when they were already approaching Borsod County that they were warned of a polio epidemic there and were advised by a fellow traveller to turn back immediately. It was too late, though, and upon arrival they were banned from leaving the county for two weeks. As her mother recounts:

It was there that we learned that my niece's classmate died from paralysis in Miskolc. We also learned there that the initial symptoms of polio are like a simple cold. When we got home, my daughter got the cold. Next day she had a fever … At the children's hospital they performed a lumbar puncture, which confirmed the positive result. After that, my husband took her to the infectious disease ward, because she could not walk anymore. She was completely paralysed, all her limbs from the neck down.[75]

The dissemination of information on the geographic spread of polio, travel bans and even the nature of the disease itself apparently ran into certain problems. Éva's case was by no means unique.[76] Many times, parents only learnt about the presence of an epidemic in their community when their child became ill.[77] While they could gather information on polio epidemics from the newspapers, radio and popular medical advisory books,[78] this information was often disregarded unless there was an immediate threat.

The responsibility for preserving children's health and keeping them safe from polio was shared between the paternal state and the parents, usually mothers, who were the primary figures of caretaking. Parents would contribute by keeping their household clean and preventing their children from over-exerting themselves, while the state would impose bans and regulations to curb contagion and supply the technologies of prevention.

---

[73] György Vargha, interview by Dora Vargha, 15 June 2008, Interview.
[74] Erzsébet Szöllősiné Földesi, interview by Dóra Vargha, 26 April 2010.
[75] Ákosné Szentgyörgyi, interview by Dóra Vargha, 12 November 2010.
[76] see for example Vargha, interview by Vargha, 15 June 2008.
[77] Dr. Vargha Jánosné Lázok, interview by Vargha, 24 June 2008.
[78] e.g. Andor Knoll, *Az Egészséges Gyermek. Nevelési Tanácsok Szülők Részére* (Székesfehérvár: Magyar Vöröskereszt Egészségkultúrális Osztály, 1958).

The domain of responsibilities did not have clear boundaries and shifted back and forth between the state and the parents, between official and private spheres. As these responsibilities shifted in the fight against polio, they created a confusing web of expectations and blame on both sides. The communist state, which so often used the tropes of family in its communications, positioning itself as the paterfamilias of the nation,[79] educated its citizens on disease prevention and called on them to join a mutual effort in curbing the epidemic.

Katherine Verdery, based on Romanian experience, identified a familial relationship between the communist state and its subjects, which she termed socialist paternalism. Verdery argued that the state 'posited a moral tie linking subjects with the state through their right to share in the redistributed social product'.[80] In her observations, in the eyes of the state, subjects are seen as grateful children who appreciate every benefit that the state provides for them.

The Hungarian case follows this pattern, especially when it comes to welfare and healthcare issues. A myriad of newspaper and magazine articles, publications and even governmental documents employ the familial rhetoric, portraying the state as the head of the family, the ultimate provider, and evoking the happiness and gratefulness that was expected from the citizens, especially the mothers, for organised childcare, workplace and public canteens, new healthcare networks and protection from polio in the form of vaccines.

Viewed through the lens of polio, the way the paternalist state worked included interaction between the parent-state (shown as a father) and nuclear families (first represented in this national discourse as mothers and parents, but very rarely fathers). In some instances, the subjects – mothers, parents – were transformed from the state's children or wards to partners in protecting and providing for the future generation.

The West German Hero

Though seemingly strong and unified, the nearly bankrupt Hungarian government had difficulties in fulfilling the role it set for itself and did not fall short of transferring its responsibility in disease prevention to parents in times of need or failure. In these exceptional circumstances, private solutions came to the forefront to solve national problems, inverting the usual dynamics. When the efforts to provide failed or were insufficient, a more complicated partnership was called upon, elevating subjects to heads of the nation-family and giving the responsibility for children's health back to parents, while the state stepped back as a mere facilitator.

---

[79] See Kligman, *The Politics of Duplicity.*
[80] Verdery, 'From Parent-State to Family Patriarchs: Gender and Nation in Contemporary Eastern Europe', 228.

The importance of this web of expectations and the ways in which responsibility was shared, negotiated and occasionally contested among the state, the medical profession and the lay citizens cannot be overstated. The notion of common responsibility for the health of the population and the state's role in providing tools for preserving it was a fundamental element in the concept of public health in the Socialist Bloc. This cornerstone of communist ideology shaped the way in which the epidemic management of polio played out in the region, allowing the Iron Curtain to open and close in striking ways in the process.

The fight against polio created a space in which existing political agendas could be temporarily overwritten. When the state was unable to provide vaccines or its supplies proved to be insufficient, preserving the health of children became a pretext on which the communist government could reach out to unlikely allies. For the sake of children, dissidents could become extended family members.

The promise of a polio-free future arrived on a small aeroplane around 8 p. m. on 13 July 1957. The scene of the vaccine's arrival was captured in a new polio short film: *Parents, be careful!* While the previous film, *Beware!*, concentrated on what parents could do to protect the health of their children, this later movie stressed the actions of the government in polio prevention.

After going through the usual hygienic advices of washing hands and keeping flies at bay, the film went on to provide details of polio care. The representation of therapy at once emphasised the grave consequences of polio (e.g. children 'have to learn to walk all over again') and soothed these images by presenting the high-quality care provided by the state ('highly nutritious, abundant meals contribute to healing in the hospital').[81] The aeroplane arrived at the film's climax, assuring parents that they need not fear this terrible childhood disease any longer, thanks to the government's heroic efforts.

As the number of polio cases grew, it was more and more clear that something drastic needed to be done. The new government, busy with solidifying its power through imprisonment and executions, deemed it necessary to show its strength and ability to tackle public health crises and protect the nation's children. Since domestic production was not possible, especially on such short notice, the government took several steps that, in light of the way we usually think about Cold War politics and communist regimes, may seem surprising. The fact that children were the population group most at risk from polio opened avenues for contradictory actions and rhetorical twists. In a peculiar period of the Cold War, and in a post-revolutionary setting, the state found itself trying to curb the outbreak with the help of strange bedfellows.

---

[81] 'Szülők, Vigyázzatok!', Health Ministry, Hungary, 1957.

Before the decision was made to import the Salk vaccine, the communist state had encouraged informal ways to ameliorate the unfolding epidemic. On 27 June 1957, Hungarians found the following announcement from the health minister and Dr Aladár Kátay, head of the epidemiology department of the ministry, in the weekly polio report of the party's daily newspaper: 'We inform those who are attempting to acquire Salk vaccine through their family members and acquaintances living abroad that the Health Ministry has contacted Customs and, as a result, they will give priority to sending the packages that arrive from abroad and contain this medicine.'[82]

The policy regarding packages arriving from the West originated in the tumultuous months of the 1956 revolution and its aftermath. Access to vital goods such as medicine was scarce, as buildings and infrastructure were severely damaged and production and trade were recovering slowly after coming to a full stop. Additionally, a good portion of Hungary's population had left the country. In late November, to facilitate aid coming from private persons – and as a supplement to help from international organisations such as the Red Cross – the Kádár government pronounced all packages containing food, clothing and medicine to be duty-free until 1 July 1957.[83]

As the polio epidemic loomed on the horizon, the package policy was widened to include expedited customs control in order to preserve the effectiveness of the delicate vaccines coming in personal packages.[84] Family members and friends had already started sending gift parcels[85] from abroad in March,[86] while some individuals chose to bring back doses personally from official trips to the West to vaccinate their own children and neighbours.[87]

What is remarkable in such a customs policy and the encouragement of personal aid from family members and friends living abroad is that through these announcements the state called on precisely the people it wanted to silence, punish or destroy: 'dissidents', who had left the country at various times since the Second World War because of the communist regime. Most

---

[82] Dr. Frigyes Doleschall and Dr. Aladár Kátay, 'Tájékoztató a Gyermekbénulásos Megbetegedésekről', *Népszabadság*, 27 June 1957, 8.
[83] 'Terjesszék Ki a Külföldi Ajándékcsomagok Vámmentességét', *Népakarat*, 5 December 1956.
[84] 'Ügyészségi Intézkedés a Külföldről Érkező Salk-Szérumról', *Népakarat*, 7 July 1957.
[85] Medical parcels coming from abroad were not isolated incidents peculiar to Hungary alone. A Czechoslovakian RFE report from 1954 writes in detail about foreign medicine parcels and remarks that the health ministry of Czechoslovakia must approve of them reaching their destination. Radio Free Europe, 'Information from Czechoslovakia. How the State Gets Hold of Foreign Drugs', in *Bulletin #625* (Budapest: Open Dociety Archives, 1954).
[86] Radio Free Europe, 'Polio in Hungary: Background Report', 1.
[87] Erzsébet Kertesi, 19 May 2009.

recently, 200,000 out of the total population of 9 million citizens had left when the revolution was suppressed. About 8,000–10,000 people returned in the early summer of 1957;[88] most emigrants, however, never went back and many spoke out ardently against the Hungarian communist regime.

At the same time, the following was published in one of the major newspapers, *Népszabadság*, penned by the Health Minister, Frigyes Doleschall, and the head of the epidemiology department, Aladár Kátay:

As of now, the Hungarian production of the Salk vaccine (the most effective vaccine against polio known today) is not possible. The Ministry tried last year and earlier this year to procure vaccine that would be enough to immunise five age groups. The hard currency needed for this was available; however, we did not succeed in importing a sufficient amount, since the Salk vaccine is not in stock, and because of its short expiration period, they only make it to order. Furthermore, it is a good drug and it is scarce all across the world. Negotiations are under way and it looks like it will be available early next year.[89]

In this statement, the ministry was clearly invested in explaining away its inability to deliver protection from polio for the population, something that could have been expected in the light of the role the state set for itself and the proclaimed universal healthcare it was theoretically providing. According to the above passage, the efforts were hindered only by outside forces – the specificity of the delicate serum's production and a market economy of shortage to which Hungarians could easily relate.[90]

It is almost certain, however, that the Health Ministry alone could not have secured the hard currency and procured the vaccine: they needed the Ministerial Council's decision and approval for an intricate process that would involve the allocation of credit, adjustment of economic plans and mobilisation of foreign trade relations.

Nor was it true that the hard currency had been available for vaccine procurement. In a report submitted to the Ministerial Council, Frigyes Doleschall, the health minister, pointed out, 'The National Planning Bureau in 1956 was unable to fulfil the Health Ministry's hard currency need for

---

[88] A detailed statistical analysis on the subject of emigrants in 1956 acknowledges the difficulty in assessing an exact number of people leaving and returning László Hablicsek, 'Az 1956-os Kivándorlás Népességi Hatásai', *Statisztikai Szemle* 85, no. 2 (Illés, Sándor): 157–72, at 159–60.

[89] Doleschall and Kátay, 'Tájékoztató a Gyermekbénulásos Megbetegedésekről'.

[90] Shortage of polio vaccine in 1957 was not unique to Eastern Europe. Britain similarly experienced lack of access to the vaccine in the face of an epidemic in Coventry. However, as Gareth Millward points out, shortage was seen in this case as a failure of the British government, which was too bureaucratic, of medical experts who were too slow to act, and of experts who did not listen to 'commonsense'. Gareth Millward, '"A Matter of Commonsense": The Coventry Poliomyelitis Epidemic in 1957 and the British Public', *Contemporary British History* (2016): 1–23.

importing Salk vaccine this year.'[91] Clearly, the Health Ministry alone was too weak to push its agenda through. Something drastic needed to be done, involving the highest level of decision-making, to succeed in importing the vaccine.

A week after notifying the public about the lack of Salk vaccine and the difficulties in securing a shipment, on 4 July 1957 at a meeting of the Ministerial Council on the polio epidemic, Jenő Baczoni, deputy minister of foreign trade, revealed a plan to secure a shipment of the vaccine. He informed the council that they had found a way to import Salk vaccine originating from Canada through Denmark. This quantity would be enough to vaccinate 150,000 children. Furthermore, they had received notice that Czechoslovakia had recently been able to import a larger amount of vaccine, from which they could borrow a portion that they would return once the Danish shipment arrived.[92] It seems that the Czechoslovakian public health management was somewhat better organised than that of the Hungarians. As preparations for local polio vaccine production began in 1956, the atypical epidemic wave in the autumn urged the Czechoslovakian government to change its original plans of starting polio vaccination with a domestic vaccine at the end of 1957. Instead, Czechoslovakia acquired a vaccine from the Canadian Connaught Laboratories and started immunisation in the spring of 1957, before the onset of the epidemic season.[93] In Hungary, as we have seen, the revolution and its consequences temporarily overrode much of the concern regarding polio epidemics and it remained this way until the shock of the new outbreak.

Now that the possibility of mass vaccination was becoming a reality, the Ministerial Council did not hesitate to revoke the generous policy on personal packages containing vaccines coming from the West.

in order to curb hysterical phenomena, the public announcement [regarding polio issues] should include a statement that calls on the population to put a stop to their individual actions, in which they are trying to bring in vaccine through relatives and acquaintances living in Western countries, because the Government provides a sufficient quantity of the vaccine.[94]

[91] Frigyes Doleschall, 'A Járványos Gyermekbénulás Elleni Védekezés Időszerű Feladatai. Elő-terjesztés a Magyar Forradalmi Munkás-Paraszt Kormányhoz', ed. Minisztertanács (Budapest: National Archives of Hungary, 1957).

[92] 'A Járványos Gyermekbénulás Elleni Védekezés Időszerű Feladatai. Vita', Budapest: National Archives of Hungary, A Minisztertanács üléseinek jegyzőkönyvei, XIX-A-83-a, 1957.

[93] Vilem Skovranek, 'Present State of Vaccination against Poliomyelitis in Czechoslovakia', in Vaccination and Immunity: Neurophysical and Neuropathological Aspects of Poliomyelitis. Vth Symposium of the European Association against Poliomyelitis, ed. H. C. A. Lassen (Madrid: Europ. Assoc. Poliomyelitis, 1959).

[94] 'A Járványos Gyermekbénulás Elleni Védekezés Időszerű Feladatai. Vita', 1957.

Regaining provider status and setting up the familial dynamics of the parent-state and child-citizens was so important to the government that even before the state was able to solve vaccination with certainty, the process of reinforcing the lines of responsibility over health protection began.

After a year of going back and forth on domestic vaccine production, the pace clearly quickened. On the same day, the Ministerial Council issued a decree that put forward a comprehensive programme of polio prevention.[95] The council ordered the health minister and the minister of foreign affairs to import sufficient vaccine for the immunisation of children from six months to five years of age. The two ministers were also instructed to import gamma globulin as needed from Czechoslovakia and the GDR. This time, the ministry of finance and the National Planning Bureau received orders from the highest ranks, in the form of a decree to secure sufficient funds and hard currency for vaccine procurement and allow the health minister access to these monies without delay. In the decree, the government also included an official announcement that called on the public to refrain from procuring vaccine by private methods. A summary of the decree was published in the newspapers the very next day,[96] assuring parents that the state was indeed in control again.

Following these initial obstacles,

By a decree of the Ministry Council, through great difficulties, the Salk vaccine has arrived . . . now everyone can have access to it for free. Vaccination has begun with the help of Red Cross activists. Parents, worry no more, now we can protect your children from infant paralysis.[97]

This route of the first official vaccine shipment is symbolic of international cooperation in the struggle against polio. The practical execution of transporting polio vaccines was an enterprise that, in its official rhetoric, challenged Cold War concepts and claimed to override geopolitical tensions in the name of science and for the benefit of children. Moreover, with the arrival of the vaccine, this rhetoric made an appearance in public in Hungary. While the description of international cooperation was carefully embedded in the much more familiar discourse of the paternal state providing for and protecting its subjects, such a carefree and positive tone, completely devoid of attacks on the West, stood out from the everyday articles and newsreels to which most Hungarians were exposed. For the sake of the health of children, instead of an imperialist spy or decadent oppressor, a West German became the cele-brated hero of the day. The nameless pilot – referred to as 'a tall, black-haired

---

[95] 'A Magyar Forradalmi Munkás-Paraszt Kormány Határozata a Járványos Gyermekbénulás Elleni Védekezés Időszerű Feladatairól', in *1062/1957/VII.6./Korm* (1957).
[96] 'A Minisztertanács Indézkedései a Gyermekparalízis Megelőzése és a Betegellátás Érdekében', *Népakarat*, 5 July 1957.
[97] 'Szülők, Vigyázzatok!', Health Ministry, Hungary, 1957.

man' – said he volunteered for the flight on his day off, when he heard that it was a much-needed shipment of vaccine for the children of Hungary. 'If only everyone was like this', wrote the vice-president of the Presidential Council in the newspaper article covering the arrival of the vaccine.[98] The government considered the vaccine to be so important, and the need to communicate its final success in securing it for the country's children so pressing, that the party newspaper was able to contradict its own rhetoric in depicting this fruitful cooperation.

As the packages of Hungarian émigrés and the romantic story of the West German pilot worthy of Hollywood films attest, preventing polio with the Salk vaccine was an issue that transcended the animosity of international relations and Cold War politics. However, there is another side to the heroic story, one that shows that the Cold War was indeed fought with vaccines as well.

The news of the severe polio epidemic made it into the international press, which in the aftermath of the 1956 revolution was very interested in Hungarian affairs.[99] Interestingly, while Hungarian sources stressed the high cost and debt that the government had taken upon itself to import the vaccine, American newspapers used the term 'aid' when describing the Salk shipment.[100]

An explanation of the difference in the representation of those credited for the Hungarian vaccination can be found in contemporary international politics. In the years following the suppression of the revolution that broke out against the communist regime in October 1956, Hungarian-American diplomatic relations were at a low point. According to the Foreign Ministry, 'Among all capitalist countries ... relations [were] the worst with the United States.'[101] The conflict between Hungary and the United States was exacerbated by the formation of a United Nations Committee set up to investigate the Soviet intervention and the actions of the Kádár government. The relationship between the two countries turned so icy that the American ambassador, Edward Wailes, was recalled in the spring of 1957 and the embassy in Budapest was left without an ambassador for the next ten years.[102] The United States, therefore, could easily have been invested in portraying the Hungarian government, which the Americans perceived to be borderline illegitimate, as needing outside help, rather than capable of solving its own problems.

---

[98] Dániel Nagy, '250 000 Köbcentiméter Salk-Vakcina Érkezett. Az Egészségügyi Minisztérium Tájékoztatója', *Népszabadság*, 14 July 1957.

[99] 'Polio Epidemic Feared', *Washington Post and Times Herald*, 5 June 1957; 'Salk Expects End of Polio Some Day', *New York Times*, 9 July 1957; 'Hungary Battle Polio', *Washington Post and Times Herald*, 2 July 1957.

[100] 'World Polio Cut by Salk Vaccine. Hungary Aided in Polio Fight', *New York Times*, 10 July 1957; 'Budapest Receives Canadian Polio Aid', *New York Times*, 14 July 1957.

[101] László Borhi, *Iratok a Magyar-Amerikai Kapcsolatok Történetéhez 1957–1967*, ed. Mária and Vida Ormos, István, Iratok a Magyar Diplomácia Történetéhez (Budapest: Ister, 2002).

[102] Ibid. 20.

Importing the Salk vaccine from the West was not a unique feature of Hungarian epidemic management in the region. Most Eastern European countries were prompted by sudden or unexpectedly severe outbreaks to act fast and reach across the Iron Curtain to provide a speedy solution in the form of the Salk vaccine. As we have seen, Czechoslovakia followed a similar route in procuring the vaccine from Connaught Laboratories in the spring of 1957. Poland began domestic production in 1957 on a small scale and mass production in the second half of 1958. The vaccination was to be covered partially by a domestic vaccine and partially by imported Salk vaccine.[103] As in many countries, an epidemic served as a motive for the Bulgarian government to introduce mass vaccination into the country in September 1957. Bulgaria used imported vaccine until 1959 (from the American Merck and Connaught Laboratories), when it switched to the Soviet-produced inactivated vaccine.[104] The East German government began vaccination with the inactivated vaccine in 1958, using the so-called 'Berna' vaccine produced by the Swiss Serum and Vaccine Institute in Bern.[105] Instead of using Salk's polio vaccine, Romania began immunisation with a different inactivated vaccine: the recently released Lépine vaccine, developed in France by the physician and biologist Pierre Lépine and manufactured by the Pasteur Institute of Paris.[106]

Relying on vaccine import in polio prevention was not specific to the Eastern European Bloc either. Domestic vaccine production could not always keep up with demand, and it was mostly Canadian and American pharmaceutical companies to which medical boards turned in their goal to immunise a critical portion of the nation. Britain, after much deliberation, imported Canadian and American Salk vaccine in 1958, when domestically produced supplies proved to be insufficient to immunise the endangered population.[107] Similarly, Sweden decided to import vaccine from the American company Eli Lilly and Co. in 1957 to complement its domestic vaccine stock.[108]

---

[103] F. Przesmycki, 'Vaccination against Poliomyelitis in Poland', in *Vaccination and Immunity: Neurophysical and Neuropathological Aspects of poliomyelitis. Vth Symposium of the European Association against Poliomyelitis*, ed. H. C. A. Lassen (Madrid: Europ. Assoc. Poliomyelitis, 1959), 40–41.

[104] I. Vaptzarov, D. Bratovanov, and Th. Kristev, 'La vaccination contre la poliomyélite en Bulgarie', in *Anti-poliomyelitis vaccinations, physio-pathology of the respiratory disorder, poliomyelitis of the 'very young child'. VIth symposium of the European Association against Poliomyelitis*, ed. H. C. A. Lassen (Munich: Europ. Assoc. Poliomyelitis, 1960), 19–23.

[105] Kukowa, 'Poliomyelitis-Schutzimpfung in Der Deutschen Demokratiscen Republik', ibid. 52–53.

[106] Anda Baicus, 'History of Polio Vaccination', *World Journal of Virology* 1, no. 4 (2012): 108–14.

[107] Lindner and Blume, 'Vaccine Innovation and Adoption: Polio Vaccines in the Uk, the Netherlands and West Germany, 1955–1965'.

[108] Axelsson, 'The Cutter Incident and the Development of a Swedish Polio Vaccine'.

However, the vaccine initially procured by the Hungarian government was still not enough to vaccinate all children. On the day following the breaking news of the vaccine's arrival, the newspaper *Népakarat* suggested that people keep their enthusiasm in check: the shipment of 250,000 cm^3 of Salk vaccine was only enough to vaccinate the most endangered age group of children, those between 1 and 2 years old.[109] A week later, the vaccination was administered in Budapest and eastern Hungary, the areas most hard hit by the disease, while other parts of the country were vaccinated the week after that. The second dose of the vaccine was to be administered four weeks after the first dose.

Since the vaccine was not enough to immunise the whole endangered population, the first shipment was soon followed by smaller donations. The first came from the World Health Organisation (WHO), which sent 40,000 doses.[110] At this time, Hungary's relationship with the WHO was not completely stable. Hungary, along with other Eastern European countries such as Czechoslovakia and Poland, had followed the Soviet Union's example by withdrawing its membership[111] in 1949.[112] However, again following in the footsteps of the Soviet Union, Hungary had started to discuss rejoining the WHO in April 1957.[113] Hungary eventually ended up as the last Eastern European state to renew its membership, in 1963.[114]

Another organisation also made a vaccine donation of an unknown amount, although from Health Ministry documents, it appears that the vaccine might have been damaged during the journey and was most probably not fit for use by the time it arrived. The donation came from the National Organisation of Actio Catholica, headed by Bishop Endrey, who received the shipment from Bern, Switzerland.[115] This was not the first shipment from a Catholic organisation. According to a report by the Katpress Catholic news agency, referenced by the Radio Free Europe report, the Austrian branch of the National Catholic

---

[109] 'Beoltják Gyermekbénulás Ellen az 1–2 Éves Gyermekeket: Külkereskedelmi Szerveink már 250 000 Köbcenti Vakcinát Szereztek', *Népakarat*, 10 July 1957; 'Gyermekparalízis Elleni Védőoltás Az 1–2 Éves Gyermekek Számára', *Népszabadság*, 10 July 1957.

[110] 'Dr. Ivanovics György Akadémikus Nyilatkozata a Genfi Gyermekparalízis-Kongresszusról, a Hazánkban Folytatott Oltások Hatékonyságáról', *Népszabadság*, 23 July 1957.

[111] The constitution of the WHO did not allow for membership withdrawal, therefore these countries were considered inactive members until they activated their membership again. See *The First Ten Years of the World Health Organization*, 80.

[112] Ibid. 79–80.

[113] 'Letter from Rodolphe L. Coigney, Director of Liaison Office with United Nations to Dr. P. Dorolle, Deputy Director-General of the World Health Organization.' Geneva: Archives of World Health Organization N52/180/2/Hungary, 1957.

[114] Javed Siddiqi, *World Health and World Politics: The World Health Organization and the UN System* (Columbus: University of South Carolina Press, 1995), 108.

[115] Kátay Aladár, 'Svájci Polio-Vaccina Használhatósága.' Budapest: National Archives of Hungary, 54047, XIX-C-2-e, 1957.

Welfare Council (NCWC) sent 2,000 doses of vaccine to the same bishop.[116] Given that the relationship of the Hungarian communist state and the Catholic Church was at its worst in the 1950s, the existence of such cooperation, reaching over the Iron Curtain, indicates another venue where the apolitical space created by children's health materialised.

Vaccinating the Nation

The Janus-faced nature of Cold War relations came to light once more in the attempt to secure further large batches of the Salk vaccine. Even while the Hungarian government was so seamlessly working together with the Catholic Church and the WHO in polio prevention, the whole vaccination campaign almost broke down because of Hungary's dire relations with the United States and the poor standing of the Hungarian government in the scene of Cold War international politics.

The arrival of a second large 500,000 cm^3 batch of Salk vaccine was very far from heroic and revealed vaccine procurement as a politically fraught process. The rhetoric on aid to Hungary continued when the Hungarian government began negotiations to procure further batches of Salk vaccine from American manufacturers. It was significantly cheaper to purchase the vaccine from the United States than from Canada, so Hungary decided to step on the minefield of severed diplomatic relations and pursue the procurement from the United States.[117] The Hungarian diplomats involved in the process were appalled by the representation of aid and benevolence from the American parties. According to the internal notes of the Hungarian Foreign Ministry, Garret G. Ackerson, the temporary chargé d'affaires of the United States Embassy in Budapest,[118] met with Hungarian colleagues to discuss the possibility of Salk vaccine procurement. In the interpretation of the Hungarians, Ackerson offered help to the Hungarian government in purchasing Salk vaccine from American companies, but when pressed for the exact nature of this help, evaded any particulars. The Hungarians informed him that they had already managed to negotiate a further 500,000 cm^3 of vaccine on their own, and while grateful for

---

[116] Radio Free Europe. 'Polio in Hungary: Background Report.' Budapest: Open Society Archives, 1957, 2.

[117] Jenő Baczoni, 'Levél Sebes István Elvtársnak, a Külügyminiszter Helyettesének.' Budapest: Magyar Nemzeti Levéltár, XIX-J-1-k USA Admin 1945–1964, 57, A Salk szérum beszerzése, 3516/1, 1957.

[118] Ackerson was the diplomat who gave refuge to Cardinal József Mindszenty, Roman Catholic primate of Hungary, after the crushing of the 1956 revolution. Lee A. Daniels, 'Garret G. Ackerson, 88, Envoy in East Europe during Cold War', *The New York Times*, 16 September 1992.

the offer, were not in need of assistance at this time.[119] In a letter to the press office of the Ministry, Károly Szigeti, the Hungarian official taking part in the meeting, noted that the Voice of America, Radio Free Europe and other Western radios had been portraying this offer as a grand gesture from the Americans and that it would be necessary to correct this misinformation through the press.[120]

The conflict soon moved from radio waves and pages of newspapers to diplomatic channels. Again, the issue of hard currency posed obstacles to closing the deal and caused delays in purchasing the vaccine. This delay was lengthened by the fact that 100,000 cm^3 of the vaccine was held up at customs in the United States, awaiting an export licence. This was particularly worrisome for Hungarians. Children had already been vaccinated with the initial Canadian batch of vaccine and were due to receive the second dose. If there was further delay, it would compromise the immunisation process and they would need to start the whole vaccination campaign again.[121] This was something they could not afford either financially, in terms of public health organisation, or for fear of losing face.

The Hungarians considered the absence of an export licence to be a diplomatic blackmailing tool on the part of the Americans. József Hamburger, head of Medimpex, the state company in charge of the vaccine import, was of the opinion that the United States would not sign the licence until the UN committee on the 1956 revolution concluded its investigation.[122] Even though members of the Foreign Trade Ministry and the Foreign Ministry were furious with the United States, they mutually agreed to save the counter-attack for later until an alternative Canadian shipment was secured.[123]

Eventually the additional Canadian shipment was not needed, nor did the Hungarians launch a public or diplomatic counter-attack. The Hungarians arranged a new meeting with Ackerson and this time took up his offer of assistance, and Ackerson honoured the request. The new shipment left the United States shortly afterwards and the Hungarian vaccination continued. If there were any further agreements in the background between the Hungarians and Americans to ensure the deal, the sources are silent on the matter. The United States did reveal that Hungary had already received 13 per cent of its

[119] Károly Szigeti, 'Feljegyzés Ackerson Tanácsos Amerikai id. Ügyvivő Látogatásáról.' Budapest: Magyar Nemzeti Levéltár, XIX-J-1-k USA Admin 1945–1964, 57. doboz, Amerikai segítség ajánlat gyermekbénulási gyógyszer vásárlásához, 19/3/h, 1957.
[120] 'Sajtóközlemény-Tervezet.' Budapest: Magyar Nemzeti Levéltár, XIX-J-1-k USA Admin 1945–1964, 57, Amerikai segítség ajánlat gyermekbénulási gyógyszer vásárlásához, 1957.
[121] László Hamburger, 'Az Amerikai Fél Által Támasztott Salk-Szérum Szállítási Nehézségei. Feljegyzés Baczoni Jenő Miniszterhelyettes E.T. Részére', ibid., 1376/B, 1957.
[122] Ibid.
[123] Jenő Baczoni, 'Levél Sebes István Elvtársnak, a Külügyminiszter Helyettesének', ibid., A Salk szérum beszerzése, 3516/1, 1957.

Salk vaccine export quota, i.e. the total Salk vaccine that the United States planned to export for the year. For this reason, they were not planning to release any more to this small Eastern European country, and warned the Hungarian government that for the further steps of their vaccination campaign, they should look elsewhere to procure the Salk vaccine.[124] With the vaccine crisis resolved, the Hungarian Foreign Ministry decided to forego any open criticism or to launch any propaganda against the United States and considered the whole affair as 'case closed'.[125]

After the first official shipment of the Salk vaccine, nationwide immunisation could begin. To ensure sufficient tools for the mass campaign, the Hungarian army lent sterilisation equipment and syringes to the Health Ministry.[126] The vaccine was free of charge, and vaccination was organised on a voluntary basis. The Health Ministry headed the distribution and administration of the vaccine, while public health stations were responsible for the local organisation. Vaccination teams consisting of physicians and technicians administered the vaccine, and in some cases, the district doctor[127] or a private practitioner[128] injected the children.

The vaccination was free and voluntary, although parents were strongly encouraged to get their children vaccinated. Parents had to take their children to the local mother and child protection facilities on a designated day according to the alphabetical order of the children's family names. Although the vaccination was organised according to permanent residence,[129] it was not limited to where families lived. For example, if someone was on holiday elsewhere or travelling during the vaccination period, they did not need to return home to receive the vaccine.[130] This aspect of how the vaccination was organised probably made sense at the time. A lot of people were travelling in the summer, especially children, who, during the summer holiday from school, were often deposited for weeks at the homes of grandparents and family members while their parents were working. However, this facilitation of

---

[124] Károly Szarka, 'Ackerson Amerikai Ügyvivő Látogatása', ibid.
[125] Jenő Baczoni, 'Salk-Szérum Beszerzése', Budapest: Magyar Nemzeti Levéltár, XIX-J-1-k USA Admin 1945–1964, 57, A Salk-szérum beszerzése, 1–00279/957, 1957.
[126] I. Benyó, 'Gyermekbénulás Elleni Folytatólagos Védőoltások Szervezése', Budapest: National Archives of Hungary, Egészségügyi Minisztérium iratai, 53.135/1957, 1957.
[127] Aladár Petrilla, The Results of Intracutaneous Poliomyelitis Vaccination in Hungary, 1957, Acta Microbiologica (Budapest: Akadémia Kiadó, 1958), 198–200.
[128] According to the report of the Microbiology Department of the Budapest Medical University, 80,000 children received vaccine through private practice by the end of the year. Ilona Szeri, Pál Földes and Szilárd Bognár, 'Adatok a Poliomyelitis Elleni Intrakután Védőoltás Kérdéséhez', Orvosi Hetilap 100, no. 38 (1959): 1364–65, at 1364.
[129] 'Csütörtökön És Pénteken Kapják Az Első Védőoltást Az 1–2 Éves Gyerekek', Népakarat, 16 July 1957.
[130] 'Július 18. És 19-Én Megkezdődik a Gyermekbénulás Elleni Védőoltás. Az Egészségügyi Minisztérium Hivatalos Tájékoztatója', Népakarat, 14 July 1957.

vaccination also contributed to later problems, when it became difficult to track down who was vaccinated and how many doses they had received.

The concept of free vaccination, administered on a mass scale, was a particular point of conflict and comparison between the two sides of the Iron Curtain. It was the ultimate representation of socialised medicine, a sign of the Red Menace in countries like the United States, the home country of Salk. His mass field trials in 1954 and the mass distribution of the vaccine the following year by the National Infantile Paralysis Foundation rang alarm bells. The fear of socialised medicine and of physicians being excluded from the vaccination process mobilised the medical profession to protest and lobby against low-cost, mass immunisation – with success.[131] Ironically, the AMA (as a tool in protecting its professional territory) was using Cold War rhetoric against a process that was organised not by the government, but by a foundation. One that, in fact, opposed any federal support or intervention in its mass trials and vaccinations for those same reasons: that it would reflect communist thinking and would be un-American.[132]

Meanwhile, in Hungary, the vaccination programme was not contested in any way, at least not on a professional and political level. This was, after all, socialised medicine, where doctors were appointed by local councils, and virology and public health departments answered to the Health Ministry. While many issues could spark battles among administrators, party officials and healthcare professionals, free vaccination on a mass scale was not one of them. However, there must have been some sort of suspicion towards the vaccine among the population, as some parents did not choose to vaccinate their children.[133] Some even went as far as to write a statement about their choice.[134] The communist government pointed fingers at an alleged counter-propaganda against vaccination, which reveals that at least a certain level of resistance among the population must have been perceived. Such a threat to the vaccination programme was taken so seriously that legal action was advised against anyone engaged in counter-propaganda against the Salk vaccine, with up to one year's imprisonment in accordance with the laws of 'criminal law protection of the democratic state order and the republic' from 1937 and 1947.[135]

Thus, it was important for the government to win the support and cooperation of parents. Leaflets titled 'What do we need to know about the vaccine

[131] Oshinsky, *Polio: An American Story.*
[132] Ibid. 200, and Colgrove, *State of Immunity*, 121–24.
[133] 'Az Egészségügyi Minisztérium Tájékoztatója a Gyermekbénulásos Megbetegedésekről', *Népszava*, 21 July 1959.
[134] Olga Ábel, 'Eddig 67 000 Gyereket Oltottak be Salk-Vakcinával a Fővárosban az Új Akció Kezdete Óta', ibid., 7 August.
[135] Benyó, 'Gyermekbénulás Elleni Folytatólagos Védőoltások Szervezése,' Insert no. 2.

against infantile paralysis?' informed parents about the vaccination process and the significance of this particular disease prevention.[136] Newspapers published photos that showed photogenic toddlers receiving the vaccine, bravely facing the needle, sometimes accompanied by personal stories of the vaccination experience.

The time is 5:55 p.m. The medical tools have been sterilised and the cherry-red Salk vaccine is sparkling in the vial. The doctor washes her hands and calls out to the nurses: The first one may come.

- What's your name, dear?
- Zsuzsika Csekő.
- How old are you, little one?
- Five – she replies bravely.

But her self-confidence lasts only until the needle touches her little arm. Then, she starts whimpering. Before she could break out crying, though, Zsuzsika Csekő has already received the first dose of vaccine against polio.
- We have inoculated three hundred children today from 8 a.m. to 4 p.m. in my district – says the doctor – Children usually take the vaccine very calmly, in my experience they discipline themselves much more in public.[137]

Stories such as the one above were aimed at convincing parents to subject their children to the painful injection. Moreover, by showing children's bravery and emphasising the feat of the doctors, the propaganda set an example and laid out expectations for parents and children in how to behave in the fight against polio. Finally, these images of healthy and beautiful children, and the stories that accompanied them, communicated an assurance by the state that they would maintain the health of children and provide healthcare and vaccine for all in need.[138]

According to a subsequent report, the vaccine was administered in 0.2 millilitre doses, into the skin.[139] While the inactivated vaccine was usually injected into the muscle, some countries chose intradermal inoculation. This was called the Danish method[140] and served the purpose of sparing doses. The vaccine needed to immunise one child could be reduced by up to 20 per cent of

---

[136] Ibid.   [137] Sz. Gy., 'Most Jöjjön a Következő...', *Népszava*, 11 February 1958, 1.
[138] At least part of the propaganda relating to the polio epidemic was the result of decisions on the highest levels. Ministerial Council meeting minutes from early July reveal an order for a 'calming' article based on statistical data that includes statements from healthcare professionals as well. 'Javaslat a Gyermekparalízisről Szóló Sajtócikk Megjelenésére Vonatkozóan. Münnich Elvtárs Szóbeli Javaslata.' Budapest: National Archives of Hungary, Minisztertanács Iratai, M-KS 288.f/33. ő.e., 9R/81, 1957.
[139] Kátay, 'Vaccination against Poliomyelitis in Hungary,' 45.
[140] Paul, *A History of Poliomyelitis*, 436.

110   Unlikely Allies

the original dose this way.[141] Since the intradermal vaccination method required special skill, vaccination brigades were set up, headed by doctors who were trained and experienced in this technique.[142]

The original decree on the vaccine import[143] set the sufficient quantity of vaccine that was needed to immunise the at-risk population at 1 million millilitres. At the same time, the decree pointed out that the shipment they were able to procure at that point would be enough to inoculate 375,000 children with two doses each.[144] However, a later decree, authorising the Foreign Ministry to issue payment for the Canadian import, referred to the same amount of vaccine as sufficient for the immunisation of 500,000 children.[145] The numbers become even more confusing if we take into account the dosage of 0.2 millilitres per injection. Using the Danish intradermal method, the initial shipment of 250,000 millilitres would have been enough to vaccinate the maximum number of 625,000 children (not taking into account the amount used for testing and the potential amount lost in transit and during administration). What we do know is that out of the 250,000 millilitres of the vaccine, 113,826 millilitres were issued for the first injections,[146] although it is not clear how much of that amount was used and how much of the remainder was reallocated to the second dose in August. As of now, it is uncertain how many children were indeed vaccinated with this initial shipment. It is also difficult to determine whether the number of injections specified by the decree was computed by the intramuscular method that required larger doses or whether the dosage in the 1960 report was inaccurate.

In August, the Health Ministry broadened the vaccination campaign. Between 9 August and 9 September, the new shipment of vaccine was to arrive from the American pharmaceutical company Parke-Davis. Together with the 250 litres of the first shipment, the ministry calculated that all children

[141] Sticchi L. et al., 'The Intradermal Vaccination: Past Experiences and Current Perspectives', *Journal of Preventive Medicine and Hygiene* 51, no. 1 (2010): 7–14, at 9. Currently, the WHO is considering using intradermal vaccination methods for the same reasons. See Martin Friede, 'Dose-Sparing by Intradermal Immunization' (Geneva: World Health Organization, 2006).

[142] Benyó, 'Gyermekbénulás Elleni Folytatólagos Védőoltások Szervezése.'

[143] Ferenc Münnich, 'A Magyar Forradalmi Munkás-Paraszt Kormány Határozata a Járványos Gyermekbénulás Időszerű Feladatairól Szóló 1062/1957/Vii.6./Korm Sz. Határozat Kiegészítéséről', in *3290/1957* (1957).

[144] Ibid.

[145] Minisztertanács, 'Gyermekbénulás Elleni Szérum Behozataláról', in *3311/1957* (Budapest, 18 July 1957).

[146] Gábor Veres, 'Kimutatás Salk Vakcina Kiadásáról És Készletéről', Budapest: National Archives of Hungary, Egészségügyi Minisztérium Állami közegészségügyi felügyelet és járványvédelmi főosztály iratai, XIX-C-2-e, 53137, 1957.

born between 1 January 1951 and 28 February 1957 could be vaccinated with two injections before the year was over.[147] All children born in 1955 and 1956 who had not received their first injection in July were to be immunised, while the others from this age group would receive their second injection. Since there was now enough vaccine to broaden the programme, the age group was also widened: children up to 6 years old were also included, along with infants born in January and February 1957. The areas most severely affected by the epidemic received priority in organising the vaccination: the eastern counties of Borsod-Abaúj-Zemplén, Hajdú-Bihar and Szabolcs-Szatmár, the cities of Miskolc and Debrecen, and the capital, Budapest.[148]

By November, over 1 million children were said to have received two doses of vaccine,[149] and by the end of the year, the number of vaccinated children was reported to be 1.2 million.[150] The Salk vaccination was deemed a success. Because the vaccine was seen to have contributed to curbing the epidemic wave, in the three-year healthcare plan and the budget allocation for 1958, the government decided to assign 30 million forints to acquiring the Salk vaccine.[151] This way, children between 0 and 6 years old would be able to receive a third injection of the vaccine in 1958.[152] Soon, however, its success would have to be re-evaluated after the second largest epidemic wave in Hungarian history hit in the summer of 1959.

In the aftermath of the political and social crisis of the 1956 revolution, the Kádár government was faced with a new one, this time in the form of a severe epidemic. The new regime was performing a delicate balancing act. On the one hand, it was in the process of solidifying its power following a major uprising that was widely supported by the population and repressed by the Soviet army. The Kádár government fortified its position with the support of the hated occupiers, therefore it needed to show its strength: revolutionaries were incarcerated, many executed. On the other hand, the government also needed to show that it was capable of dealing with a major public health crisis and able to

---

[147] Benyó, 'Gyermekbénulás Elleni Folytatólagos Védőoltások Szervezése', Budapest: National Archives of Hungary, 1957.
[148] Ibid.
[149] 'Egymillió Gyerek Kapott Idén Védőoltást', *Népakarat*, 27 November 1957; 'Egymillió Gyerek Kapott Idén Védőoltást. Megkezdődtek a Magyar-Szovjet Orvosi Napok', *Népakarat*, 27 November 1957.
[150] Szeri, Földes, and Bognár, 'Adatok a Poliomyelitis Elleni Intrakután Védőoltás Kérdéséhez', 1959.
[151] 'Magasabb Összeg Egészségügyre – 30 Millió Salk-Vaccinára. Az Egészségügy Hároméves Tervéről és Jövő Évi Költségvetéséről Tárgyalt az Országgyűlés Szociális és Egészségügyi Bizottsága', *Népakarat*, 15 November 1957.
[152] Benyó, 'Gyermekbénulás Elleni Folytatólagos Védőoltások Szervezése', Budapest: National Archives of Hungary, 1957.

protect an important group upon which the communist regime centred much of its propaganda: children. The memories of the bloody uprising were too fresh to risk public discontent. Demonstrating incompetence in the face of a danger that affected the families, friends and acquaintances of children, or in other words most of the population, on a very personal level was not an option.

The fact that the disease mostly affected children and that the image of the child occupied a central part in the Communist Party's imagery of the future of the country prompted surprising steps from the government. It was for the same reason that these actions were relatively uncontested. For the sake of the children, the West German pilot could become a hero in the coldest days of Cold War Hungary; the paternal state could pass its self-proclaimed role of caretaker to citizens (actual parents); scientists could criss-cross Europe in a quest for domestic vaccine production, a project that would span three consecutive governments; and enemies new and old could become temporary allies in the common fight against an invisible, but powerful, enemy. Because it was for the good of children, in response to the concern of mothers and for the future of a healthy and strong nation, the holes that opened up in the Iron Curtain and the policies and practices that went against domestic politics and ideology seemed justified.

The holes in the Iron Curtain and alliances were, of course, temporary. They lasted while there was imminent threat of a dreaded disease. With the nation's vaccination, this threat disappeared: the light went dark, policies were withdrawn and rhetoric hardened as the epidemic wave of 1957 withered and died away. The communist state could be secure in its capabilities; it demonstrated its power and efficiency at home and to the world, albeit using a Western technology, with vaccinations carried out in the Eastern framework of the providing state. The citizen-children and child citizens were under threat of disease no more and they had the state to thank for that. Or at least that was the plan until 1959.

4   Local Failure in a Global Success

At first, it seemed that the unprecedented cooperation between emigrants, international organisations, the Catholic Church and the communist government of Hungary was fully successful. Medimpex, the state company that imported the vaccine in the summer of 1957, received an award for its efforts.[1] The following year there was no epidemic and the government celebrated the feat.[2]

However, a new and severe outbreak in the summer of 1959, when almost 2,000 children fell prey to the disease, prompted the state and the medical profession to re-evaluate their success. How could such a severe epidemic happen when a high number of children were supposed to have been protected by the Salk vaccine? What went wrong? Who was to blame? Public health officials, parents, ministers and doctors tried to work out the reasons for what appeared to be a complete failure. They engaged in a conversation on effectiveness and prevention by using and producing medical data in various ways, clashing lay and medical experiences, and revealing a broad set of expectations.

The introduction of the Salk vaccine, its perceived success and eventual failure was an overtly political issue that manifested in the pages of medical journals and daily newspapers, during visits to the doctor and in private conversations. The uncertainties of knowledge and practice in polio vaccination brought to the fore sweeping, high-stakes problems at all levels of governance and daily life.

The controversy that followed the 1959 epidemic provides a glimpse into the way a new vaccine, introduced worldwide over the course of a few years, played out locally, raising the question of the extent to which vaccination with a particular vaccine in different locales could be interpreted as the same. When

---

[1] 'Letter to Jenő Incze Foreign Trade Minister', Budapest: National Archives of Hungary, Egészségügyi Minisztérium Állami Közegészségügyi Felügyeleti és Járványvédeli Főosztály, XIX-C-2-e, 54304/1957, 1957.

[2] András Faludi, '1958 Örvendetes Eredményeket Hozott a Gyermekbénulás Elleni Küzdelemben', Népszabadság 1959, 4.

113

we think of vaccination on a global scale, we often consider vaccines as objects moving across countries and continents. However, they also move from clinical trials to the field, from national to transnational use and are translated from scientific debates to vaccination policy, and onto parents and vaccinees. If we interrogate the key moments when scientific research moves on to public health intervention and across political dividing lines, cultures and societies, vaccines are revealed to be part of a larger conceptual framework and, as medical technologies, something that cannot be divorced from local expectations and interpretations created in the process.

While the Hungarian story of the Salk vaccination failure adds to a growing scholarship that questions the seeming universality of biomedical technologies such as vaccines,[3] the discussions and debates brought to light by an epidemic crisis also reveal the very tangible consequences of international medical and political rivalries. At the end of the 1950s, the Salk vaccine's efficacy was under debate at poliomyelitis conferences and in the pages of medical journals. Several methods for using the vaccine existed and there was no international standard set out for the vaccine's application. Knowledge about the disease and its prevention was in flux, complicated by the personal agendas of rival scientists and situated in a Cold War world built on antagonism and contest. In the face of scientific uncertainties, medical data gained political meaning and vaccination campaigns became political acts. As is usually the case with vaccine evaluation, determining the Salk vaccine's success or failure in Hungary in the 1950s was far from a merely medical affair. There was plenty of blame to go around for the epidemic of 1959. Citizens distrusted the state, the state was disappointed by the lack of compliance of citizens, physicians were dissatisfied with the chaotic centralisation of medical supplies and methods, and everyone was frustrated by the scientific certainties of the disease in a time of epidemics and revolutions.

This chapter follows the evaluation of the Salk vaccine in Hungary between 1957 and 1960 and analyses how a new epidemic wave affected the scientific and political discourse on polio. The way in which vaccine efficiency was determined over time shaped subsequent vaccine policies in the country and

---

[3] Jeremy Greene's work on the generic drug market explores problems in sameness and similarity in therapeutics, see Jeremy A. Greene, *Generic: The Unbranding of Modern Medicine* (Baltimore: Johns Hopkins University Press, 2014). A collection on HPV vaccines edited by Keith Wailoo, Juiie Livingston, Robert Aronowitz and Steven Epstein provide a global, comparative view of vaccine reception, use and its meaning in Keith Wailoo et al., eds., *Three Shots at Prevention: The HPV Vaccine and the Politics of Medicine's Simple Solutions* (Baltimore: Johns Hopkins University Press, 2010). Studies on vaccine development and vaccination and highlight the role of the state in the different way the 'same' vaccines play out across the globe in Stuart Blume, Paul Greenough, and Christine Holmberg, eds., *The Politics of Vaccination: A Global History*, Studies for the Society for the History of Medicine (Manchester: University of Manchester Press, 2017).

contributed to Hungary's path-breaking role in polio eradication. Moreover, changes in the evaluation of the Salk vaccine highlighted broader problems in the relationship between the government and its citizens and between the efficiency of production and the organisation of the state.

Defining Success

Aladár Kátay, director of the epidemiology department at the Health Ministry and head of the poliomyelitis section of the Hungarian Microbiology Society, published one of the first comprehensive accounts of the 1957 epidemic wave in an article in *Népegészségügy*,[4] the public health journal of the Health Ministry. Titled 'Our current situation and tasks in epidemiology', Kátay's article discussed Salk vaccination and its evaluation.

Regarding the efficacy of the administered vaccination, we have to state first and foremost that given the time needed to gain relative protection, we did not expect any direct result in the peak of the epidemic as a result of the vaccine. We did expect, however, the ameliorating effect in the last section of the epidemic wave and we are expecting children of the most endangered age to be protected in the epidemic waves of the coming years. The effect of the vaccination on [1957's] epidemic cannot be measured yet. It is a fact that the epidemic wave receded drastically sooner, already in September. However, *this alone is no proof.*[5]

Kátay stressed that further studies were needed to determine vaccine efficiency – an epidemiological-statistical analysis of morbidity among the vaccinated and non-vaccinated population and an immunological study of blood samples taken from vaccinated children. This opinion did not gain much publicity. Again, there was no space for uncertainty or doubt regarding the feat of importing and distributing the precious vaccine.

The sudden decline of the epidemic wave did come up, however, in further scientific evaluations, some of which provided different explanations: for instance, that the decline could have been caused by other factors, such as the particular pattern of the epidemic in 1957. In a report by the State Hygienic Institute in *Népegészségügy*, Dr Ottó Rudnai pointed out that compared to the polio epidemics of the past, the wave of 1957 was unusual. The curve of polio cases increased and also decreased much more drastically than before, creating a much sharper spike in the diagram than previous epidemics. The temporal layout of the epidemic wave was also peculiar: polio usually reached its peak

[4] Aladár Kátay, 'Járványügyi Helyzetünk És Feladataink', *Népegészségügy* 8, no. 10–11 (1957): 247–58.
[5] Ibid. 253–54 (emphasis mine).

in August, and only three times in the past twenty-five years had it peaked in July, as it did in 1957.[6] Strangely enough, Rudnai decidedly left issues of vaccine evaluation out of the report. The only time he mentioned the vaccine at all was in relation to the changes in the affected age groups after the end of the epidemic: 'We do not wish to address the issue or the efficacy of the vaccine here, but . . . the decline in polio incidence among children under 6 years old in the fourth quarter [of 1957] is probably due to the effect of the vaccine.'[7] Thus, a more cautious evaluation of the vaccination's effect on the epidemic detects a possible change months after the epidemic wave was over.

By April 1958 the Health Ministry was presenting the vaccination process as a clear success. Nationwide vaccination with the brand-new vaccine was a costly enterprise, especially for an Eastern European country like Hungary struggling with debt and difficulties in accessing hard currency. Therefore, it was important to demonstrate that it had actually worked. In the context of polio, the moment of the vaccine import marked a turning point in the ability of the state to gain control of the unpredictable and chaotic situation that the epidemic waves had caused and to return to its role as a providing and protective parent.

On the pages of *Népszava* in June 1958, Dr Frigyes Doleschall, the Hungarian health minister, evaluated the success of vaccination:

We began vaccination in July 1957, that is, during the epidemic: The epidemic wave quickly started to recede and by October it ended. Thus, it finished before we could apply the three doses of vaccine that are needed to achieve optimal immunity. *This alone proves the efficiency of the vaccine.*'[8]

The interpretation of the Health Ministry, therefore, was that even one dose of the vaccine was enough to curb polio and cause a sudden decline in the epidemic wave. For this, the decline of the epidemic served as proof.

In scientific publications, there was also a shift towards the emphasis on a marked success in the vaccination campaign, although with more reserved enthusiasm. As virologist Aladár Petrilla points out in his report of 1958 in the journal *Acta Microbiologica*, a scientific evaluation of the vaccination was indeed a difficult task. First of all, vaccination started at the peak of the epidemic rather than preceding it, making it difficult to pinpoint the efficacy

---

[6] Otto Rudnai, 'Az 1957. Évi Poliomyelitis Járvány. Közlemény az Országos Közegészségügyi Intézet (Főigazgató: Bakács Tibor Dr.) Járványügyi Osztályáról (Osztályvezető: Petrilla Aladár Dr.)', ibid. 39, no. 5–6 (1958): 121–27, at 124.

[7] Ibid. 127.

[8] 'Dr. Doleschall Frigyes Miniszter Nyilatkozata a Népszavának az Egészségügy Hároméves Tervéről, a Salk-Oltásokról és a Gyógyszerfogyasztásról', *Népszava*, 17 June 1958, 1–2, at 2 (emphasis in original).

of the vaccine. Secondly, it seemed that many children eligible for the vaccine did not receive any injections, while many outside the age group set by the Health Ministry managed to be immunised all the same.[9] Unfortunately, Petrilla does not elaborate on how the latter was achieved, nor does he reveal the source of his information. Thirdly, around 80,000 children were vaccinated in private practice, with a different method and different dosage.[10] Instead of the intradermal method used in the state vaccination campaign, these children received a higher dose intramuscularly. Their results would therefore complicate the overall evaluation.

However, in the overall evaluation Petrilla states: 'The effect of the vaccination was satisfactory.'[11] He lists six factors that can serve as proof of the success of the vaccine – none of which had been communicated by the health minister in the newspaper. As there was no control group and, in May 1958 when the article was submitted to the journal, no way of knowing if a new epidemic had been prevented or not, Petrilla turned to alternative comparisons to analyse the effects of the vaccine.

First, he pointed out that the incidence rate in the autumn months was much lower than in previous epidemic years, which could be a result of the vaccination campaign. The second piece of proof was a comparison with neighbouring countries Austria and Romania, where there was no mass vaccination, at least according to the information of the Hungarian State Institute of Hygiene. While Romania seemed to suffer an even more severe epidemic that lasted longer than Hungary's, the curve was quite similar, whereas Austria's epidemic produced a much more gradual curve, staying well below the Hungarian one except for the months of October and November. The example of these two countries and the comparison with Hungary was left without analysis and conclusion, as Petrilla moved on to points three and four, both emphasising the decrease in the ratio of polio cases among the 0–6 age group compared to children older than six. The fifth piece of evidence was the difference in incidence rate between unvaccinated and vaccinated (either one or two doses) children in the months of October to December 1957. By this time, the vaccine should have taken effect. Petrilla found that the incidence rate of the non-vaccinated children was double that of those vaccinated once and five times the rate of children vaccinated twice. Petrilla admitted that these numbers were based on months with an overall low incidence rate (following the outbreak), which made evaluation difficult. For instance, the low number of cases in Budapest (nine in total over the course of three months) made it impossible to produce statistically relevant results.[12] Petrilla's last piece of evidence is the difference in the way the epidemic wave receded for children born between

[9] Petrilla, *The Results of Intracutaneous Poliomyelitis Vaccination in Hungary, 1957.*
[10] Ibid. 307.   [11] Ibid. 300.   [12] Ibid. 304–05.

1955 and 1956 and for children born between 1951 and 1954. The younger
population (one-year-olds) had received their vaccinations one month earlier
than the three-to-six-year-olds, and the case numbers among the former started
falling earlier than among the latter. Petrilla pointed out that the evaluation of
the effect on two-year-olds was not possible, since the report cards only
contained the age of the children, not the birth years, and thus there was no
way of knowing whether two-year-olds were born in 1954 or 1955 and
therefore to which vaccination group they would belong.[13] Other possible
reasons for the difference in age groups (e.g. comparison to age patterns in
previous epidemics) were not discussed.

In his summary, Petrilla used an even more cautious tone. Whereas he had
claimed at the beginning of the article that the effects were satisfactory, he now
changed his evaluation, saying, 'The efficacy of the vaccination could not be
determined exactly.'[14] He further confused his analysis by first admitting that
the unvaccinated population included vaccinated children who had received
vaccine through private practice, and then that he considered the 'unvaccinated
group' as a control group for the evaluation of the vaccination.

These evaluations of the Salk vaccine seemed to fall in line with what Tibor
Bakács, director of the State Hygienic Institute from September 1957, wrote in
his memoir in the 1970s: 'During the sectarian years [the pre-1956, Stalinist
era], it was an institutional directive that 'research is only allowed with the
certainty of success.' Those who could not show results in time in their
research were reprimanded and not only on the scientific level.'[15] Bakács
saw this attitude and distrust in scientific research, which was still prevalent
in 1957, as one of the main challenges he faced as director. It is hardly
surprising that scientists therefore did not have much choice but to produce
results and success, especially in a case of such national importance as the Salk
vaccination.

Meanwhile, the vaccination campaign continued, as further age groups were
included in the immunisation programme in February 1958. The Health
Ministry raised the age limit from 6 to 18 years and covered the broadened
vaccine needs by importing further batches of vaccine. The vaccination campaign was organised in state homes for mothers and infants,[16] kindergartens
and health centres. Older children were vaccinated in high schools and vocational schools.[17] However, the age group of 14 to 18 was apparently not very
enthusiastic about receiving vaccination. According to a newspaper article in

---

[13] Ibid. 306.   [14] Ibid. 308.
[15] Tibor Bakács, *Egy Életrajz Ürügyén* (Budapest: Kossuth Könyvkiadó, 1978).
[16] Single mothers would be admitted to the former, while orphans and state wards were accom-
modated in the latter.
[17] 'Tizennyolc Éves Korig Adnak Gyermekbénulás Elleni Védőoltást – Február 10-én Kezdődik
az Új Oltási Kampány', *Népakarat*, 28 January 1958, 3.

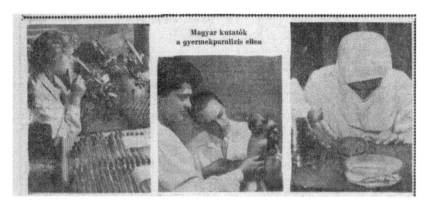

Figure 4.1 *Hungarian researchers against poliomyelitis.* Népakarat,
18 September 1957, 2, no. 218, 1. Credit: Arcanum Digitecha. **This image is
protected by copyright and cannot be used without further permissions
clearance.**

Népszava in April, the majority did not show up at the immunisation points.
Therefore, they were called upon by the newspaper to attend their vaccination
before the epidemic months of the summer began.[18]

In the spring of 1959, polio vaccination became compulsory and was
administered through a continuous vaccination programme. The process had
begun a year before, in March 1958, when Vilmos Kapos, director of the
Public Health and Epidemiology Station of Budapest, had proposed implementing continuous immunisation for children instead of the method of vaccination campaigns that had hitherto been applied. Kapos argued that at many
points during the campaigns there had been some kind of epidemic in place,
e.g. flu or polio, which set back vaccination processes. Moreover, many
children specified by the respective age groups of certain vaccination programmes were in daycare (*bölcsőde*), where infectious diseases were a constant feature, therefore often barring whole communities from taking part in a
campaign. These children then would have to be vaccinated in the next
campaign, joining the ones who were regularly scheduled. This produced a
serious strain on authorities providing and distributing the vaccine.[19]

Continuous vaccination would serve as a solution to these problems, since
individual children could be vaccinated at the moment they reached the

---

[18] Moldován, 'Aki Még Nem Kapott – Áprilisban Jelentkezzék Gyermekbénulás Elleni Védőoltásra', *Népszava*, 16 April 1958.
[19] Vilmos Kapos. 'A Kötelező Védőoltások Folyamatos Végrehajtása a Főváros Területén',
Budapest: National Archives of Hungary, Egészségügyi Minisztérium Állami közegészségügyi
felügyelet és járványvédelmi főosztály iratai, XIX-C-2-e 1959, 51453, 1958.

required age or recovered from their current illness. Until then, polio vaccinations had been organised in biannual campaigns, in which children of certain age groups were vaccinated over the course of several days. In April, the Humán Vaccine Production and Research Institute assured the Health Ministry that in terms of vaccine distribution, continuous vaccination was indeed possible.[20] The next month, plans were afoot: the Health Ministry authorised the experimental implementation of continuous immunisation along with the diphtheria-pertussis-tetanus and smallpox vaccines. Budapest was to report on the progress of the test run every six months.[21]

The government issued the decree on mandatory immunisation against poliomyelitis in September 1958,[22] to become effective in 1959.[23] Children between 6 months and 17 years old were to receive compulsory polio injections with the Salk vaccine. In cases of epidemic outbreaks, the health departments of city or county councils had the authority to order additional mass vaccinations against the disease.[24] It was parents' responsibility to appear with their children before the vaccinating doctor, and everyone who was obliged to be vaccinated would receive an immunisation card on which the physicians could record vaccinations and control examinations.[25] Although the continuous immunisation programme was still in its experimental phase in Budapest, Kapos assured the Health Ministry that they would be able to conform to the new regulation, despite the extra strain it placed on their infrastructure.[26]

The use of the Salk vaccine was thus established and became fixed in the legal system. In this environment, there was little space for doubts or the circulation of alternative views, especially on a public level. The subjects of vaccination policies and their parents and guardians were not consulted at any point of the process. Instead, vaccination and the evaluation of its success were centrally decided. After all, the epidemic had receded, the summer panic was over and the main task remaining was to reach as many children as possible with the vaccination programme to try to avert another attack. For this project, emphasising that the efficacy of the vaccine had been confirmed was crucial. Soon, however, the immunisation programme would be put to the test in the

---

[20] Oltóanyagtermelő és Kutató Intézet Humán. 'Kötelező Védőoltások Folyamatos Végrehajtása a Főváros Területén', ibid. 51918.

[21] Aladár Kátay. 'Folyamatos Védőoltások a Fővárosban.' Ibid. Magyar Oszágos Levéltár, 52417.

[22] 'Rendelet a Kötelező Védőoltásokról', *Népakarat*, 17 September 1958.

[23] *A Magyar Forradalmi Munkás-Paraszt Kormány 1027/1958 (VIII. 3.) Számú Határozata a Gyermekbénulás Elleni Védekezésről*, 1958.

[24] *Az Egészségügyi Miniszter 5/1958. (IX. 16) Eü. M. Számú Rendelete a Védőoltásokra Vonatkozó Jogszabályok Végrehajtásáról* (1958), 1.

[25] Ibid. 2.

[26] Vilmos Kapos. 'A Folyamatos Védőoltások a Fővárosban', Budapest: National Archives of Hungary, Egészségügyi Minisztérium Állami közegészségügyi felügyelet és járványvédelmi főosztály iratai, XIX-C-2-e 1959, 51250, 1959.

face of a new epidemic – one that would prove to be tragic for thousands of children and their families.

An Unexpected Epidemic: Polio in 1959

Another summer came – the second since vaccination against polio had begun. Again, as two years previously, the heat rose in early June, compelling 37,000 people in Budapest to go to the baths and swimming pools on the first hot Sunday of the year. To the relief of many, beer production had been well prepared for the summer and Budapesters consumed 1.6 million glasses of beer in one day alone – along with hundreds of kilograms of ice cream.[27] National plans for children's summer holidays were also underway: The National Council of Trade Unions was to take 30,000 schoolchildren on holiday, while the Pioneer movement planned summer camps for 200,000 children.[28]

As the summer progressed, the temperature kept rising every day. Swimming pools and outdoor baths were increasingly packed at weekends, with children and adults basking in the sun. But despite renewed assurances in the newspaper about the beer and ice cream supply in recreational places,[29] clouds of fear grew in the summer sky.

On 21 July readers of *Népszava* found the all too familiar health minister's report on the back page of the newspaper. The minister called attention to the growing number of poliomyelitis cases in Budapest and informed the public about the decree of the Health Ministry, which brought forward all scheduled polio vaccinations due in the autumn of 1959 and even in the spring of 1960.[30] Ten days later, Vera Szekeres, a paediatrician, wrote a newspaper article warning parents to avoid crowds and swimming pools and not to tire children with either games or studying during the holidays.[31] Polio was back.

Soon, more and more cases were reported in Budapest, and the epidemic started spreading to Kecskemét, Szeged, Mohács and towns in Pest County.[32] While the number of cases was lower than in the severe epidemic of 1957, it climbed higher than any other year before. In July 1959, 252 cases of paralytic polio were registered, which was surprisingly high compared to

[27] 'Rekordforgalom Az Első Meleg Nyári Vasárnapon', *Népszava*, 9 June 1959.
[28] 'Harmincezer Iskolásgyermeket Üdültet a SZOT, Kétszázezer Gyerek Megy Úttörőtáborba', *Népszava*, 4 June 1959.
[29] 'Kánikulai Jelentés a Strandokról, a Közlekedésről és a Vasárnapi Előkészületekről', *Népakarat*, 11 July 1959.
[30] 'Az Egészségügyi Minisztérium Tájékoztatója a Gyermekbénulásos Megbetegedésekről', *Népszava*, 21 July 1959, 8.
[31] 'Megkezdték a IV. Salk-Védőoltás Beadását', *Népszava*, 31 July 1959.
[32] 'Az Egészségügyi Minisztérium Tájékoztatója a Gyermekbénulásos Megbetegedésekről', *Népszava*, 2 August 1959, 11.

122   Local Failure in a Global Success

those of previous years. In July 1958, the number had been 21; in 1956, 145; in 1955, 83; and in 1954, 198. Only the stunningly high number of 705 cases from July 1957 surpassed the number in 1959.[33] In August, the epidemic escalated, climbing up to 761 cases, well above the 487 of August 1957 and four times as many as the average number of cases in the August of previous epidemic years.[34]

Again, as two years previously, an intensive vaccination campaign was quickly organised. A report on the Budapest campaign in July 1959 reveals the details:

Vaccination in the capital is executed by the 73 Mother and Infant Protection Agencies. Children under 5 years are summoned with personalised request cards. The request cards for [those] under 2 years old include punitive measures; the ones for above 2 year olds do not. Nurses and Red Cross activists visit the homes of children who do not appear for vaccination despite the request.[35]

While vaccination took over as the primary mode of prophylaxis, as the numbers continued to creep up, other, more traditional steps were also taken to soften the blow of the epidemic. Children could no longer seek refuge from the summer heat in swimming pools or on the banks of the Danube; epidemic areas were closed off from holiday travels organised for children; tonsillectomies were postponed[36] in order to reduce the number of children with a weakened immune system and a wound in the gateway of the disease – the gastrointestinal system – exposed to polio; daycare centres in which outbreaks had been registered were shut down and disinfected.[37]

In exceptional cases, children in the immediate environment of polio patients could also receive gamma globulin. As an article in *Orvosi Hetilap* pointed out: 'Gamma globulin has ceased to be a mass tool of poliomyelitis prophylaxis, but in certain cases, we cannot renounce the protection it offers.'[38] Doctors would prescribe the serum to those who 'due to their age or other reasons could not be

[33] 'Az Egészségügyi Minisztérium Tájékoztatója az Ország 1959. Évi Július Havi Járványügyi Helyzetéről', *Népegészségügy* 40, no. 9 (1959): 252.
[34] 'Az Egészségügyi Minisztérium Tájékoztatója az Ország 1959. Évi Augusztus Havi Járványügyi Helyzetéről', *Népegészségügy* 40, no. 10 (1959): 279–80.
[35] Gábor Vastagh and Ottó Rudnai. 'Jelentés a Fővárosi Poliomyelitis Elleni Védőoltások Ellenőrzéséről', Budapest: National Archives of Hungary, Országos Közegészségi Intézet Járványügyi és Mikrobiológiai Főosztályának iratai, XXVI-C-3-e, 5450/1959, 1959.
[36] Ottó Rudnai. 'Heti Fertőzőbeteg Jelentés 1959. 30. Hét', Budapest: National Archives of Hungary, Országos Közegészségügyi Intézet iratai, XXVI-C-3-e, 5421/1959, 1959.
[37] *Az Egészségügyi Miniszter 8200–4/1953. Eü. M. Számú Utasítása a Fertőző Betegségek Megelőzéséről Szóló 61/1953 (XII.20) M. T. Számú Végrehajtása Tárgyában.* 3.sz. melléklet a 8200–4/1953. Eü. M. számú utasításhoz.
[38] Pál Földes and Szeri Ilona, 'A Gamma-Globulin Prophylaxis Szerepe a Poliomyelitis Elleni Küzdelem Jelenlegi Helyzetében', *Orvosi Hetilap* 100, no. 3 (1959): 115–17 at 116.

vaccinated previously'.[39] The vaccine would be distributed free of charge by the local public health and epidemiology station.[40]

The epidemic wave started to recede in the autumn. While 509 cases were registered in September, the number fell to 199 in October and 96 in November.[41] These numbers were still much higher than the respective data from the previous epidemic year,[42] 1957, although in that year, as we have seen in the previous section, the epidemic curve was unusually spiky, beginning and ending sooner than in an average epidemic year.

About 25 per cent of cases were reported in the capital and the surrounding Pest County in the peak month of August. Other epidemic areas were Bács-Kiskun, Szabolcs-Szatmár, Győr, Sopron, Veszprém, Heves, Fejér and Békés Counties. The incidence rate was highest in Pest County, at 21.6 per 100,000.[43] At the peak of the epidemic, the disease truly spread across the whole country; there was no county or region in Hungary that was not affected.[44]

In total, 1,830 people, mainly children, fell ill with paralytic polio, making 1959 the second largest epidemic year in Hungary after 1957, with its 2,334 cases. Pest County continued to remain at the epicentre throughout the epidemic wave, reaching an incidence rate of 30.9 per 100,000, while the average rate was 18.3 nationwide. Similarly to 1957, it was Type I poliovirus that spread across the country that year. This type was more virulent than Types II and III, which had been the culprits in the epidemic years preceding 1957 and could have accounted for the severity of the previous two epidemics.[45]

Something else was also different from previous epidemics. There was a statistically significant change in the age groups afflicted by the disease. The ratio of affected children between 1 and 2 years of age fell, while the number of cases among infants under one year and children between 3 and 5 years grew.[46] Public health officials and epidemiologists like Bakács and Rudnai

[39] 38/1958. (VI.10.) Korm. Számú Rendelet a Védőoltásokról Szóló 60/1953. (XII.20.) M.T. Számú Rendelet Kiegészítéséről.
[40] Barnabás Göllner, 'Gamma-Glonulin Felhasználása Fertőzőbetegségek Megelőzésére', Budapest: City Archives of Budapest, Budapest Fővárosi Tanács VB Egészségügyi Osztályának iratai, XXIII.115.a/34. kisdoboz, 180788–1959, 1959.
[41] Aladár Kátay, 'Járványügyi Adatok Közlése az Egészségügyi Világszervezettel', Budapest: National Archives of Hungary, Egészségügyi Minisztérium Állami Közegészségügyi Felügyelet és Járványvédelmi Főosztály iratai, XIX-C-2-e, 57370, 1959.
[42] In November 1957, 45 cases of poliomyelitis were registered in Hungary, while in 1959 the number was over double with the 96 cases. Ibid.
[43] 'Az Egészségügyi Minisztérium Tájékoztatója az Ország 1959. Évi Augusztus Havi Járványügyi Helyzetéről', 1959.
[44] Gábor Vastagh, 'Az Országos Közegészségügyi Intézet Járványügyi Tájékoztatója 1959. Augusztus Hóról.' Budapest: National Archives of Hungary, Országos Közegészségügyi Intézet Járványügyi és Mikrobiológiai Osztályának iratai, XXVI-C-3-e, 5571/1959, 1959.
[45] Ottó Rudnai, The 1959 Poliomyelitis Epidemic in Hungary, Acta Microbiologica (Budapest: Academiae Scientiarum Hungaricae, 1960).
[46] Ibid. 439.

explained that this was the effect of the Salk vaccination. According to their argument, the reason for the increase among the two age groups was that infants had not been fully vaccinated (they started receiving vaccine from the age of six months, often even later), while in the cases of older children, the vaccine had lost much of its protective effect. Children between 1 and 2 years old had mostly received all their injections and had been vaccinated relatively recently.[47]

'The 1959 epidemic was, to some extent, unexpected. It was hoped that the Salk vaccination, carried since 1957, would protect the otherwise most endangered age groups, which have been vaccinated most systematically', wrote Ottó Rudnai in a report on the 1959 epidemic.[48] Tibor Bakács similarly voiced puzzlement, and perhaps disappointment: 'In the light of ... the fact that from 1957 to 1959, 70 to 90 percent of the population under 20 years of age had been vaccinated with Salk vaccine, it was difficult to explain how the 1959 epidemic had come about.'[49]

Placing the Blame

Who or what was to blame for this unexpected epidemic? Were parents irresponsible for not having their children vaccinated? Was it the state that failed to organise immunisation effectively or secure adequate supplies? Was it the fault of physicians, who undermined the success of vaccination with doubts and alternative views? Or perhaps did blame lie with the vaccine itself, which had given a false sense of security to the nation?

The epidemic of 1959 changed the game. In the search for explanations, the success story of the Salk vaccine in Hungary was re-evaluated. The state blamed the parents who neglected their children and acted irresponsibly in not taking their children to be vaccinated. Doubts formed about the intracuteanous method in the medical community. Bitter parents pointed fingers at the state, as a persistent conspiracy theory took hold among them. Administrators pointed out deficiencies in organisation, adding that medical supplies had also failed to reach the standard required for a successful immunisation. Finally, the Salk vaccine, which was slowly losing the battle against the rising live-virus vaccine of Albert Sabin, came under scrutiny. The following section analyses these circles of blame in order to unravel further the expectations and responsibilities shared among the multiple actors of state, medical profession and parents.

[47] See ibid. and Dr Tibor Bakács, 'Poliomyelitis Prophylaxis in Hungary', ibid. VII, no. 3: 329–37.
[48] Rudnai, *The 1959 Poliomyelitis Epidemic in Hungary*, 442
[49] Dr Tibor Bakács, 'Poliomyelitis Prophylaxis in Hungary', ibid. VII, no. 3: 329–37 at 331.

The Parents: Irresponsibility and Neglect

It seems that there were definitely issues with the organisation of the vaccination process from the beginning. A side note on an internal draft version of the ministerial instructions for the August–September vaccination campaign in 1957 reveals that 'the preparation and announcement of the vaccinations in July were flawed in many instances'.[50] Sándor Tóth's opinion might have informed the minister's unfavourable view of the vaccination campaign. Tóth, the managing hospital director in Debrecen, the second largest city in the country and home of the regional medical centre, submitted a report that listed several problems he had observed in his region.[51] One of the recurring problems was that many parents did not turn up at the vaccination points to have their children immunised. This issue became central very early on in the outbreak of the new epidemic and served as a context in which all public communication about polio was framed.

As the previous section shows, there were many similarities between the epidemics of 1957 and 1959. The type of the virus, intensity of the epidemic and age groups afflicted during these two events all stood out in comparison to previous epidemics. The 1959 epidemic was also extraordinary for another reason. This time, the nation was supposed to have been vaccinated. This epidemic, especially with such vehemence, should not have happened.

The paternalist state, which had invested so much in reclaiming its role as the provider by importing the Salk vaccine in 1957 and was then so intent on proving its efficacy, could neither afford a loss of face in 1959, nor could it admit to a failure or claim responsibility for this tragic turn of events. For two years, virtually every public communication had discussed polio in the context of the government's achievement in securing the Salk vaccine and saving Hungary's children from the crippling disease.

While the government was consistent in emphasising its own heroic role in the fight against polio throughout 1959, the new epidemic did bring about a change in viewpoint on the rate of vaccination. Up until the outbreak in the summer of 1959, one of the achievements emphasised frequently in newspapers was the success in immunising the masses with the vaccine. In November 1957, in a talk delivered at the Hungarian–Soviet Medicine meeting, the Hungarian vice-minister of health demonstrated the success of implementing the great pillar of Soviet healthcare – prevention – by stating that one million

---

[50] Benyó, 'Gyermekbénulás Elleni Folytatólagos Védőoltások Szervezése', Budapest: National Archives of Hungary, 1957.
[51] Sándor Tóth, 'Gyermekbénulás Elleni Védőoltásokkal Kapcsolatos Felmerült Problémák', Debrecen: National Archives of Hungary, Egészségügyi Minisztérium Állami Közegészségügyi Felügyeleti és Járványvédeli Főosztály, XIX-C-2-e, 53137, 1957.

children had been given the Salk vaccine.[52] In June 1958, the health minister boasted that 'two and a half million people, that is, one fourth of the population, has been immunised against polio'.[53] The same number was cited in the report titled 'The results of 1958 in Hungarian healthcare and its plans for 1959', assembled in early 1959 by Health Minister Doleschall Frigyes and submitted to the president of the Ministerial Council, Ferenc Münnich, on 9 January 1959.[54] Where vaccination rates did not reach a high percentage, as was the case in Budapest, public health officials pointed to the proliferation of privately imported and implemented vaccines that could have reached as many as 80,000 people.[55]

However, the evaluation of the vaccination rate changed quickly in official communications when the first signs of an epidemic started to show. In the summer of 1959, newspaper readers wishing for more information about the spread of the disease looked in vain for the weekly reports of the Health Ministry, as they had done in 1957. While in the summer of 1957 the Health Ministry had issued a report every week on polio in major newspapers, eight in total, only two reports appeared in 1959. The reports had become scarce and less informative about the number of cases and infected areas.[56] Instead, they concentrated on vaccination issues, and most of all, on scolding parents for neglecting their duties.

The first report barely gave any information about the cases and geographical spread of the disease: almost half consisted of an overview of previous prevention efforts and the success of immunisation before offering details of the growing number of polio cases and naming parents as responsible for this unfortunate turn of events.

In the summer of 1956 the number of polio cases in Budapest was unusually high; on a national scale the highest number of people contracting the disease was in 1957. The number of new cases already started falling in the three months after vaccination was introduced and the epidemic ceased completely. In 1958 reports of the disease were scarce from all over the country. The number of cases stayed low in the summer months

[52] 'Egymillió Gyerek Kapott Idén Védőoltást. Megkezdődtek a Magyar-Szovjet Orvosi Napok', *Népakarat*, 22 November 1957, 1.
[53] 'Dr. Doleschall Frigyes Miniszter Nyilatkozata a Népszavának Az Egészségügy Hároméves Tervéről, a Salk-Oltásokról és a Gyógyszerfogyasztásról', *Népszava*, 17 June 1958, 1–2.
[54] Frigyes Doleschall, 'A Magyar Egészségügy 1958. Évi Eredményei És 1959. Évi Terve.' Budapest: National Archives of Hungary, Doleschall Frigyes egészségügyi miniszter iratai, XIX-C-2-q, 1959.
[55] I. Ferencz, 'The Results of Mass Poliomyelitis Vaccination Program Carried out in 1957 in Hungary', in *Vaccination and Immunity, Neurophysical and neuropathological aspects of poliomyelitis. Vth Symposium of the European Association against Poliomyelitis*, ed. H. C. A. Lassen (Madrid: Europ. Assoc. Poliomyelitis, 1959).
[56] 'Az Egészségügyi Minisztérium Tájékoztatója a Gyermekbénulásos Megbetegedésekről', *Népszava*, 21 July 1959, 8, and 'Az Egészségügyi Minisztérium Tájékoztatója a Gyermekbénulásos Megbetegedésekről', *Népszava*, 2 August 1959, 12.

as well, and never before had so few cases been reported nationally than in that year. The situation remained favourable nationally in the first half of this year as well, but recently the number of polio cases has been rising in Budapest. Based on examinations so far, it appears that this increase is primarily caused by the fact that many children were not taken to get immunised in Budapest. There are also many children who only received one or two out of the three shots.[57]

Other articles, such as the one titled 'All our responsibility', published in *Népszabadság* in July 1959, placed the blame more directly:

Who wouldn't remember the anxiety with which we looked at news about poliomyelitis cases two years ago, and what a weight had been lifted off the shoulders of worried parents, when the good news spread: the aircraft bearing the first batch of Salk vaccine has landed on Ferihegy airport? We gave news almost every day about steps taken to prevent the further spread of the disease, among them the credit of millions of forints, with which the government secured vaccine for the most endangered age groups. The greatest wish of all parents was to have their children protected against the dangerous disease that often leaves severe marks for life. All the more surprising is it that according to information recently published by the Health Ministry, a lot of children in the capital had not been taken to be immunised and based on examinations it can be said: the rising number of cases ... are caused by exactly this.[58]

The argument thus was simple and outright: the government had done everything in its power to curb the disease, and through great sacrifice provided protection for the children. But it was the parents who had neglected their duties and with their irresponsible behaviour caused a new epidemic.

What is particularly interesting in this latter account of events is the ambivalent relationship between the state and its citizens. On the one hand, the state and parents together comprised an all-encompassing family, creating a unit in which all members were responsible for working for the benefit of all. On the other hand, the actions of the state were completely removed from this unit; the credit that was needed to buy vaccine was presented as the sole sacrifice of the government, giving the impression that the debt of the country would not affect citizens in any way and therefore they need not be concerned.[59]

But by 'a lot' of unvaccinated or only partially vaccinated children, how many were meant? Was participation in the vaccination campaigns against polio really a problem throughout? Or was the citing of low vaccination rates instead a tool of the government, used to point at a scapegoat to take the blame?

---

[57] 'Az Egészségügyi Minisztérium Tájékoztatója a Gyermekbénulásos Megbetegedésekről', *Népszava*, 21 July 1959, 8.

[58] Jenő Faragó, 'Mindannyiunk Felelőssége', *Népszabadság*, 24 July 1959.

[59] This remote concept of a country's debt, removed completely from the lives of the people inhabiting the country, came to be a persistent attitude towards state debt in later years, and only surfaced as a major problem in the eyes of citizens after 1989.

The number of children to be vaccinated in each age group was set according to data provided by the Central Statistical Office (CSO). Vaccine distribution was then calculated based on the number of local eligible children, and so was the vaccination result. According to an official evaluation of the Public Health Control and Epidemiology Department of the Health Ministry (PHCED) from early 1958, a total of 983,000 children were eligible in Hungary for vaccination during the campaigns of 1957. This number does not include the number of children in Budapest, since the data was still missing when the evaluation was compiled.[60] Of the almost 1 million children born between 1 January 1951 and 28 February 1957 (between 6 months and 6 years old), 792,000 were vaccinated twice, while 190,000 were not vaccinated at all. This means that, at least officially, at the beginning of Salk vaccination in Hungary, 80 per cent of the population under 6 years old were vaccinated. The evaluation remarks that some children in the 'non-vaccinated' group in fact received a first dose at the time when the rest were having their second dose, so the overall number of vaccinated children is likely to have been higher.[61]

A report from 1957 on Pest County, the region that suffered the highest incidence rate in the 1959 outbreak, reveals that in at least some cases, the data from the Statistical Office did not match local reality. The county's public health and epidemiology station reported that 70 per cent of eligible children had been vaccinated in August 1957 (most of them twice), while 10 per cent were ill at the time of the campaign. The director therefore deemed the campaign rather successful. Moreover, he argued, the ratio was probably even higher since 'the number of children belonging to the age groups assigned for vaccination is significantly lower, according to local data, than what is shown by the CSO'.[62]

In the report from Debrecen mentioned at the beginning of this chapter, Sándor Tóth, for one, saw deficiencies in the way the campaign was announced and the public informed about it. He pointed out that there was very little time in July to advertise the campaign adequately. In addition to posters and radio news, the local PHCED tried to disseminate information by employing Red Cross and party activists and even literally 'drumming up' eligible families in railway stations: a drummer shouted out the details of the campaign during the rush hours of dawn and late evening, when agricultural

[60] If the report on Budapest was ever completed, it is lost from the archives of the Health Ministry.
[61] Aladár Petrilla, 'Jelentés a Poliomyelitis Ellenes Védőoltások Előzetes Eredményeiről', Budapest: National Archives of Hungary, Román József egészségügyi miniszter iratai, XIX-C-2-e, 1958.
[62] Sándor Sólyom. 'Augusztus Hónapban Végzett Gyermekbénulás Elleni Védőoltásokról Jelentés', Budapest: National Archives of Hungary, Egészségügyi Minisztérium Állami közegészségügyi felügyelet és járványvédelmi főosztály iratai, XIX-C-2-e, 53935, 1957.

and factory workers commuted to and from their workplaces. However, participation in the vaccination did not reach the desired quantity. Other counties were more optimistic about their efficiency and did not report problems of any kind. The PHCED station of Somogy County, for instance, remarked that 'the vaccination in the whole of the county has been executed smoothly and according to plans'.[63] The report of Vas County recounted even bigger success: 'The result of the vaccination is 105 percent. This number proves that as an outcome of the good work in providing information, the population of the whole county understood the significance of the vaccination and complied gladly to our request'.[64]

Unfortunately, such reports from later months in 1958 and 1959 are missing from the archives. It is therefore difficult to tell if there was a significant change in participation in vaccination as time went by, or if the records of 1957 can be taken as representative of the full period of Salk vaccination. It is also unknown whether the numbers and accounts of the campaign's sweeping success were results of wishful thinking rather than fastidious data collection, or to what extent such reports were tools for the personal advancement of local medical directors and PHCED stations. However, since the 1959 polio outbreak was peculiar in that it was roughly equally severe all across the country and not one county escaped the disease, it is possible to conclude that differences in vaccination rates, if there indeed were notable differences, did not significantly affect the outbreak of polio.

The only available public health document that chided parents for not taking their responsibility of vaccinating their children against polio seriously was a report submitted to the Health Ministry by the city council of Budapest in June 1959 on the health status of the capital's citizens.

Since the administration of the vaccine concerns nearly 100,000 children, it places a great burden on the vaccinating apparatus; therefore it is very important that the parents comply in time with the vaccination requests. Although vaccination discipline has recently improved, nevertheless in the case of many parents we need to revert to the disfavoured tools of fining, in order to get their children vaccinated in time.[65]

One explanation could be that Budapest was unique in that its parents disregarded their duties both as guardians and as citizens and that the vaccination rates were indeed lower than in other parts of the country. Alternatively, in a progress report from one political authority to another, blaming parents for

---

[63] Pál Lakos. Ibid., 53885.
[64] László Balló, 'Salk Védőoltások a Megye Területén', ibid., 54099.
[65] 'Budapest Fővárosi Tanács Végrehajtó Bizottsága Határozati Javaslata a Főváros Egészségügyi Helyzetének További Javítására', Budapest: National Archives of Hungary, Egészségügyi Minisztérium Vilmon Gyula miniszterhelyettes iratai, XIX-C-2-p, 1959.

any past or future faults in the vaccination campaign could well have been a strategy the council wanted to pursue.

What the evaluations and reports do reveal is that apart from the above instance, the responsibility of the parents and the excessive blame present in the public discussion of the 1959 epidemic was almost completely absent in the internal papers of the Health Ministry and the State Hygienic Institute. Officially, therefore, there was hardly any foundation for the extent of finger-pointing that the government exercised in the public media. On the contrary, an article published in *Orvosi Hetilap* in 1961 stated that 'according to the Health Ministry, by 1959, 90 per cent of the population under 18 years old was vaccinated three times with the Salk vaccine'.[66]

Furthermore, there is no sign that the issue of a low vaccination rate contributing to a new epidemic was further explored by the government after the summer of 1959. The recognition of the problem was localised to public discourse and also to the narrow temporal segment of the summer of 1959. The blame on parents was mostly laid through newspapers, not in scientific or in administrative literature. In a society where the working class had allegedly won the class struggle, it was ideology that took the place of socio-economic factors in placing blame. In a time of unexpected epidemic outbreak, blaming parents became a political tool for the government to preserve its image as a provider and successful protector of the nation's children.

Quality: Organisation and Supplies

While the internal papers of the Health Ministry did not blame parents outright for the epidemic of 1959, they did raise issues that might have contributed to the unsuccessful immunisation of the nation. These problems mainly had to do with organisation, material supplies and the implementation of instructions and regulations.

The uncertainty about numbers that became apparent in the reports mentioned above originated from the lack of a clear registration system of vaccination. This might sound astonishing, given our preconceptions about the way a state socialist regime would work, but it seems from the documents of the Health Ministry that the state did not actually know who was vaccinated or how many doses they received. The numbers that local PHCED stations submitted to the ministry referred to the number of doses administered only, in order to calculate the amount of vaccine that needed to be distributed for the next campaign.

---

[66] György Losonczy et al., 'A Salk Vakcináció és a Poliomyelitis Klinikai Lefolyásának Össze-függése', *Orvosi Hetilap* 101, no. 16 (1961): 733–35 at 733.

In 1957, the State Hygienic Institute sent out inquiries to local PHCEDs in order to ascertain how many polio patients were vaccinated and thereby to evaluate the effectiveness of the vaccine.[67] By the end of the 1959 epidemic, there was written proof of vaccination in certain cases;[68] however, the registration system was still in its test phase in July 1959.[69]

Since 1955, it had been the local registrar's duty to issue vaccination cards at birth, along with the birth certificate.[70] The vaccinating authority issued vaccination cards for older citizens.[71] All compulsory vaccinations had to be recorded on the card, with dates and the sequence of doses (e.g., Salk I, II and III). The card was the responsibility of the person receiving the vaccination or their guardian; they had to take it to the vaccination point with them and check that it had been filled in by the doctor or nurse correctly. However, in 1956 there was still no 'unified vaccination registry and appropriate vaccination system'[72] in place.

Parallel to the individual cards, beginning in 1958, the lists containing the names of people eligible for immunisation were compiled locally. These lists were made in accordance with a decree of the Health Ministry. The lists, compiled by the city councils' public health departments and village district physicians, contained not only the number of injections that each person received but also permission for delaying vaccinations (e.g. illness) or indication of absence without proper reason.[73] The documents were meant to be kept for twenty years in their respective archives.[74] In actuality, after each campaign came to a close, the lists were usually transferred to a general file-storage space, where it was 'impossible to find them after 1–2 years'. Therefore, in 1959 the State Hygienic Institute recommended that district physicians keep these files separately for easy access in the future. However, it seems that the system of lists was not nationally applied. In some places, like Stalin City

[67] Petrilla. 'Jelentés a Poliomyelitis Ellenes Védőoltások Előzetes Eredményeiről', Budapest: National Archives of Hungary, 1958.
[68] Bakács, 'Poliomyelitis Prophylaxis in Hungary', 0.
[69] Aladár Petrilla. 'Védőoltási Kimutatások Módosítása', Budapest: National Archives of Hungary, Országos Közegészségi Intézet Járványügyi és Mikrobiológiai Főosztályának iratai, XXVI-C-3-e 1.d., 5331/1959, 1959; 'Jelentés a Poliomyelitis Ellenes Védőoltások Előzetes Eredményeiről.' Budapest: National Archives of Hungary, 1958.
[70] 'Az Egészségügyi Miniszter 8200–5/1953. Eü.M. Számú Utasítása Védőoltásokról Szóló 60/1953. (XII.20.) M.T. Számú Rendelet Végrehajtása Tárgyában', in *38/1958. (Eü. K. 19)*, ed. Egészségügyi Minisztérium (Budapest, 1958).
[71] *Az Egészségügyi Miniszter 5/1958. (IX. 16) Eü. M. Számú Rendelete a Védőoltásokra Vonatkozó Jogszabályok Végrehajtásáról*, 1958.
[72] 'Budapest Főváros Lakossága Egészségügyi Ellátásának 1956. Évi Fejlesztési Terve.' Budapest: City Archives of Budapest, Budapest Fővárosi Tanács VB Egészségügyi Osztályának iratai, XXIII. 115.a. 214. box, 1956.
[73] 'Az Egészségügyi Miniszter 8200–5/1953. Eü.M. Számú Utasítása Védőoltásokról Szóló 60/1953. (Xii.20.) M.T. Számú Rendelet Végrehajtása Tárgyában', 1958.
[74] Ibid.

(*Sztálinváros*), a system of individual vaccination registration was introduced to keep track of immunisation in place of lists. This system was actually favoured by the head of the SHI over the official system set by the decree, as it meant that when a document disappeared it was only one person's data that was lost, as opposed to the data of a whole list of people.[75]

The lack of a clear and organised administrative system posed challenges for scientific inquiries. Shortly after the epidemic in 1959 broke out, the State Hygienic Institute contacted hospital directors in larger Hungarian cities to collect blood samples for the examination of immunity against poliomyelitis and the effect of the Salk vaccine. Blood would have to be collected from children staying in hospitals with non-polio cases and without fever. Vaccination histories would need to be taken 'based on vaccination cards or the account of the parents'.[76] Instead of choosing to leave children without written vaccination records out of the study, the institute simply chose to ask the parents. This suggests that either they were afraid that the required amount of samples could not otherwise be collected or that they were happy to take the words of the parents as the equivalent of written proof when it came to vaccination. In any case, the presence of vaccination cards was clearly not a fixed or given reality in the eyes of the SHI.

Another problem was the registration of polio cases. The PHCED station was supposed to collect reports and forward them to the State Institute of Hygiene. However, the reporting was often belated, as records of new cases were held up at the district physician's office. A recurring problem seemed to be that many hospitals would not report the children with polio in their care, even though they were obliged to report to the PHCED station via telephone as soon as a case came in.[77]

Furthermore, paralytic polio cases were not connected to vaccination information; when a polio case was reported, the information about when and how many doses of vaccine the child received (if any) was not included in the form. Therefore, to determine how many children were indeed vaccinated out of those who had since come down with polio, a separate data collection was necessary. This system stayed in place through the whole period of Salk vaccination, with only the minor difference that the additional questionnaire form in use since 1957 was submitted for revision and update at the end of the 1959 epidemic.[78]

[75] 'Védőoltási Kimutatások Módosítása.' Budapest: National Archives of Hungary, 1959.
[76] 'Polio Elleni Védőoltások Immunológiai Ellenőrzése', Budapest, 5416, 1959.
[77] Ottó Rudnai, 'Jelentés a Szabolcs-Szatmár Megyei Köjál Epidemiológiai Munkájának Ellenőrzéséről', Budapest: National Archives of Hungary, Egészségügyi Minisztérium Állami Köze-gészségügyi Felügyeleti és Járványvédeli Főosztály, XIX-C-2-e, 56593/1959, 1959.
[78] Bakács. 'Poliomyelitis Betegek Védőoltására Vonatkozó Adatgyűjtés', Budapest: National Archives of Hungary, 1959.

The fact that it was difficult to establish a link between polio cases and vaccination histories did not cause problems only for the Health Ministry and the SHI. For children who contracted polio despite being vaccinated and their families, it was particularly vexing that they were not able to track their own vaccination.

I was vaccinated. I don't know how many doses, though. This is such a problem as well. My mother went [to the local health centre] to ask about my vaccination, about the card. They said that they don't have it. One would think that these things, this information would be important to know for the treatment later on.[79]

While being vaccinated – but not being able to check their immunisation history and details – caused concern and frustration about the illness and damaged trust in the treatment for some of those who came down with polio and suffered paralysis, others faced grave consequences because of the lack of clear directives and a national registration system. Katalin Parádi was particularly unlucky in being a rare case of someone who contracted polio *twice*. She came down with polio and was paralysed in the arm in 1944, and then again after being vaccinated in the summer of 1959: 'The vaccination was organised in my high school. I told them I already had polio and therefore do not need the vaccine. They did not care and made me get the vaccination. It was not open for discussion.'[80]

Katalin's story shows that vaccination outside the most endangered group of those under 3 years old was not entirely voluntary, as the law and the newspapers made it out to be. Of course, 'voluntary' did have a particular meaning in this period, as Stakhanovites all over the country did overtime in factories voluntarily, while thousands of people demonstrated voluntarily in support of the Communist Party, Lenin and Stalin. Moreover, in the case of schools, parents were more often informed about, rather than involved in, decisions about education, extracurricular tasks and, as Katalin's case shows, health. In an already complicated and rather imperfect system of vaccination registration, such arbitrary mini-campaigns would make keeping track of individual immunisation history even more difficult.

Apart from organisational issues, the quality of equipment used in the campaigns also raised concern. A grave material problem that Sándor Tóth pointed out in his report on Debrecen was most probably an issue throughout the country: apparently, the needles supplied by the Health Ministry for the vaccination were of such bad quality that it was impossible to be certain if adequate doses could be administered. Simply put, the needles were leaking. 'Even after exchanging the [faulty] needles, they were not perfect, therefore it

[79] Zoltán Török, interview by Dora Vargha, 8 September 2011.
[80] Parádi, interview by Vargha, 27 January 2010.

was not possible to verify the quantity of vaccine in each case.'[81] As a solution, many doctors started using their own needles. However, that went against the idea of a centrally organised and executed vaccination, in which the methods, quantities and tools used were standardised and controllable.

The ministry did react to Tóth's observation and ordered a 'better quality check at the time of receiving the needle shipment from the manufacturer'.[82] However, Tóth's report was handed in after the second campaign in August, which means that by the time the problem was pointed out to the ministry, the 'most endangered' age group had already received two doses of the vaccine. If some of these doses had been incomplete, that would have undermined the whole campaign.

Apart from vaccination issues, there seemed to be further problems with compliance with laws and regulations regarding the polio epidemic. A complaint from 1957, written by the PHCED station director in Nógrád County, reveals that although children's travel was restricted by law and children's organised holidays put on hold in times of epidemics (see Chapter 2), the execution of the law was another matter altogether.

> We learned by accident that a group of schoolchildren from Budapest had holiday[ed] in Hasznos village, without informing the district physician ... the directors of the respective schools organised this through correspondence ... and the Station only learned about it well afterwards ... In our investigation we have found that not a single holiday-organising authority complied with what is set out in the law. The teachers were sent to locations without previous physical examinations. But an even bigger mistake was that they all brought their own kitchen staff with them, who were not examined either.[83]

The director went on to mention five instances in which groups of children were brought to the county for holidays despite the ban on travel.

The ministry archives are lacking in evidence of any steps taken to strengthen enforcement of the law restricting child travel for future epidemics. Perhaps faith in the vaccination meant that this problem had low priority among any upcoming issues. Therefore, it is quite possible that similar incidents did happen in the next epidemic year of 1959.

Inadequate reporting, the absence of a clear (and functioning) vaccination system, deficiencies in equipment and the lack of strict law enforcement could all have contributed to the new epidemic in 1959. The confusion over numbers, data collection and reporting also complicated vaccine evaluation.

---

[81] Tóth, 'Gyermekbénulás Elleni Védőoltásokkal Kapcsolatos Felmerült Problémák', Debrecen: National Archives of Hungary, 1957, 1.
[82] Handwritten note on ibid.
[83] Imre Ádám, 'Az Ifjúság Csoportos Üdültetése.' Budapest: ibid., 54228/1957.

These questions of quality were, however, overshadowed by issues of quantity: the amount of vaccine used throughout the campaigns.

Quantity: The Method

Not all physicians were convinced that the intracutaneous method was the best utilisation of the vaccine or that it would provide the same protection as the intramuscular method. The amount of vaccine used also came under debate. According to Tóth, the 'vaccination brigades' were fully committed to the method and quantity chosen by the Health Ministry, but in 'larger places', by which he probably meant cities with hospitals and health centres, alternative opinions and doubts voiced by doctors may have caused concern and suspicion among the public. This last issue was perhaps the most persistent problem in the course of polio vaccination with the Salk vaccine.

An article published in *Orvosi Hetilap* shows that there was, indeed, a heated if not very visible debate about the intracutaneous method for years. Among the reports published regarding the vaccination campaign of 1957, only one reveals laboratory testing of the Salk vaccine, published by the Microbiology Institution of the Budapest Medical University.[84] The aim of the study was to test the effects of the intracutaneous vaccination as practised in the mass campaign. This meant, as explained in Chapter 2, that vaccines were administered into the skin rather than the muscles. This method made it possible to cut down significantly the amount of vaccine needed for one injection, thereby stretching the available shipments in order to reach more people.

After vaccinating fifteen children with two consecutive injections, the study found that while Danish, British and Czech studies had found that Salk vaccination with this method provided 30 per cent less protection against Type I polio, the Hungarian case did not show such a difference. This test could have been the proof that Rudnai needed to declare the success of the vaccination, but at the end of the article, he wrote: 'Our data are not suitable to draw conclusions for the efficacy of the 1957 vaccination campaign. This is because the mass vaccination was not executed with the same vaccine used in our study.' This statement is puzzling for more than one reason. First of all, according to Petrilla, 'The bulk of the vaccine used in the campaign was prepared by three laboratories: Connaught; Eli Lilly and Co.; Parke-Davis and Co. Smaller quantities manufactured by other laboratories were also used.'[85] If such a study was planned to test the vaccine and the vaccination method, why did this particular group of scientists not have access to the

[84] Szeri, Földes, and Bognár, 'Adatok a Poliomyelitis Elleni Intrakután Védőoltás Kérdéséhez'.
[85] Petrilla, *The Results of Intracutaneous Poliomyelitis Vaccination in Hungary, 1957*, 298.

vaccines used in the mass campaign? The article was published in 1959, so perhaps at the time of the study the vaccine batches had all been used or were not accessible for such testing. But then why would such a study, executed with an unknown vaccine batch and therefore seemingly irrelevant to the vaccination campaign, be worth publishing in a renowned journal two years after the vaccination campaign had started? The last sentence of the article reveals the answer: the laboratory testing 'strengthened the trust in intracutaneous vaccination'.[86]

Two years after vaccination with the Salk vaccine began, the method still needed 'strengthening'. The question still unanswered was whether the intracutaneous vaccination method was as effective as the intramuscular method. The former could be administered with a fraction of the full dose for the latter, making it possible to save a significant amount of vaccine – and money. Was this method to be blamed for the epidemic in 1959? Did the Hungarian state, in the end, compromise the health of its children in its efforts to save resources?

As mentioned in the previous chapter, the method used by the Hungarian authorities was called the Danish method. Denmark served as a model in the quest to curb polio in Hungary: it produced its own Salk vaccine (in the laboratories that the three Hungarian scientists visited on their study trip in 1956), was at the forefront of free mass vaccination, and could show significant results in both prophylaxis and polio treatment. In a report presented at the Fourth International Poliomyelitis Conference, the Danish delegation described its vaccination process. According to the delegates, 99 per cent of children between 9 months and 14 years had been vaccinated by 1957, and 93 per cent of 15–19-year-olds and 85 per cent of 19–35-year-olds had received the vaccine. Vaccination was voluntary and free of charge for citizens. Intradermal (intracutaneous) injections were administered with a domestically produced Salk vaccine. The dosage was 0.3 millilitres per injection in three doses. The population under 18 years also received a fourth booster injection of one millilitre, administered intramuscularly.[87]

There had been no significant epidemic waves in the previous three years in Denmark, and the annual average incidence rate dropped from 15 per 100,000 before vaccination to 0.65 after 1955. However, the Danish delegation was wary of drawing conclusions as to the efficacy of the vaccination. Since such a high percentage of the population was immunised, there was no control group to make a scientific observation possible.[88] They pointed to the fact that there

---

[86] Szeri, Földes, and Bognár, 'Adatok a Poliomyelitis Elleni Intrakután Védőoltás Kérdéséhez', 1365.

[87] Henningsen, 'Poliovaccination in Denmark'.

[88] 'Poliomyelitis. Papers Presented at the Fourth International Poliomyelitis Conference', 30.

had been no epidemic outbreak for six years, noting their resulting temptation to announce that their immunisation campaign had worked, but 'even if it [was] longer than the intervals formerly observed between bigger outbreaks, nobody can tell whether the immunity in the population is obtained by the 1952–1953 epidemics or by the vaccination.'[89]

Hungarians definitely used less vaccine in each individual injection than did their counterparts in Denmark. Also, Hungarian scientists and politicians were much bolder in drawing conclusions about the efficiency of the vaccination than their Danish colleagues. While Denmark's vaccination method and results were defined as a success and a model for one country, on an international scale there was no clear agreement on what constituted successful immunisation programmes and how efficiency could be evaluated on a national scale.

The question of the vaccination method was not settled while Salk vaccination was in use in Hungary. A letter from the Health Ministry to the head of the PHCED, containing detailed instructions regarding vaccination in March and April 1959, reveals that in at least some cases, the intramuscular method made a comeback, which also brought about changes in the quantity of vaccine used.

Children born between 1 September 1957 and 30 September 1958 are legally obliged to be vaccinated. The first vaccination in March needs to be administered with 1 ml, the second in April with 0.5 ml vaccine . . . In the case of the compulsory vaccination of 6–18 months old [children], the vaccine has to be administered intramuscularly.[90]

The reason for the decision to change the method of administering the vaccine in the spring of 1959 is unclear. It is also puzzling why only one particular age group was included in this change. Nor did it fit into the method described by the Danish delegates, whose system Hungary was allegedly using. However, the seemingly arbitrary switch from intracuteanous to intramuscular vaccination does demonstrate that despite the internal and external communication of the Health Ministry, there was no clear, unanimous agreement on the method in the national vaccination campaign.

The State: A Conspiracy Theory

Physicians and health officials were not the only ones looking for a reason for the severe epidemic wave of 1959. The debates and uncertainties regarding the

---

[89] 'Poliovaccination in Denmark', 26.
[90] Béla Tóth, 'Gyermekbénulás Elleni Védőoltások 1959. Március És Április Hónapban', Budapest: City Archives of Budapest, Budapest Fővárosi Tanács VB Egészségügyi Osztályának iratai, XXIII.115.a/34. kisdoboz, 181.476, 51.070/1959 V/3, 1959.

required amount of vaccine to establish immunity filtered down from the medical profession and surfaced as rumour among the population, while distrust in the vaccine and, most of all, in the state led to bitter explanations.

It is common belief among Hungarians living with polio today that the reason for the 1959 epidemic (in which many of them contracted the disease) was that the state halved the required dosage during the vaccination campaigns with the Salk vaccine.[91] According to this explanation, quantity won over quality, as was the case in most cases of production and services in the communist era. The state could not afford (or rather chose not to spend the money) to purchase enough vaccine, and because it was irresponsible, or simply did not really care about its citizens, decided to stretch out its supply and give lower doses than needed.

Uncertainties about the quantity of vaccine used could have originated from the medical profession itself. As Tóth also remarked, the doubts voiced by physicians could have affected vaccination rates; something about the vaccine and its quantity most probably circulated among the public. Moreover, even today, the belief in the state's culpability in deliberately halving the vaccine is shared by some health workers as well.[92] Another source for this widely held interpretation of events could be the state itself. As shown in Chapter 3, the Health Ministry made efforts to curb the public's expectations by emphasising that the initial vaccine would not be sufficient to immunise all children.[93] Moreover, in the article 'Fight against infectious diseases', Tibor Bakács, director of the State Hygienic Institute, brought up the issue of the vaccination method in public:

I consider it necessary to note here: international research of the latest years has established that 0.2 ml vaccine injected intradermally (into the skin) and 0.5 ml vaccine injected intramuscularly (into the muscle) are basically equal in effect. Among the great specialists of the vaccines against infant paralysis, the Danish [von] Magnus refers to this result. Our comparative epidemiology research also confirms this.[94]

A combination of unexplained changes in the method of vaccine administration, the circulating alternative views of local physicians and the often confusing information lay people could read in the pages of newspapers could very well have served as fertile ground for the view that something was amiss in the organisation and execution of the vaccine campaigns.

[91] Based on conversations at the National Heine-Medin Convention of the Hungarian Organization of Disabled Associations (Meosz), 6 November 2010.
[92] Dékány Pálné, interview by Vargha, January 11, 2008; Mészáros, interview by Vargha, 11 January 2008.
[93] 'Beoltják Gyermekbénulás Ellen az 1–2 Éves Gyermekeket: Külkereskedelmi Szerveink Már 250 000 Köbcenti Vakcinát Szereztek', Népakarat, 1957.
[94] Tibor Dr. Bakács, 'A Fertőző Betegségek Elleni Küzdelem', Népszabadság, 26 August 1959.

Whatever the origins of the conspiracy theory might be, as of now there is no evidence in the governmental archives that proves a premeditated plan to 'halve' the vaccine. It is more likely that in search of an explanation, parents, health workers and polio patients identified the state as the entity to blame, as a responsible actor in the unexpected tragedy.[95] This was hardly surprising in an environment in which the state blamed parents for misconduct and failed to deliver any other explanation for the epidemic, while parents helplessly watched their often fully vaccinated children come down with the paralysing disease.

One can only guess, therefore, where this rumour (as the information at this point cannot be termed more than a persistent rumour) originated. What it does reveal, however, is something very important in the relationship and mutual expectations among the state and its citizens. People did expect the state to provide protection, especially for their children, against polio. It was the state itself that set up this expectation, through its rhetoric of paternal roles and through propaganda emphasising the importance of care for mother and child.[96] However, people also expected poor quality, insufficient quantity and corruption in the distribution of any product or service provided by the state. Moreover, the state was by no means perceived as a friend by many – especially just a year after the revolution. So a wilful deception that endangered children was not wholly unimaginable.

The Salk Vaccine: From the Saviour of Children to an Imperfect Technology

In 1960, based on the blood samples and information collected after the epidemic wave had settled, Bakács of the State Hygienic Institute estimated that '35.4 per cent of those who contracted poliomyelitis in 1959 had a written record of vaccination with 3 doses and an additional 2.7 per cent certainly remembered having been subjected to vaccination.'[97] Over one third of the people – mainly children – who came down with polio in 1959, therefore, had been fully vaccinated. In a study conducted by the infectious disease hospital in Budapest (László Hospital), 53.3 per cent of polio patients had received two

---

[95] No doubt subsequent events, such as a feeling of abandonment by the state after the mid 1960s, or the drastic changes in the health-care and welfare system in the post communist era, all feed into an often bitter and disappointed perception of the Salk vaccination. I argue, however, that the particular set of expectations explored in this section have existed in the 1950s as well as throughout the communist era – and in many cases, even today.

[96] See e.g. László Buga, *Hogyan Gondoskodik Államunk a Dolgozó Anyáról és Gyermekéről* Útmutató Városi És Falusi Előadók Számára (Budapest: Művelt Nép könyvkiadó, 1953); Gyula Surányi, *Egészséges Anya – Egészséges Gyermek* Útmutató Városi és Falusi Előadók Számára (Budapest: Művelt nép könyvkiadó, 1953).

[97] Bakács, 'Poliomyelitis Prophylaxis in Hungary', 332.

or more doses of Salk vaccine beforehand, and 37.3 per cent were fully vaccinated with three or four doses, including the 'reminder' injection.[98] Both evaluations stated that these ratios were in accordance with international experiences of the Salk vaccine.

Until the epidemic in 1959, there was no mention in Hungary of the efficacy rate of the Salk vaccine in international experience. Not one newspaper article, not one governmental or ministerial document pointed to the fact that the vaccine would not protect the whole population even if everyone received the full dosage. However, in the thick of the epidemic wave, the blaming of parents gave way to the rather detached and objective citing of efficacy rates of the vaccine. In August, the official line of the State Hygienic Institute was that the efficacy of the Salk vaccine was between 70 per cent and 80 per cent in Hungary, which, they argued, fell in line with the experiences of socialist and capitalist countries. These figures were published in the daily newspaper *Népszabadság*.[99] A joint evaluation by the institute and László Hospital from 1961 then modified these numbers to between 60 per cent and 70 per cent.[100]

Experiences with the Salk vaccine on a global scale had far been from uniform. The WHO's Expert Committee on Poliomyelitis pointed out in their third report in 1960 that:

The review of national experiences clearly shows that in most areas the protection afforded had been the greatest where the degree of vaccination had been high. This experience, however, had not been universal and some unsatisfactory rates of protection have been reported. The reasons for these variations in experience are not clear, although vaccine potency and mode of administration have been suggested as possible factors.[101]

In fact, the effectiveness and long-term protection of the Salk vaccine had been the focus of investigations and international comparisons for the last three years of the 1950s. It appeared that the Salk vaccine had failed to fulfil the hopes and dreams of other countries as well. In a paper presented at the Fifth International Poliomyelitis Conference, Alexander Langmuir described the rising trend of polio cases in the late 1950s as 'a sobering experience'.[102]

---

[98] Losonczy et al., 'A Salk Vakcináció és a Poliomyelitis Klinikai Lefolyásának Összefügg-ése', 734.

[99] Dr Bakács, 'A Fertőző Betegségek Elleni Küzdelem', *Népszabadság*, 1959.

[100] Losonczy et al., 'A Salk Vakcináció és a Poliomyelitis Klinikai Lefolyásának Összefügg-ése', 733.

[101] Expert Committee on Poliomyelitis, 'Expert Committee on Poliomyelitis. Third Report', in *Technical Report Series*, ed. World Health Organization (Geneva: World Health Organization, 1960), 4.

[102] Alexander D. Langmuir, 'Inactivated Virus Vaccines: Protective Efficacy', in *Poliomyelitis. Papers and Discussions Presented at the Fifth International Poliomyelitis Conference Copenhagen, Denmark, July 26–28, 1960*, ed. International Poliomyelitis Congress (Philadelphia and Montreal: J. B. Lippincott Company, 1961), 105–13, at 105.

At the same time, based on data collected through the National Poliomyelitis Surveillance Program, Langmuir determined the effectiveness of the Salk vaccine to be '80 per cent for 3 or more doses and 90 per cent or better for 4 or more doses'.[103] His Canadian colleague, F. P. Nagler, recounted similar experiences, with 85–90 per cent of the Canadian population being fully protected against paralytic poliomyelitis after three injections.[104] Czechoslovakian virologists were not so enthusiastic, however. In a report to the Fifth International Poliomyelitis Conference, they measured a 66–74 per cent efficacy rate following two intradermal injections in 1957, and, based on epidemiological data and serologic investigations, concluded: '[W]e do not feel justified in concluding that the inactivated vaccine ... could ensure a long-term prevention of epidemics of poliomyelitis in our country.'[105]

The Hungarian failure of epidemic prevention with the Salk vaccine was widely acknowledged and was taken into account when the WHO's Expert Committee on Poliomyelitis assessed polio vaccine efficacy and global applicability.

The review of national experiences with inactivated poliovirus shows that in most countries where this vaccine has been widely used the order of protection that it was originally expected to give on the basis of controlled field trials has been maintained. However, in the USA and Canada, localized outbreaks have occurred in which unvaccinated sections of the population were particularly affected. Failure to obtain protection on a satisfactory national basis appears only to have been experienced in Hungary and possibly in Israel.[106]

Israel experienced a severe outbreak following Salk vaccination. In the outbreak of 1958 the main victims of the disease were children who had received two injections with the inactivated vaccine. However, Israeli virologists were reluctant to draw conclusions about efficacy; they found a number of factors that made the evaluation problematic, among them variations in the antigenicity of the vaccine, uneven geographic distribution of cases, difference in age-specific rates and the fluctuation of epidemic waves.[107]

These accounts revealed that differences between efficacies as measured in various locales could be significant. As renowned polio expert Herdis von

[103] Ibid. 106.
[104] F. P. Nagler, 'Protective Efficacy of Inactivated Poliovirus Vaccines in Canada', ibid. 122.
[105] V. Skovranek, 'Investigations of the Effectiveness of Inactivated Vaccine against Poliomyelitis in Czechoslovakia', ibid. 136.
[106] Expert Committee on Poliomyelitis, 'Expert Committee on Poliomyelitis. Third Report', 51.
[107] Natan Goldblum, 'Efficacy of Poliomyelitis Vaccine in Israel during the 3-Year Period 1957–1959', in *Poliomyelits. Papers and Discussions Presented at the Fifth International Poliomyelitis Conference, Copenhagen, Denmark, July 26–28, 1960*, ed. International Poliomyelitis Congress (Philadelphia: J.B. Lippincott Company, 1961), 138–42.

Magnus pointed out, '[M]any countries have made observations which indicate that the inactivated polio vaccine has yielded a 60 to 90 per cent protection against paralytic disease.'[108] For some, an important factor in the varying efficacy rate of the Salk vaccine was to be found in the lack of standardisation. There was no 'universally available reference vaccine' and several countries set different requirements for the type of test to be used when determining vaccine potency.[109] Standardisation of this procedure was seen as urgent, in order to find 'a reliable basis for any comparison to be made between vaccines'.[110]

Other sources reveal that vaccines were not necessarily at hand when needed, which could have interfered with vaccination campaigns and their results. Britain, for instance, had to put vaccinations on hold between the second and third injections, owing to 'an unhappy chapter of accidents' in procuring a Canadian vaccine: monkeys needed for the vaccine production fell sick, live virus was found in one of the vaccine batches, another batch failed the antigenic potency test and, finally, a sudden increase in local demand reduced the available vaccine export supplies.[111]

Of course the accounts and measurements, and their representations by the leading public health officials and virologists of the respective nations, cannot be divorced from professional and political agendas. The United States had invested significantly in the Salk vaccine, which had been heralded as one of the most important medical interventions of the time. Canada was one of the largest suppliers of Salk vaccine to the global market. Both nations had much to lose if the Salk vaccine was not as efficient as initial laboratory results and field trials showed. Conversely, Czechoslovakia was already heavily invested in the development and testing of the live polio vaccine by the end of the decade and had pitted the low results of the Salk vaccination against the preliminary data from the Sabin trials. Hungary's efficacy evaluation was formed in this context of interests and justifications, as well as a moment of transition as virologists and public health decision-makers tried to make sense of the 1959 epidemic.

The growing disillusionment with the Salk vaccine in 1959 is especially striking, since it was that year that Hungary finally managed to start experimental mass production of the vaccine. Newspapers had already announced

---

[108] Herdis von Magnus, 'Present Knowledge About Duration of Sero-Immunity after Vaccination with Inactivated Polio Vaccines', in *Poliomyelitis. Papers and Discussions Presented at the Fifth International Poliomyelitis Conference Copenhagen, Denmark, July 26–28, 1960*, ed. International Poliomyelitis Congress (Philadelphia and Montreal: J. B. Lippincott Company, 1961), 155.

[109] Roderick Murray, 'The Standardization of Potency of Poliomyelitis Vaccine', ibid.

[110] P. L. Bazeley, 'Standardization of Polio Vaccine Potency', ibid. 186–95.

[111] 'Poliomyelitis Vaccine', *The British Medical Journal* 1, no. 5078 (1958): 1053.

the start of Salk vaccine production in 1958,[112] but mass production of the vaccine did not begin until a year later. Virologist Sándor Koch, a participant in the Danish study trip in 1956, headed the process at the State Institute of Hygiene.

We made the vaccine because it was an interesting technological task, but I was not excited about the routine production of it. A good friend of mine, Dr Pál László, head of department at László hospital, told me one day: 'Come and see us.' So I went. In several rooms, children with paralysed limbs were playing and laughing, and then, as if it was by accident, he took us to another room, where about twenty children from infant[s] to teenagers were lying in iron lungs. My good friend told me: 'You know, these children will never be able to breathe spontaneously in their life, because their respiratory system is paralysed by polio . . . so tell me, are you going to produce the vaccine or not?' It was this visit that made me realise that I have to keep on going and produce the vaccine.[113]

A batch of the domestically produced vaccine was then tested in Copenhagen at the Stetens Seruminstitut before it was distributed to Hungarian children.[114] Following Danish approval of the vaccine, the fourth, booster injections administered during the 1959 epidemic were partly covered by domestic vaccine production.[115]

The lack of an epidemic in 1958 was also re-evaluated. While prior to the 1959 epidemic, the quiet year of 1958 was considered to be the clear result of immunisation with the Salk vaccine, by 1960 a virological coincidence was named as the reason for the lack of a polio epidemic that year. Apparently in 1958 there had been an outbreak of Bornholm disease (named after the Danish island where it was first reported), a Coxsackie B virus, which most probably interfered with the poliovirus and, as Bakács argued on the pages of *Orvosi Hetilap*, obstructed the spread of polio.[116]

Similar to polio, Coxsackie B viruses are enteroviruses. The interaction between the two groups of viruses began to be explored in the early 1950s,

---

[112] Moldován, 'Aki Még Nem Kapott – Áprilisban Jelentkezzék Gyermekbénulás Elleni Védőoltásra', *Népszava*, 1958; 'Dr. Doleschall Frigyes Miniszter Nyilatkozata a Népszavának az Egészségügy Hároméves Tervéről, a Salk-Oltásokról és a Gyógyszerfogyasztásról', ibid., 17 June 1958, 1–2.

[113] Mezei, '. . .Isten Van, Az Ember Történik.' *Koch Sándor Virológussal Beszélget Mezei Károly*, 24.

[114] Sándor Koch, 'Szubjektív Virológia', *Természet Világa* 130, no. 2 (1999): 60–62.

[115] Aladár Kátay, 'The Active Immunization against Poliomyelitis in Hungary and Its Three Years' Results', in *The Control of Poliomyelitis by Live Poliovirus Vaccine. Studies on Mass Vaccinations in Hungary, in the USSR, in Czechoslovakia and the German Democratic Republic. Papers Presented at the Hungarian-Soviet Medical Conference September 24–30, 1960*, ed. J. Weissfeiler (Budapest: Publishing House of the Hungarian Academy of Sciences, 1961), 71–84.

[116] Dr. Tibor Bakács, 'Az Eddigi Poliomyelitis Vaccinatio Eredményeinek Értékelése', *Orvosi Hetilap* 101, no. 20 (1960): 685–91.

when it was unclear whether they mitigated or exacerbated each other's effects.[117] Soon, the interference of the two viruses and Coxsackie's 'sparing effect' on polio became a theory represented quite well in international medical literature.[118] This meant that people who caught the much milder Coxsackie B virus could not be super-infected with polio at the same time. Bakács argued that the outbreak of Bornholm disease coincided with the usual time of polio in the summer and that this greatly contributed to the lack of a polio epidemic in 1958.

In light of the 1959 epidemic, the vaccine was quickly transformed from the saviour of Hungarian children to an imperfect technology. This process was further sped up by the appearance of a new vaccine in the Soviet Union. As early as August 1959, newspapers were starting to write about the coming of the new vaccine, claiming it would be even more effective than the Salk vaccine: 'a vaccine that was developed based on research by the American Sabin and the Pole Koprowski'.[119]

In 1960, the *Orvosi Hetilap* published the translation of Chumakov's article on the mass immunisation of the population of the Soviet Union with the Sabin vaccine.

Today we cannot consider the Salk vaccine, despite all its advantages, to be a tool in liquidating polio in a range of countries ... Post-vaccinated immunity is not complete either ... The virus keeps circulating in the population and the danger of poliomyelitis epidemics remains ... Neither the intracutaneous nor the intramuscular methods are suitable for immunising tens of millions of children, which would be needed to build immunity against poliomyelitis in the whole of the population.[120]

Scarcely six months had passed between the unquestionable celebration of the Salk vaccine and the publication of such a statement as a valid view in Hungary. A few months later, Bakács, leading virologist of the State Institute

[117] Gilbert Dalldorf, 'The Sparing Effect of Coxsackie Virus Infection on Experimental Poliomyelitis', *Journal of Experimental Medicine* 94, no. 1 (1951): 65–71.

[118] See e.g. Erik Lycke, 'Interference between Poliomyelitis Virus and Coxsackie B or Echo Viruses', *Archives of Virology* 8, no. 3 (1958): 351–59; N. F. Stanley, 'Attempts to Demonstrate Interference between Coxsackie and Poliomyelitis Viruses in Mice and Monkeys', *Proceedings of the Society for Experimental Biology and Medicine*, no. 81 (1952): 430–33; Gilbert Dalldorf and Robert Albrecht, 'Chronologic Association of Poliomyelitis and Coxsackie Virus Infections', *Proceedings of the National Academy of Sciences USA* 41, no. 11 (1955): 978–82. The question of the virus interference of Coxsackie B and poliomyelitis, however, remained far from being settled until the 1960s. Richard L. Crowell, 'Specific Viral Interference in Hela Cell Cultures Chronically Infected with Coxsackie B5 Virus', *Journal of Bacteriology* 86, no. 3 (1963): 517–26.

[119] Dr Bakács, 'A Fertőző Betegségek Elleni Küzdelem'.

[120] M. P. Csumakov et al., 'A Lakosság Poliomyelitis Elleni Tömeges Per Os Immunizálása a Szovjetúnióban Sabin Attenuált Törzseiből Készített Élő Vakcinával', *Orvosi Hetilap* 101, no. 4 (1960): 109–17.

of Hygiene, reiterated this assertion as vaccination began with the new Sabin vaccine in Hungary.[121]

The Hungarian experience tells a peculiar story about polio prevention with the Salk vaccine. The overwhelming majority of polio histories, especially those on polio in the United States, follow the narrative of the introduction of the Salk vaccine as a watershed event in blocking the return of a major epidemic and marking the beginning of the end of polio. The 1959 epidemic in Hungary, however, shows that this story cannot be universally extended. Rather, the experience with Salk vaccination in this particular Eastern European state highlights how scientific uncertainties pertained to the disease throughout the 1950s. There was and still is no clear answer why the vaccination did not work. No clear standards guided the campaigns and, apart from the initial controlled trial in the United States in 1954, there was no proof of efficacy on the level of a population for a vaccine against an epidemic that did not occur every year.

The scientific uncertainties of the disease and the preventive technology magnified the political and social forces at work in the vaccination process. The expectations of researchers and their role in producing progressive scientific results, of the state and its role as provider and protector, and of the citizens and their role as compliant and grateful were challenged and contested. Inefficiencies in state and healthcare organisation became apparent, as haphazard reporting and data management made scientific and political evaluations and decision-making difficult. Physicians resisted the overruling of their professional judgement, while some parents defied the intervention of the state in their decisions about their children's health.

The Hungarian Salk vaccination also highlighted changes that took place in the two years between the epidemics. The coming of a new epidemic soured the initial enthusiasm for this Western technology and triggered changes in medical discourse, in the perception of citizens and the state, and in the technology itself. Medical data changed in meaning. The interpretations of statistics on vaccine efficacy in the population produced in the early autumn of 1957 changed drastically over the next two years: from being inadequate evidence in 1957, they became the ultimate proof of efficacy by 1958, only to turn into numbers signifying an epidemiological coincidence to explain away the new outbreak in 1959. In the eyes of the state, parents transformed from thankful beneficiaries in non-epidemic times to ungrateful and irresponsible citizens who neither appreciated nor deserved the sacrifices of the state,

---

[121] Dr Tibor Bakács, 'Az Eddigi Poliomyelitis Vaccinatio Eredményeinek Értékelése', ibid., no. 20: 685–91.

and who even brought the epidemic on themselves. Furthermore, the Salk vaccine of early 1959 was not the same as the Salk vaccine of six months later. The former was the saviour of children and a symbol of the state's commitment to the health of future generations, while the latter was an imperfect technology to which Hungary had temporarily reverted until a better option became available.

5   Sabin Saves the Day

In December 1959, Hungary became one of the first countries in the world to begin nationwide mass vaccination with the Sabin polio vaccine. Though not often recognised as a player in the history of public health, this Eastern European state introduced the vaccine to its national immunisation programme four years before the United States – the country where the vaccine was developed. This campaign put Hungary at the frontline of polio vaccination along with the Soviet Union and Czechoslovakia, where the Sabin vaccine was tested. The Hungarian model of annual intensive mass vaccination campaigns became one of the bases on which the WHO built its global strategy of polio eradication in the late twentieth century.[1]

The development and implementation of the live poliovirus vaccine in Hungary is in many ways an unusual Cold War story: one in which scientists all over the world, among them American and Soviet researchers, worked together and shared results that led to the immunisation of millions of children in national mass vaccination programmes. The scientific cooperation surrounding polio seems to have reached its climax in the development of the Sabin vaccine, revealing global cooperation that arched over conventional Cold War hostilities. Polio could clearly no longer be defined as 'an American story'.[2]

In order to plan and execute prevention methods, develop vaccines and provide state-of-the-art treatment for a new epidemiological phenomenon, scientific communities needed to be constantly in touch with each other, share new experiences and knowledge and cooperate in figuring out the next step.

---

[1] Harry F. Hull et al., 'Progress toward Global Polio Eradication', Journal of Infectious Diseases 175, no. Supplement 1 (1997), S4–S9, at S4.

[2] In his fundamental work, David Oshinsky focuses on the development of Salk and Sabin vaccines and presents the process as an American story. He argues that 'the polio crusade . . . remains one of the most significant and culturally revealing triumphs in American medical history.' David M. Oshinsky, *Polio: An American Story* (Oxford and New York: Oxford University Press, 2005), 7. While I am not debating here the important role of polio in American politics, culture and public health, I wish to broaden the spectrum of the history of polio vaccines and argue that especially in the case of the Sabin vaccine, polio research and vaccine development quickly became a global project with universal goals.

The lack of widely accepted standard procedures and the presence of intense debates in the fields of virology, medicine and public health ensured that a space for exchange and cooperation existed continuously, and it was one that ignored barriers erected after the Second World War between the East and West.

At the same time, the evaluation and introduction of this new vaccine was highly determined by the Cold War itself. Cold War frustrations and preconceptions permeated the scientific debate over the efficacy and safety of the new vaccine. The countries' choices to introduce the new vaccine were largely shaped by the relations between the national public health structure, the government and its infrastructure and the vaccines, which, in turn, were mostly determined by being part of the 'capitalist' or 'communist' regime.

Hungary's encounter with the Sabin vaccine presents a microcosm of global Cold War politics. Hungary's choice of the Sabin vaccine over the Salk vaccine, and the country's participation in the network of field trials, had much to do with being part of the Eastern Bloc and having a healthcare system that favoured mass vaccination programmes. Moreover, the particular ways in which the introduction of the Sabin vaccine and the success of eliminating polio from the country's epidemiology reports gained political significance show the dynamic nature of the Iron Curtain. In an effort to prevent the epidemic, gaping holes opened through which the two sides connected, only to close again when the East and West realigned along conventional Cold War lines.

Drawing the Iron Curtain: Development of Live Poliovirus Vaccines

Hungary's experiences with polio vaccines and the government's decision to switch from Salk to Sabin were nested in a broader process of vaccine development. While the laboratory work of the development of live virus vaccines has a fascinating history in itself, it is the human experiments and field trials that provide the most compelling insights into the Cold War political context of vaccine development. Research groups headed by three different scientists tested three different vaccines across the globe, spanning South America to South East Asia and Africa to Eastern Europe. By 1959, according to the WHO's report,[3] at least fifteen countries had conducted field trials with live poliovirus vaccines. The international cooperation in organising the trials and coordinating the evaluation of the new vaccines was unprecedented in this formative decade of international public health.

---

[3] 'Summary of Conference on Live Poliovirus Vaccines', Geneva: World Health Organization, WHO/Polio/43, 1959, 3.

Although the live poliovirus vaccine, developed by Albert Sabin, made its official debut in national vaccination programmes in 1959 and 1960, its story in fact began much earlier. The concept of live virus vaccines had been known for decades before live poliovirus vaccine development started, and work on the live vaccine ran parallel to Salk's research on the inactivated vaccine.

Live virus vaccines had been in use for more than 100 years in the case of smallpox and for over twenty years in the case of yellow fever.[4] The concept, therefore, was not new, and many thought that a live vaccine would be more effective than the killed one to begin with, in that it would work quicker and probably provide a more lasting protection since it followed the pattern of a natural infection.[5] Most importantly, those vaccinated would put the attenuated virus back into the environment through their stools, creating a chance to immunise others indirectly.[6] The challenge of the live, attenuated polio vaccine was to find a strain of virus that would not cause paralysis, but would provide immunity nonetheless. This method took considerably longer than Salk's process of finding a way to kill the virus and preserve it.

It was Max Theiler, developer of the yellow fever vaccine, who introduced the idea of a live attenuated poliovirus. In 1946, after passing poliovirus continuously through mice, he reported having produced a strain that immunised monkeys without causing paralysis in them.[7] Theiler did not pursue this research further, but several of his peers did: in the 1950s Hilary Koprowski, Albert Sabin and Herald Cox took on live polio vaccine development.

Koprowski was born in Warsaw to a Jewish family and left Poland in 1939 after the Nazi occupation. From working with the Rockefeller Foundation in Brazil on yellow fever, he arrived at the Lederle Laboratories in the United States, where he started to work on the live polio vaccine. Albert Sabin, the most well-known of the three, was of Russian descent, also from a Jewish family, and worked on the polio vaccine at the University of Cincinnati. H. R. Cox, an American scientist, became head of the Virus and Rickettsial Research Department at Lederle Laboratories in 1946 and, for a while, worked with Koprowski there.

The first researcher to conduct experiments with live poliovirus vaccine was Koprowski. In 1947, he was his own first experimental subject; three years later he moved on to experimenting on mentally disabled children in a state institution in New York's Hudson Valley.[8] In light of the Nuremberg Code of 1947, this was an ethically dubious experiment at the least even by contemporary standards. Koprowski received much criticism when he presented his

[4] Paul, *A History of Poliomyelitis*, 441.
[5] 'Attenuated Poliomyelitis Vaccines', *British Medical Journal* 1, no. 4961 (1956): 284.
[6] Oshinsky, *Polio: An American Story*, 244–45.   [7] Paul, *A History of Poliomyelitis*, 441.
[8] Oshinsky, *Polio: An American Story*, 135.

results in 1951 to a round table convened by the National Foundation of Infantile Paralysis. Reservations about his methods softened as time went on, and his experiment on 'volunteers' became represented as a brave first step in the development of a new and successful vaccine.[9]

In 1956 a new opportunity presented itself for Koprowski to test his vaccine, this time in Belfast, Northern Ireland.[10] Koprowski, therefore, also became the first to take his vaccine abroad. The trial, however, turned out to be a disappointment for Koprowski's Irish counterpart: the strain used by Koprowski proved to be unsuitable as a vaccine, since it regained its cytophatic power, turning virulent in the volunteers' bodies. It was thus deemed unsafe.[11]

Korpowski, Sabin and Cox turned to field trials outside the United States in part because the Cutter incident had raised suspicions against polio vaccines. In the spring of 1955, almost 200 patients in the United States (mostly children and family members) had contracted paralytic polio from a faulty batch of the Salk vaccine produced by the Cutter laboratories.[12] This incident had a tremendous impact: it shook public trust in the vaccine and changed vaccine regulation and control in the United States.[13] Furthermore, by the time Sabin's vaccine required mass testing in order to establish its efficacy, the Salk vaccine had become widespread in the United States. Millions of children were now immunised with the killed-polio vaccine, making it impossible to test and evaluate a new vaccine against the same disease.

Not everyone shared the excitement over this international project, however. United States health officials did not uniformly accept vaccine testing on foreign ground. In a congressional hearing on polio vaccines in 1961, Alexander Langmuir, chief epidemiologist of the Department of Health, Education and Welfare and founder of the Epidemic Intelligence Service, found it important to note that 'it is not as though they [Koprowski, Sabin and Cox] went elsewhere to test. They went to the place to test that would give the best tests, but all of the questions were started and worked on in this country before any overseas activity.'[14] In a scientific race between East and West, the fact that such an important vaccine was first widely tested and produced outside the United States needed explanation and emphasis that all, indeed, were first

[9] Ibid. 135–37.
[10] Lindner and Blume, 'Vaccine Innovation and Adoption: Polio Vaccines in the Uk, the Netherlands and West Germany, 1955–1965', 438.
[11] D. S. Dane et al., 'Vaccination against Poliomyelitis with Live Virus Vaccines. I. A Trial of Tn Type II Vaccine', *British Medical Journal* 1, no. 5010 (1957): 59–65.
[12] Offit, *The Cutter Incident*; National Heine-Medin Convention of the Hungarian Organization of Disabled Associations (Meosz), 6 November 2010.
[13] Oshinsky, *Polio: An American Story*, Offit, *The Cutter Incident* and Colgrove, *State of Immunity*.
[14] *Polio Vaccines*, 16 March 1961, 108.

developed on American soil. Cooperation may have characterised live vaccine development, but Cold War frustrations gave context to its presentation. From 1958, international live poliovirus trials accelerated, due to a report published by the World Health Organisation (WHO). That year, a severe polio epidemic outbreak in Singapore provided the first opportunity for a trial of Sabin's vaccine. The WHO's Second Expert Committee Report on Poliomyelitis recounted that eleven weeks into the epidemic, the Singapore government decided to introduce the vaccine.[15] The report stated that 'there would appear to be sufficient justification for initiating at this time trials of the currently-available tested lots of attenuated poliovirus vaccine in increasingly large numbers of people.'[16] This was the green light for which live virus researchers had been waiting. Proponents of live vaccine field trials trumpeted the report's recommendations that a large-scale trial of attenuated vaccine should be attempted in the face of an emerging epidemic, and in a place where polio was endemic. Sabin agreed to the trial on the condition that 'adequate laboratory control could be assured'.[17] Almost 200,000 children were vaccinated on a voluntary basis.

Koprowski also kept working on his vaccine after he left the Lederle Laboratories and relocated to the Wistar Institute at the University of Pennsylvania. In early 1958, he conducted a mass-vaccination trial in the Ruzizi Valley in Belgian Congo.[18] The idea of an animal trial in the Congo came up in personal conversations during Koprowski's participation in a rabies conference organized by the WHO in 1955 in Kenya. The trial, involving chimpanzees and their carers, was soon broadened to include a total of 244,596 people living in the Belgian Congo and Ruanda-Urundi.[19] It is not clear how volunteers were recruited, or if the people living under colonial rule had a choice about, or full understanding of, the trial for which they were enlisted. In any case, this time there was no protest by fellow scientists on ethical grounds.[20] In the end, the project was inconclusive, and was discontinued as

---

[15] 'Expert Committee on Poliomyelitis', in *Technical Report Series*, ed. World Health Organization (Geneva: World Health Organization, 1958).

[16] Ibid. 25.

[17] J. H. Hale et al., 'Large-Scale Use of Sabin Type 2 Attenuated Poliovirus Vaccine in Singapore during a Type 1 Poliomyelitis Epidemic', *British Medical Journal* 1, no. 5137 (1959): 1541–48, at 1541.

[18] Hilary Koprowski, 'Historical Aspects of the Development of Live Virus Vaccine in Poliomyelitis', ibid. 2, no. 5192 (1960): 85–91, at 90.

[19] Allan M. Brandt, 'Racism and Research: The Case of the Tuskegee Syphilis Study', *The Hastings Center Report* 8, no. 6 (1978): 21–29.

[20] Medical experiments on vulnerable populations were not unknown to public health practice of the midtwentieth century. See Susan M. Reverby, '"Normal Exposure" and Inoculation Syphilis: A PHS "Tuskegee" Doctor in Guatemala, 1946–1948', *Journal of Policy History* 23, no. 1 (2011): 6–28, and 'Washington Conference on Live Poliovirus Vaccines', *British Medical Journal* 2, no. 5146 (1959): 235–36, at 236.

efforts for independence from colonial rule generated political and social upheaval in the country.[21]

Lederle Laboratories also continued with vaccine development and conducted field trials of their own in Central America in 1959, using a vaccine developed by Herald Cox in Colombia, Nicaragua and Costa Rica.[22] The mass immunisation campaigns in the latter two countries produced disappointing results, as the number of polio cases did not fall significantly after vaccination.[23] However, a controlled trial in Minnesota[24] with the same vaccine reported 'excellent antibody responses'.[25]

Koprowski's strains were later widely tested in Finland and Poland. In Poland, the introduction of Koprowski's vaccine followed that of the Salk vaccine by one year.[26] During the five months between October 1959 and April 1960, more than 7 million children were immunised,[27] including roughly 80 per cent of the population between 6 months and 15 years of age.[28] In 1961, the country reverted to the Salk vaccine after an increase of polio cases following the oral vaccination with Koprowski's Type III attenuated strain over the previous two years.[29]

It is not clear how Koprowski was able to conduct such a large field trial behind the Iron Curtain. He was born in Poland, certainly, but as an immigrant living in the United States, his experimentation on Polish youth with American-made vaccines could easily have made him a suspect rather than a friend. Contemporary reports and articles never addressed the issue of Koprowski's access to an Eastern European country's children for field trials. Perhaps one of the reasons is that another influential and large field trial diverted attention from Koprowski's endeavour: one that was not only conducted behind the Iron Curtain, but in the grounds of the arch enemy itself. This was Albert Sabin's vaccine in the Soviet Union.

[21] 'Fifth International Poliomyelitis Conference', *British Medical Journal* 2, no. 5197 (1960): 533–34, at 534.

[22] Expert Committee on Poliomyelitis, 'Expert Committee on Poliomyelitis. Third Report', 14.

[23] 'Live Poliovirus Vaccines', *British Medical Journal* 2, no. 5193 (1960): 202–3, at 203.

[24] Robert N. Barr et al., 'Use of Orally Administered Live Attenuated Polioviruses as a Vaccine in a Community Setting', *Journal of the American Medical Association* 170, no. 8 (1959): 893–905.

[25] 'Washington Conference on Live Poliovirus Vaccines', 235.

[26] Jan Kostrzewski. 'Poliomyelitis in Poland.' Geneva: World Health Organization Library, World Health Organization VIR/Polio/69.2, 1969.

[27] 'European Association against Poliomyelitis', *British Medical Journal* 2, no. 5257 (1961): 951–52.

[28] H. Koprowski. 'Preliminary Report as of September 1960 of Mass Vaccination in Poland with Koprowski's Strains of Attenuated Virus.' Geneva: World Health Organization Library, Study Group on Requirements for Poliomyelitis Vaccine (Live, Attenuated Virus), 1960.

[29] Kostrzewski, 'Poliomyelitis in Poland'.

The new vaccine was the result of an exceptional cooperation between Russian and American scientists, Mikhail Chumakov and Albert Sabin, at a particular moment of the Cold War. The slight thaw that followed Stalin's death opened up new opportunities for exchange. Khrushchev's secret speech against Stalin's rule had significant effects for the biomedical sciences as well.[30] Historian Saul Benison argues that it was the increase in the incidence of polio that convinced Soviet authorities that 'it was costly socially and economically not to take advantage of the great breakthroughs in American biomedical research vis-à-vis polio'.[31] For the first time since the Second World War, medical cooperation between the two superpowers started to become a reality.

In early 1956, a Soviet medical mission arrived in the United States, led by Mikhail Chumakov, his wife and colleague Marina Voroshilova and Anatoli Smorodintsev.[32] This visit was significant enough for Hungarian newspapers to keep the public informed about it, from the arrival of the Soviet scientists to their engagement with American colleagues.[33] The delegation studied the production of the Salk vaccine and ongoing research in epidemiology. During the trip, they also visited the laboratory of Albert Sabin. This visit turned out to be the beginning of a decade-long exchange. Sabin returned the favour in June 1956, spending a month touring the Soviet Union for talks and laboratory visits. Scientists, specimens and vaccine vials crossed the Iron Curtain in both directions as cooperation intensified between American and Soviet virologists, especially between Sabin's and Chumakov's groups. This cooperation had the blessing of both the FBI and the State Department, despite warnings from the Department of Defense that the materials and research involved could be used in making biological weapons.[34] Scientists' foreign travel was not strictly controlled only on the Eastern side of the Iron Curtain. In the 1950s, many American scientists in other fields ran into difficulties or were denied passports for political reasons when applying (600 passport applications were rejected on political grounds in the 1950s up until 1958).[35] Sabin's relative freedom in travelling, therefore, was not entirely typical of his time.

[30] Konstantin Ivanov, 'Science after Stalin: Forging a New Image of Soviet Science', *Science in Context* 15, no. 2 (2002): 317–38.
[31] Benison, 'International Medical Cooperation: Dr. Albert Sabin, Live Poliovirus Vaccine and the Soviets', 465.
[32] Ibid. 467.
[33] 'Megérkezett New Yorkba M. Csumakov Vezetésével a Szovjet Orvostudós-Küldöttség', *Szabad Nép*, 20 January 1956, 4; M. P. Csumakov, 'Harc a Gyermekbénulás Ellen', ibid., 10 April 1956.
[34] Oshinsky, *Polio: An American Story*.
[35] Jessica Wang, *American Science in an Age of Anxiety: Scientists, Anticommunism and the Cold War* (Chapel Hill and London: University of North Carolina Press, 1999), 276–77.

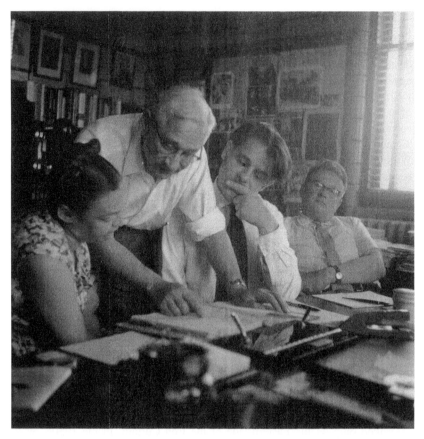

Figure 5.1 *From left to right: Marina K. Voroshilova, Albert B. Sabin,*
Mikhail P. Chumakov, Anatolii A. Smorodintsev. Undated. Miscellaneous,
Assorted Letters and Photographs. Box 01. File 05 (Assorted Professional
Photographs, 1950s–1960s). University of Cincinnati. Hauck Center for the
Albert B. Sabin Archives. **This image is protected by copyright and cannot**
be used without further permissions clearance.

In the broader context of scientific cooperation between the two sides in the
Cold War, the exchange of knowledge and specimens among Sabin and
Chumakov was a rare, albeit not unique, phenomenon. While the American
and Russian virologists shared virus strains, production and testing methods in
developing the live polio vaccine, the post-Stalin era gave way to various
collaborative projects. The International Geophysical Year (IGY), held
between 1957 and 1958, and the Antarctic Treaty proclaiming Antarctica to
be a 'continent dedicated to peace and science' were heralded as symbolising

the universality of science and international cooperation.[36] At the same time, the IGY and the Treaty reflected deeply ingrained Cold War hostility and the concerns over the Space Race.[37] Attenuated poliovirus strains were also not the only biomedical specimens to circulate the globe in the 1950s. From the immediate post-war years onwards, blood samples were collected around the world to determine the frequency of blood groups,[38] and with the rise of serological epidemiology, serum banks were organised under the auspices of the WHO to collect and freeze blood for epidemiological surveillance and 'for as yet unknown' uses.[39]

The exceptional quality of the scientific exchange between Sabin and Chumakov was that it resulted in a tangible product that would be widely used and considered successful in both the East and West: the polio vaccine used today in eradication efforts. Their cooperation led to the largest field trial in the history of polio, involving over 16.5 million people across the Soviet Union.[40] As soon as Sabin finished selecting the optimal strain for creating the vaccine, he sent samples to Smorodintsev in Leningrad. Field trials with the strain started in 1957 on a very small scale, with the vaccination of sixty-seven children. This number gradually grew to 150, then to 2,010, and finally to 20,000 in 1958.[41] Parallel to Smorodintsev's trials, another field trial, initiated by Chumakov, then director of the Poliomyelitis Research Institute in Moscow, took off in greater proportions. Chumakov asked Sabin to send

---

[36] Roger D. Launius, James Rodger Fleming, and David H. DeVorkin, *Globalizing Polar Science: Reconsidering the International Polar and Geophysical Years*, 1st edn, Palgrave Studies in the History of Science and Technology (New York: Palgrave Macmillan, 2010). For more on the International Geophysical Year, see Colin P. Summerhayes, 'International Collaboration in Antarctica: The International Polar Years, the International Geophysical Year and the Scientific Committee on Antarctic Research', *Polar Record* 44, no. 231 (2008): 321–34; Elena Aronova, Karen S. Baker, and Naomi Oreskes, 'Big Science and Big Data in Biology: From the International Geophysical Year through the International Biological Program to the Long Term Ecological Research (LTER) Network, 1957–Present', *Historical Studies in the Natural Sciences* 40, no. 2 (2010): 183–224.

[37] Adrian John Howkins, 'Frozen Empires: A History of the Antarctic Sovereignty Dispute between Britain, Argentina, and Chile, 1939–1959' (PhD thesis, University of Texas at Austin, 2008).

[38] Jenny Bangham, 'Blood Groups and Human Groups: Collecting and Calibrating Genetic Data after World War Two', *Studies in History and Philosophy of Biological and Biomedical Sciences* 47, Part A (2014): 74–86.

[39] Joanna Radin, 'Unfolding Epidemiological Stories: How the Who Made Frozen Blood into a Flexible Resource for the Future' ibid. 62–73; 'Serum as Sentinel: How Cold Blood Became a Resource for Population Health', *Limn*, no. 3 (2013), www.limn.it/articles/serum-as-sentinel-how-cold-blood-became-a-resource-for-population-health/ (Last accessed 11 June 2018).

[40] M. P. Chumakov et al., 'Some Results of the Work on Mass Immunization in the Soviet Union with Live Poliovirus Vaccine Prepared from Sabin Strains', *Bulletin of the World Health Organization* 25, no. 1 (1961): 79–91.

[41] A. A. Smorodintsev et al., 'Results of a Study of the Reactogenic and Immunogenic Properties of Live Anti-Poliomyelitis Vaccine', ibid. 20 (1959): 1053–74.

him 'the greatest possible amount' of vaccine for testing and producing. Sabin sent enough to vaccinate 300,000 children.[42] Chumakov started the trial with 20,000 and, following its initial success, was able to conduct the largest field trial to date in the history of polio vaccines.

By the end of 1959, over 15 million people, spanning fourteen republics of the Soviet Union, were vaccinated in the trial. Smorodintsev and his team immunised more than 1.5 million of the subjects; the rest received the vaccine from Chumakov's lab in the Institute for Poliomyelitis Research in Moscow. The Soviet Union's Minister of Health issued an order on 16 December 1959 for the mass immunisation of the whole population between the ages of 2 months and 20 years by July 1960. This meant vaccinating 77 million people in a matter of months.[43] The *British Medical Journal* deemed this campaign a 'Blitzkrieg against poliomyelitis'.[44]

Parallel to the Soviet campaign, smaller but equally important trials were conducted in Czechoslovakia and Hungary. Both countries had seen severe outbreaks of polio in the 1950s[45] and already had a strong interest in live poliovirus vaccines. Moreover, the use of live poliovirus vaccine and its potential to eliminate the wild virus from the environment fitted well with socialist medicine's emphasis on prevention and an interventionist approach to the environmental causes of illness and disease, as heralded by Czechoslovakian[46] and Hungarian[47] public health professionals.

Collaboration in the trials and mass vaccination with the Sabin strain did not occur in Eastern Europe suddenly, nor did it come through the Soviet Union. Sabin had been in touch with Hungarian and Czechoslovakian scientists for years by the end of the 1950s, sharing views, data and methods, mostly on vaccine production and efficacy. His impressive correspondence attests to an extensive professional network that fostered scientific exchange and personal ties within and across the Iron Curtain. Scientists from East and West met not only at international conferences, but collaborated in laboratory

---

[42] Albert B. Sabin, 'Role of My Cooperation with Soviet Scientists in the Elimination of Polio: Possible Lessons for Relations between the U.S.A. And the U.S.S.R.', *Perspectives in biology and medicine* 31, no. 1 (1987): 57–64, at 61.

[43] Chumakov et al., 'Some Results of the Work on Mass Immunization in the Soviet Union with Live Poliovirus Vaccine Prepared from Sabin Strains', 1961.

[44] 'Mass Immunization with the Live Poliovirus Vaccine in the Soviet Union', *British Medical Journal* 1, no. 5187 (1960): 1729–30, at 1729.

[45] for Czechoslovakia see Karel Žáček et al., 'Mass Oral (Sabin) Poliomyelitis Vaccination. Virological and Serological Surveillance in Czechoslovakia, 1958–59 and 1960', ibid., no. 5285 (1962): 1091–98.

[46] Moore, 'For the People's Health: Ideology, Medical Authority and Hygienic Science in Communist Czechoslovakia'.

[47] László Cserba, 'Az Egészségügy Gazdasági Helyzete 1957. Évben', *Népegészségügy* 38, no. 4 (1957): 87–89.

work, shared publication drafts,[48] circulated specimens,[49] advised each other
on methods and kept each other up to date on the latest results. Sabin's own
research no doubt benefited from this intensive exchange, as he had direct
and instant access to work conducted in laboratories across Eastern Europe.
Conversely, Hungarian and Czechoslovakian virologists gained easier access
to publication opportunities in international journals[50] and later received
help, through invitations and scholarships, in facilitating study trips to the
United States.[51]

This collaboration and the personal connections between virologists in the
East and West rested on long-standing ties. Hungarian publications on polio,
published between the world wars, demonstrate an extensive knowledge of
contemporary epidemiological research and place findings in the context of up-
to-date data and theories published by German, French, Romanian, Swedish,
American and British colleagues.[52] Many further ties were established in the
interwar era. The Rockefeller foundation had a significant role in setting up
public health institutions and providing fellowships for study in the United
States for researchers and public health officials in both countries.[53] Grants
from the Rockefeller Foundation continued to be available to individual

[48] Albert B. Sabin, 'Letter from Sabin, Albert B. To Domok I. Dated 1961–02-01.' Cincinnati:
Hauck Center for the Albert B. Sabin Archives, Sabin Archives. Correspondence, OPV
International, Box 02 File 09 (Hungary – 1960–67), 1961; 'Letter from Rethy, Lajos to Sabin,
Albert B. Dated 1961–03-06.' Cincinnati: Hauck Center for the Albert B. Sabin Archives, Sabin
Archives. Correspondence, OPV International, Box 02 File 09 (Hungary – 1960–67), 1961.
[49] Albert B. Sabin, 'Letter from Sabin, Albert B. To Ivanovics, G. Dated 1955–03-03.' Cincinnati:
Hauck Center for the Albert B. Sabin Archives, Correspondence, Individual, Box 13. File 09
(Ivanovics, George – 1954–60), 1955.
[50] 'Letter from Sabin, Albert B. To Clegg, H.A. Dated 1961–02-01.' Cincinnati: Hauck Center for
the Albert B. Sabin Archives, Sabin Archives, OPV International, Box 02 File
09 (Hungary – 1960–67), 1961.
[51] See e.g. Albert B. Sabin. 'Letter from Sabin, Albert B. to Vaczi, L. Dated 1963–10-16.'
Cincinnati: Hauck Center for the Albert B. Sabin Archives, Sabin Archives. Correspondence,
Individual, Box 09. File 18 (Geder, Laszlo – 1963–68), 1963.
[52] Barla-Szabó, 'A Heine-Medin-Kór Kezelése Lyssa Ellenes Oltásokkal'; Hainiss, 'A Heine-
Medin-Betegség Kóreredete és Kezdeti Szakaszának Jelentősége'; Székely, 'A Poliomyelitis
Anterior Acuta (Heine-Medin) Serumtherapiájáról'.
[53] Moore, 'For the People's Health: Ideology, Medical Authority and Hygienic Science in
Communist Czechoslovakia', 125, Erik Ingebrigtsen, 'Priviliged Origins: "National Models"
and Reforms of Public Health in Interwar Hungary', in Imagining the West in Eastern Europe
and the Soviet Union, ed. György Péteri, Pitt Series in Russian and East European Studies
(Pittsburgh: University of Pittsburgh Press, 2010). Gábor Palló, 'Make a Peak on the Plain: The
Rockefeller Foundation's Szeged Project', in Rockefeller Philanthropz and Modern Biomedicine: International Initiatives from World War I to the Cold War, ed. William H. Schneider
(Bloomington: Indiana University Press, 2002), 87–106; Grósz Emil, 'A Rockefeller Foundation Magyarország Közegészségügyéért', Orvosi Hetilap 68, no. 51 (1924): 910–1110. More
broadly on the Rockefeller Foundation and Eastern Europe in the interwar era, see Paul
Weindling, 'Public Health and Political Stabilisation: The Rockefeller Foundation in Central
and Eastern Europe between the Two World Wars', Minerva 31, no. 3 (1993): 253–67.

158   Sabin Saves the Day

researchers due to its shift from public health to grants in medical research and education in the immediate post-war years;[54] it greatly fostered connections in polio vaccine development, and, indirectly, affected the politics of polio research in the United States. For instance, returning from one of his Eastern European trips, Sabin served as an intermediary for the Czechoslovakian Dionyz Blaskovic, who had worked closely with Jonas Salk and Thomas Francis on a Rockefeller Grant in obtaining freeze-dried blood serum specimens.[55]

The relatively large field trials in Czechoslovakia were organised by the Hygiene and Epidemiological Service in 1958 and 1959, with vaccines prepared from the Sabin strains by the Institute of Sera and Vaccines in Prague and additional batches acquired from Chumakov in the Soviet Union.[56] While personal relationships provided the basis for the endeavour, the Czechoslovakian scientists requested Sabin's assistance through the WHO.[57] Sabin personally aided the bureaucratic process of shipping the strains from Cincinnati to Prague in the spring of 1958 and kept a close eye on the trials.[58] The trials were conducted in four regions (Ústi nad Labem, Liberec, Juhlava and Ostrava)[59] and in total 140,000 children between 2 and 6 years of age were vaccinated.[60]

Finding the serological results favourable, Vilem Skovranek, head of the Hygienic Services, had already laid out a potential plan to extend the vaccination to a broader, national scale in early 1959, but was discouraged by the

[54] John Farley, *To Cast out Disease: A History of the International Health Division of the Rockefeller Foundation (1913–1951)* (Oxford: Oxford University Press, 2004).
[55] Albert Sabin, 'Letter from Sabin, Albert B. to Pillemer, L. Dated 1957–06–10.' Cincinnati: Hauck Center for the Albert B. Sabin Archives, Correspondence, Individual, Box 02. File 21 (Blaskovic, D. – 1957–69), 1957. Blaskovic returned to the United States and was repeatedly supported by The Rockefeller Foundation in '*Annual Report, 1960*' (New York: The Rockefeller Foundation, 1960).
[56] Karel Žáček et al., 'Mass Oral (Sabin) Poliomyelitis Vaccination. Virological and Serological Surveillance in Czechoslovakia, 1958–59 and 1960', *British Medical Journal*, no. 5285 (1962): 1091–98.
[57] A. M. Payne. 'Letter from Payne, A. M. to Sabin, Albert B. Dated 1958–05–27.' Cincinnati: Hauck Center for the Albert B. Sabin Archives, Sabin, Albert B., 1906–1993 – Correspondence, Sabin Archives. Correspondence, OPV International. Box 02. File 03, 1958, Albert B. Sabin, 'Letter from Sabin, Albert B. to Rivers, Thomas M. Dated 1958–10–06', in *Correspondence, NFIP* (Cincinnati: Hauck Center for the Albert B. Sabin Archives, 1958).
[58] Albert B. Sabin, 'Letter from Sabin, Albert B. to Raska, Karel Dated 1958–09–25', in *Correspondence, OPV International* (Cincinnati: Hauck Center for the Albert Sabin Archives, University of Cincinnati, 1958).
[59] D. Slonim et al., 'History of Poliomyelitis in the Czech Republic – Part III', *Central European Journal of Public Health* 3, no. 3 (1995); Vilem Skovranek, 'Letter from Skovranek, Vilem to Sabin, Albert B. Dated 1958–11–10', in *Correspondence, OPV International* (Cincinnati: Hauck Center for the Albert B. Sabin Archives, 1958).
[60] Vilem Skovranek and Karel Zacek, 'Oral Poliovirus Vaccine (Sabin) in Czechoslovakia. Effectiveness of Nation-Wide Use in 1960', *JAMA* 176, no. 6 (1961).

uncertainty of the vaccine supply at the time.[61] Based on studies by mostly Soviet scientists,[62] the vaccination programme was eventually extended to a nationwide campaign in 1960. By the use of domestically produced vaccine from Sabin strains and also vaccine imported from the Soviet Union,[63] 93 per cent of Czechoslovakia's child population was vaccinated, totalling roughly 3.5 million children between the ages of 2 months and 14 years.[64] The mass vaccination was deemed to be an instant success: no confirmed poliomyelitis cases developed in the territory of Czechoslovakia in the first two epidemic seasons after the beginning of the campaign.[65]

Although less widely known than the field trials and early mass immunisation programmes in the Soviet Union and Czechoslovakia, Hungary was also among the Sabin vaccine pioneers. Hungarian virologists and public health authorities had been following oral vaccination trials closely throughout the year. They met with Chumakov, Sabin and Smorodintsev in Moscow in May, along with virologists from Czechoslovakia and Poland.[66]

A turning point in the development of serious interest came with the epidemic of the summer of 1959. In September the State Hygienic Institute hosted an international congress on microbiology, at which one of the focus points was the issue of live polio vaccines. Chumakov delivered the keynote address about the Russian findings,[67] while Albert Sabin's presentation was read in his absence. Vilem Skovranek, deputy minister of health in Czechoslovakia and a key player in the Czechoslovakian field trials, also presented a paper on the live polio vaccine.[68] He soon recounted his experiences at the conference to Sabin in a letter, and added that 'both in Hungary and

---

[61] V. Skovranek. 'Letter from Skovranek, V. To Sabin, Albert B. Dated 1959–01-22.' Cincinnati: Hauck Center for the Albert B. Sabin Archives, Sabin, Albert B., 1906–1993 – Correspondence, Box 02. File 03, 1959.

[62] Ibid.

[63] Vilem Skovranek, 'Present State of Poliomyelitis after Nation Wide Vaccination with Live (Oral) Vaccine in Czechoslovakia', in *Programs of Vaccination, encephalitis and meningitis in enteroviral infections, virological and clinical problems. VIIth symposium of the European Association against Poliomyelitis*, ed. H. C. A. Lassen (Oxford: Euro Assoc. Poliomyelitis and Allied Diseases, 1962).

[64] Vilém Škrovánek and Karel Žážek, 'Oral Poliovirus Vaccine (Sabin) in Czechoslovakia. Effectiveness of Nation-Wide Use in 1960', *Journal of the American Medical Association* 176, no. 6 (1961): 524–26.

[65] Skovranek, 'Present State of Poliomyelitis after Nation Wide Vaccination with Live (Oral) Vaccine in Czechoslovakia.'

[66] M. P. Chumakov. 'Letter to Albert B. Sabin Dated 1959–04-18.' Cincinnati: Hauck Center for the Albert B. Sabin Archives, Sabin, Albert B., 1906–1993 – Correspondence, Box 3. File 09 (Soviet Union – 1959–68), 1959.

[67] Domokos Boda, '50 Years Ago: Polio Epidemics, Immunisation, and Politics', *BMJ* 340 (2010): b5297.

[68] 'A Gyermekbénulás Elleni Élő Oltóanyagról Tárgyal a Mikrobiológiai Kongresszus', *Népszava*, 23 September 1959.

160   Sabin Saves the Day

[Czechoslovakia] a mass vaccination with live vaccine is planned for the beginning of 1960'.[69]

In fact, Hungarians did not wait until the following year to introduce the Sabin vaccine. György Ivánovics, a virologist, informed Sabin in October that they were intending to begin vaccination in a limited section of the country in November and would later extend it to the whole of Hungary.[70] Trials began in Győr-Moson-Sopron County in 1959 on 3 and 4 November, during which the population between the ages of 3 months and 15 years[71] was vaccinated. Virologists reported the average acceptance rate of the vaccine to be 96 per cent.[72] The trial was short, and little time was spent on the evaluation of the results. The State Hygienic Institute analysed 127 stool samples before and after the trial to investigate the presence of the attenuated virus after vaccination, but the overall evaluation of the vaccine and the decision to introduce it nationally were based on the large-scale field trials conducted by the Soviet Union, as well as the experiences of Czechoslovakia and Singapore with the Sabin, and Poland and the Belgian Congo with the Koprowski strains.[73]

'There Is No Cold War'

While international meetings gave a frame to scientific collaboration and served as a venue to discuss problems and display trial results, national policies regarding science funding and research directions also contributed to collaboration in polio research. The moment of political thaw that made the global cooperation of live poliovirus vaccine development possible coincided with several turning points in scientific research conditions on both sides of the Iron Curtain. The United States had recently increased federal financial support for scientific research, and Washington became more receptive to international cooperation in the field.[74] American scientists had more resources and support

[69] V. Skovranek, 'Letter from Skovranek, V. to Sabin, Albert B. Dated 1959–05-10.' Cincinnati: Hauck Center for the Albert B. Sabin Archives, Sabin, Albert B., 1906–1993 – Correspondence, Box 3, File 09 (Soviet Union – 1959–1968), 1959.

[70] G. Ivanovics, 'Letter from Ivanovics, G. to Sabin, Albert B. Dated 1959–10-26.' Ibid., Box 13, File 09 (Ivanovics, George – 1954–1960).

[71] 'Az Egészségügyi Minisztérium Tájékoztatója az Ország 1959. Évi November Havi Járványügyi Helyzetéről.' Budapest: National Archives of Hungary, Egészségügyi Minisztérium Állami közegészségügyi felügyelet és járványvédelmi főosztály iratai, XIX-C-2-e, 57370/1959, 1959.

[72] I. Dömök, Elisabeth Molnár, and Ágnes Jancsó, 'Virus Excretion after Mass Vaccination with Attenuated Polioviruses in Hungary', British Medical Journal 1, no. 5237 (1961): 1410–17. 1410.

[73] Bakács, 'Az Eddigi Poliomyelitis Vaccinatio Eredményeinek Értékelése', 690.

[74] See Benison, 'International Medical Cooperation: Dr. Albert Sabin, Live Poliovirus Vaccine and the Soviets', 465, and Oshinsky, Polio: An American Story, 251.

to work together with foreign colleagues. In fact, research opportunities widened on a massive scale for both superpowers, fuelled by intense political, economic and military rivalry.[75] Ironically, then, antagonistic Cold War objectives helped open opportunities for cooperation across the Iron Curtain.

At the same time, in the Soviet Union, scientific discourse was changing, gradually breaking with Stalinist concepts of the superiority of a particularly Soviet form of science and medicine.[76] According to Sabin, the vice president of the Soviet Academy of Sciences made this change clear when, in defence of Sabin at a lecture in the Soviet Union, he stated, '[W]e have now reached a stage in Soviet science where we cannot and should not any more speak of Soviet genetics, Western genetics or American genetics. There is just one kind of genetics, the kind that gives reproducible results.'[77]

As shown in Chapter 1, polio began to create a unique space in Cold War politics preceding the thaw, mainly due to the involvement of children's health and the threat of disabling future generations amid post-war recovery. The internal changes and new avenues in both American and Soviet scientific environments, together with a more general thaw in Cold War policies, further widened this space to produce a hitherto unprecedented medical cooperation between the two arch-enemies.[78]

The global effort to put a stop to polio epidemics created a community of scientists who transcended Cold War barriers and defied the world order. Scientists and national public health authorities shared results of field trials from all over the world with three different live virus vaccines, along with updates on vaccine use and epidemiological data, in the pages of major scientific journals and at international conferences.

For instance, at a symposium and conference in Moscow in May 1960, in addition to the 300 specialists from the Soviet Union, 73 foreign scientists from 19 countries took part in eight working sessions. During the three days of the conference, '23 reports and communications results were summarized of the mass application of live poliovirus vaccine in 9 republics

[75] Mark Solovey, 'Science and the State during the Cold War: Blurred Boundaries and a Contested Legacy', *Social Studies of Science* 31, no. 1 (2001): 165–70.
[76] Loren R. Graham argues that the issue of Lysenkoism, the Soviet alternative to theoretical genetics, served as early steps in going against the regime for dissidents of the regime, like Zhores Medvedev and Andrei Sakharov in the early 1960s. Loren R. Graham, *What Have We Learned About Science and Technology from the Russian Experience?* (Stanford: Stanford University Press, 1998), 34–35.
[77] Benison, 'Albert Sabin Reminisces', interview, 3 June 1976, 2–5. Cited in Benison, 'International Medical Cooperation: Dr. Albert Sabin, Live Poliovirus Vaccine and the Soviets'.
[78] The significance of such cooperation is shown by present day interpretations of the development of the oral polio vaccine. An article in *Science* magazine from 2010, for example, refers to the cooperation between the USSR and the US as an example to follow in resolving conflict among the US and the Islamic world through 'vaccine diplomacy'. Peter J. Hotez, 'Peace through Vaccine Diplomacy', *Science* 327 (2010): 1301.

of the Soviet Union, as well as in Poland, Hungary, China, Bulgaria, Sweden and the USA.'[79] The success of the new vaccines ignited a scientific euphoria, strengthening the sense that science, as putatively objective and universal, could serve as a tool to stop the Cold War and unite humanity in a common bond. Opening the Sixth Symposium of the European Association of Poliomyelitis in 1959 in Munich, the organisation's president referred to the participating scientists, from twenty-five different countries, as 'members of our polio family'.[80] Going a step further, at the Fifth International Poliomyelitis Conference in 1960 in Copenhagen, Basil O'Connor (who was president of the American National Foundation for Infantile Paralysis) celebrated the achievements of the cooperation in his opening speech:

This is a council, not of war, but of victory. Together we have successfully created weapons against a common enemy that bring within our reach a triumph for all mankind, the coming elimination of epidemic-paralytic poliomyelitis. We meet now to compare notes on what we have created, to report our experiences and help each other in reaching decisions on the most effective use of those weapons. Your very presence here, from the East, from the West, is proof to the world that in your high calling, in search for the truth that frees man from disease, there is no cold war.[81]

This feeling of unity marked the end of a decade in which other domains of public health had been hindered by Cold War tensions. For much of the 1950s, the Soviet Union, along with most Eastern European countries, remained outside the WHO as a sign of protest against the agency's politics. Since the founding document of the WHO did not permit the unjoining of the agency, the Eastern European countries were termed *inactive*. The Soviet Union returned to the international agency in 1957 along with Bulgaria, Albania, Poland and Romania.[82] Other states rejoined later, with Hungary being one of the last countries from the Eastern Bloc to rejoin in 1963.

Although the development of the live vaccine was the result of intensive cooperation that reached across the Iron Curtain, its implementation followed Cold War fault lines. Several major points of conflict emerged, all of which had significant effects on polio prevention in Hungary and worldwide. Convictions and reservations about the efficacy and safety of the Sabin vaccine

---

[79] 'The Main Results of the IV Scientific Conference of the Institute and the International Symposium on Live Poliovirus Vaccine and the 1st Soviet–American Discussions of Problems Relating to the Control of Poliomyelitis' (paper presented at the IV Scientific Conference of the Institute and the International Symposium on live poliovirus vaccine and the 1st Soviet–American Discussions of Problems Relating tto the Control of Poliomyelitis, Moscow, 1960).

[80] H. C. A. Lassen, 'Eröffnungsansprache', in *VIth Symposium of the European Association of Poliomyelitis* (Brussels: European Association of Poliomyelitis, 1959), 6.

[81] O'Connor, 'The Setting for Scientific Research in the Last Half of the Twentieth Century'.

[82] *The First Ten Years of the World Health Organization*, 80.

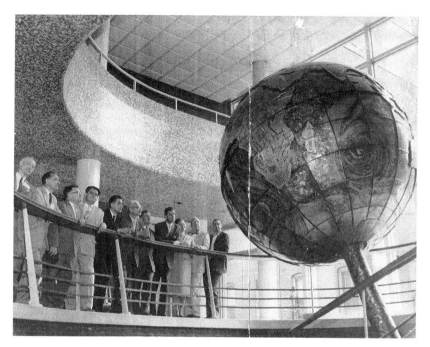

Figure 5.2 *First International Conference on Oral Polio Vaccine at PAHO headquarters in Washington, 1959. Miscellaneous, Assorted Letters and Photographs. Box 02. File 02 (1950's). University of Cincinnati. Hauck Center for the Albert B. Sabin Archives.* **This image is protected by copyright and cannot be used without further permissions clearance.**

divided the East and West, while varying healthcare and economic structures had a direct effect on the choice of the vaccine (i.e. to stick with the hitherto-used Salk vaccine or change to Sabin), as well as the speed of introduction and licensing. Furthermore, differences in welfare systems and socialised medicine, a sensitive point in Cold War concerns, influenced the efficiency of vaccine application.

National Mass Vaccination

The introduction of the Sabin vaccine in Hungary in 1959 could not have been more different from that of the Salk vaccine two years before. In the case of the killed-virus vaccine, the state was slow to move in vaccine production. In addition, it faced challenges in its acquisition and ran into significant problems in the vaccination campaigns. Meanwhile, in the introduction and dissemination of the brand-new Sabin vaccine, Hungary was quick to adopt it following field trials and became the first country in the world to organise a nationwide mass vaccination with the oral vaccine. While countries like the Soviet Union and Czechoslovakia had immunized millions of children through their trials, introducing a vaccine in a national programme with the aim of protecting each and every one of a nation's children was a significant step, regardless of population size.

Shortly after the vaccine trial in Hungary, the national weekly newsreel quickly broke the news about the live poliovirus vaccine and the experiences of children in Győr-Moson-Sopron County.

A new polio vaccine has arrived from the Soviet Union, the Sabin vaccine ... Its protective effect is stronger than that of the Salk vaccine ... The new vaccine was warmly welcome all throughout Győr county ... and will make its way to every part of the country and we hope that with it we will take another step forward in preventing polio.[83]

Barely two weeks after the Hungarian field trials started, the government announced a nationwide vaccination campaign starting in mid-December 1959.[84] A year later, an estimated 2.4 million children had been immunised with the live vaccine imported from the Soviet Union.[85]

This quick acceptance of the brand-new vaccine in Hungary was very different from the scepticism voiced about the Salk vaccine back in the mid-1950s. In connection with the Cutter incident, a Hungarian newspaper article in 1955 (based on an article in the French newspaper *L'Humanité*) had argued: 'The effectiveness of a new vaccine can be established only after a long time and numerous experiments. It is a dramatic fact that due to such negligence many thousands of children became the guinea pigs of the savage protectors of free enterprise.'[86] Four years, two epidemics and a revolution later, the Hungarian press was not so squeamish about time and the number of experiments. There was a greater need for vaccination that actually worked.

Concern over the safety of the Salk vaccine was ameliorated over the years by the growing number of success stories from Europe and the United States. While knowledge about the rate of efficacy and recommended dosage remained in flux, by 1957 the Hungarian government could rely on a wide-ranging international experience of two years, reported in the pages of medical journals and at international polio conferences.

[83] 'Új Oltóanyag', Magyar Filmhíradó és Dokumentumfilmgyár, Hungary, 1959.
[84] 'December 14-én Kezdődnek a Gyermekbénulás Elleni Sabin-Féle Védőoltások', *Népszava*, 22 November 1959, 1.
[85] Chumakov et al., 'Some Results of the Work on Mass Immunization in the Soviet Union with Live Poliovirus Vaccine Prepared from Sabin Strains', 82.
[86] 'Halálos Áldozata Van az Amerikában Felfedezett Gyermekparalízis Elleni Védőoltásnak', *Szabad Nép*, 1955.

In the case of the Sabin vaccine, the context could not have been more different. There were no comparable international experiences or clear success stories that could reassure Hungarian scientists and the political leadership. Not one country had begun national mass vaccination in the autumn of 1959, and due to the novelty of the vaccine, there were no long-term observations to determine the percentage of the population who would be protected against the three polio strains. It was just two large-scale trials, albeit involving millions of vaccinees, that provided evidence of the efficacy and safety of the new product.

However, this time the trials were all conducted on home ground, that is to say, on the 'right' side of the Iron Curtain. Intensive scientific cooperation among the Eastern European countries and the Soviet Union, fostered greatly during the years of inactive membership of the WHO between 1949 and 1957,[87] made it possible for Hungarian scientists to keep an eye on live polio vaccine trials in the Eastern Bloc from the very beginning, and to gain direct information about the results from participating scientists on personal visits.[88]

While proximity and the role of the East in the vaccine trials played a large part in the quick adaptation of the Sabin vaccine, these cannot serve as the sole explanations. As the story of the introduction of the Salk vaccine demonstrates, Hungarian scientists had access to onsite visits to manufacturing labs in the West and were participants in the increasingly intensive circulation of scientific knowledge about polio. Also, by the late autumn of 1959, Salk vaccine production in Hungary had already started for the following year.

Moreover, as Hungarian paediatrician Domokos Boda's memoir[89] shows, the Cold War divide could have surprising effects: namely, trust in Western and distrust in Eastern technology. Boda was part of the delegation sent to Moscow to investigate the new vaccine and to inform the Hungarian government's choice between the Salk and Sabin vaccines and saw that enthusiasm over the new Sabin vaccine was not shared by everyone in the Soviet Union. He recounted meeting a group of Soviet virologists on his arrival; they were

---

[87] During these years, Eastern European countries signed bilateral agreements to advance scientific cooperation in health-related issues and epidemic control. See for instance 'A Magyar Népköztársaság Kormánya és a Csehszlovák Köztársaság Kormánya Között Az Egészségügyi Együttműködésre Vonatkozóan Létrejött és Budapesten 1955. Április 28. Napján Aláírt Egyezmény.' Budapest: National Archives of Hungary, A Minisztertanács üléseinek jegyzőkönyvei, XIX-A-83-a, 1957. junius 8., 1957; *The First Ten Years of the World Health Organization*.

[88] The efficiency and safety of live virus vaccines were highly debated on the pages of medical journals all over the world, as were the doubts of efficiency of the Salk vaccine. Fears of an attenuated virus turning virulent, questions of how vaccine efficiency is measurable in the case of a disease that follows patterns of ebb and tide, and issues of the method of comparison between dead and live virus vaccines formed discussions among virologists and public health specialists before, during and after vaccine tests.

[89] Boda, *Sorsfordulók*.

ardently against the introduction of the new vaccine to the Soviet Union. They argued that the Salk vaccine could be considered safe, since the Americans tested it on their own people. The Sabin vaccine was a solution with which the Americans did not wish to experiment on their own society; therefore, it must be potentially dangerous. As Boda remembered, some even went so far as to consider the introduction of the Sabin[25] vaccine part of a scheme by the Americans to destroy millions of Soviet children, cutting future generations short and thereby weakening the nation.[90] With these sentiments, the Soviet scientists were expressing the general frustrations that often arise with the appearance of new vaccines: the potential to cause disease and harm.

'My colleagues and I were in a difficult situation,' Boda wrote. 'It would be impossible to use the Sabin vaccine in Hungary if the official Soviet view was known. After agonising, we recommended the Sabin vaccine and kept quiet about the controversy.'[91] The fact that the Sabin vaccine arrived from the East, therefore, cannot alone explain the speedy implementation and fast decision-making of the Hungarian government. A more plausible explanation is that the communist government could not afford another demonstration of the limits of its power by a new epidemic that would be decidedly out of their control. After the summer of 1959, it became clear that Salk vaccination did not fulfil the hopes of curbing polio in the country. The government needed to act fast. To this end, rapidly introducing a new vaccine that promised to eradicate polio seemed the only choice.

There were changes not only compared to 1955, but compared to the previous discourse of the Salk vaccination as well. In this new rhetoric of polio vaccination, the state rehabilitated parents as allies in the fight against polio and appealed to them for cooperation in a very different tone compared to just a few months previously. 'Certainly there would be no negligent parents who would endanger children to be exposed to illness by missing vaccination,' wrote *Népszava*, in a friendlier voice, in its first article informing the public about the upcoming Sabin vaccination.[92]

Parents received a letter along with the details of the vaccinating site and time, explaining that the outbreak that summer was due to the inadequate protection the Salk vaccine provided: 'in [the] long run the protection yielded by the Salk vaccine did not prove to be satisfactory', but researchers had 'finally succeeded in preparing a material of higher protective value', the Sabin vaccine. The Public Health and Epidemiology Centre also made it clear that the cooperation of parents was essential in bringing polio under control. 'Every

[90] Interview by Dora Vargha, 18 November 2009.
[91] '50 Years Ago: Polio Epidemics, Immunisation, and Politics'.
[92] 'Tizennégy Éves Korig Minden Gyermek Kap a Gyermekbénulás Ellen Védő Új, Nagyobbhatású Gyógyszerből', *Népszava*, 18 November 1959, 1.

parent's duty is to protect children from the eventual illness. Make sure to take your child (or send your older ones) on the date fixed for vaccination to the vaccination centres', the letter instructed.[93]

Official communications in newspapers re-evaluated the state's role in vaccine procurement. In the case of the Salk vaccine, the government was portrayed as a hero, which, in spite of all hardships and even debt, had managed to go out and attain much-needed protection for children. This time, Father Russia decidedly stole the show: according to daily newspaper *Népszava*, the Hungarian government 'asked for the help of the Soviet Union and not without result: we were granted 2.5 million doses of vaccine.'[94] There was no talk of cost or debt or the achievement of the state required to import the vaccine.

National mass vaccination started on the same day, 14 December 1959, throughout the whole country, and immunisation with each type of virus had to be completed within one week. Type I virus vaccine was distributed from 14 to 19 December 1959, Type III strain from 21 to 27 January 1960 and Type II from 23 to 27 February 1960.[95] Vaccination with the Sabin vaccine in the form of drops was mandatory for children between three months and two years; for all other age groups up to the age of 14, immunisation was voluntary.[96] Vaccination was organised in Mother and Infant Protection Offices by district paediatricians. Parents received leaflets informing them about the Sabin vaccine and the campaign, which also served as their registration document. Children were also vaccinated in day-care centres, kindergartens and schools,[97] which renders the term *voluntary* dubious.

There were also clear differences in the level of organisation between the Salk and Sabin campaigns. The Ministry of Health seemed to have learnt a lesson from resistance among physicians to the Salk vaccination method, and now took care to inform the medical profession of the vaccination programme well in advance. In November the Ministry of Health organised a conference for the counties' chief hygienists, the directors and epidemiologists of the Public Health and Epidemiological Stations, and the leading paediatricians of the country, in order to acquaint them with the details of the mass

---

[93] 'Letter from the District Public Health and Epidemiological Centre Dated 1960–1967?'. Cincinnati: Hauck Center for the Albert B. Sabin Archives, Sabin, Albert B., 1906–1993 – Correspondence, Box 02, File 09 (Hungary – 1960–1967), 1959.

[94] 'Tizennégy Éves Korig Minden Gyermek Kap a Gyermekbénulás Ellen Védő Új, Nagyobbhatású Gyógyszerből', *Népszava*, 1959, 1.

[95] Kátay, 'The Active Immunization against Poliomyelitis in Hungary and Its Three Years' Results', in The Control of Poliomyelitis by Live Poliovirus Vaccine. Studies on Mass Vaccinations in Hungary, in the USSR, in Czechoslovakia and the German Democratic Republic. Papers Presented at the Hungarian-Soviet Medical Conference September 24–30, 1960.

[96] 'Budapesten December 14–15-16-án Kapják a Gyerekek a Gyermekbénulás Ellen Védő Sabin-Oltóanyagot', *Népszava*, 26 November 1959, 1.

[97] Ibid.

vaccination. Later in the month, similar conferences involved physicians and health experts at the local level.[98]

Notifying the public and disseminating information about the vaccine began well in advance of the campaign. This time, Hungarians could read about the research on the new polio vaccines of Koprowski and Sabin in the newspaper by August 1959,[99] three months in advance of the campaign, while parents were provided with detailed news about the approaching campaign a month before it started. The above-mentioned news broadcast portrayed the swift and painless vaccination more than a month prior to the start of the national campaign on 14 December 1959. Red Cross and trade union activists, the Communist Youth Association and the Women's Council all took part in informing the public about the new vaccine, its benefits and its painless application method.[100] Nor did their activities stop at public education in advance of the campaign. Once vaccinations started, every evening Red Cross activists visited the homes of those who had failed to appear before the vaccination brigades.[101]

The vaccine administration also seemed to have gone more smoothly in the Sabin campaign. The Sabin drops definitely required less technical knowledge to administer than the Salk injections, in terms of administration. The faulty needles addressed in Tóth's letter were in the past: all that was needed this time was a spoon. Parents were called on to bring their own spoons in order to facilitate the vaccination process.[102]

'Many of the little ones still get scared of the doctor; but see, no need to be afraid of the horrible needle, because they can take the vaccine against polio with sweet tea',[103] news broadcasters soothed the to-be-vaccinated children – and their parents – in advance of the campaign. A ministerial report from 1959 remarked that parents did not usually have a problem with the number of vaccinations: it was the number of injections that kept them away from vaccination.

---

[98] 'The Active Immunization against Poliomyelitis in Hungary and Its Three Years' Results', in The Control of Poliomyelitis by Live Poliovirus Vaccine. Studies on Mass Vaccinations in Hungary, in the USSR, in Czechoslovakia and the German Democratic Republic. Papers Presented at the Hungarian-Soviet Medical Conference September 24–30, 1960.

[99] Géza Dr. Petényi, 'Új Módszerek a Gyermekbénulás Elleni Védekezésre, Több Légzőszervi, Ideg- és Bélbetegség Vírus Eredetű, Új Műszerek a Veleszületett Szívhibák Pontos Megállapítására', Népszava, 16 August 1959, 5.

[100] 'Budapesten December 14–15-16-Án Kapják a Gyerekek a Gyermekbénulás Ellen Védő Sabin-Oltóanyagot', ibid., 26 November, 1.

[101] 'Élet egy Kanál Teában. Fővárosszerte Gyorsan és Szervezetten Folyik a Sabin-Oltás', Népszava, 15 December 1959, 1.

[102] 'Hétfőn Kezdődik 500 000 Budapesti Gyerek Védőoltása', Népszava, 11 December 1959, 2.

[103] 'Új Oltóanyag', Magyar Filmhíradó és Dokumentumfilmgyár, Hungary, 1959.

Of course, in practice, the campaign still had its hiccups. Interestingly, we can identify these problems from a newspaper article titled 'Sabin vaccination in the capital is progressing in a fast and well-organised manner'.[104] Many parents failed to bring their vaccination cards, and many had lost their 'invitation', the written request by the city council to appear for vaccination. The article also mentions 'distrustful' mothers who claimed that their children had a fever in order to avoid having to take the vaccine.

While the organisation of the Sabin vaccination was by far more effective than the previous years' attempts with the Salk vaccine, the result was well below the expectations of the government. For instance, in Budapest alone, they planned to vaccinate half a million children in three days.[105] However, they only managed to vaccinate 300,000. According to *Népszava*, many of the 'invitations' did not arrive with families in time because of the high workload of the Hungarian Post with the approach of Christmas and New Year's Eve. Furthermore, they also blamed the foggy, cold weather for making many children ill with colds, who could not take the vaccine while they had a fever. For these reasons, the city extended the vaccination period by three extra days.[106]

One of the reasons for the quick response to the problem of the low vaccination rate and for the relatively intensive campaign was the particularity of the Sabin vaccine. Although the Sabin drops were easier to administer, their expiration time was significantly shorter than that of the Salk vaccine. Hungary received the shipment frozen, and the vaccine was thawed in the State Institute of Hygiene, where they tested it before distributing it to the vaccination points.[107] Once the vaccine had been thawed, it needed to be used in the space of about a week.[108] This small window of usage might explain why the government (the Health Ministry and the SHI) invested such effort into the organisation of the Sabin vaccination.

While the acceptance and application of the vaccine was remarkably fast, the Health Ministry did wish to evaluate the vaccine. For this reason, the minister ordered every hospital director to report any confirmed or potential polio cases and all cases of any contagious disease that attacked the central

---

[104] 'Élet egy Kanál Teában. Fővárosszerte Gyorsan és Szervezetten Folyik a Sabin-Oltás', *Népszava*, 15 December 1959, 1.
[105] 'Budapesten December 14–15-16-Án Kapják a Gyerekek a Gyermekbénulás Ellen Védő Sabin-Oltóanyagot', *Népszava*, 26 November 1959, 1; 'Hétfőn Kezdődik 500 000 Budapesti Gyerek Védőoltása', *Népszava*, 11 December 1959, 2.
[106] 'A Hét Végéig Meghosszabbították a Sabin-Oltások Határidejét', *Népszava*, 17 December 1959, 2.
[107] 'Új Oltóanyag', Magyar Filmhíradó és Dokumentumfilmgyár, Hungary, 1959.
[108] 'Budapesten December 14–15-16-án Kapják a Gyerekek a Gyermekbénulás Ellen Védő Sabin-Oltóanyagot', *Népszava*, 1959, 1.

nervous system, whether accompanied by paralysis or not. These cases were to be reported via telephone to the PHCED as well.[109] By February 1960, 92.4 per cent of the population under 14 years of age had received immunisation with the Sabin vaccine.[110] In a matter of three months, Hungary had vaccinated 2.5 million people, more than the total number in two years of Salk vaccination.[111] The country thus joined the Soviet Union and Czechoslovakia in being among the first countries in the world to organise national mass vaccination with the new, live poliovirus vaccine.

Cold War Fault Lines

Mass vaccination with live polio vaccine quickly spread in Eastern Europe. In Bulgaria in 1960, around 2 million children between 2 months and 14 years of age were targeted;[112] in Romania in 1961, the vaccine was administered to the whole population under 30 years of age, around 10 million people.[113] Yugoslavia carried out a small field trial with the Sabin vaccine from January to May 1960, involving about 8,000 pre-school children in the city of Kragujevac, and, following a relatively severe epidemic in 1960, began mass vaccination in 1961.[114]

East Germany conducted a field trial of the Sabin vaccine in April 1960, citing the favourable results of the Soviet Union, Czechoslovakia, Hungary and Poland as the basis for their own trial. The vaccination was free and voluntary, and German virologists reported a very favourable acceptance from the population, with around 86 per cent of people between the ages of

---

[109] 'Sabin Oltások Eredményességének Értékelése', Budapest: City Archives of Budapest, Budapest Főváros Tanács VB Egészségügyi Osztályának iratai, XXIII. 115.a. 215 kisdoboz, 188.197/1959, 1959.

[110] Kátay, 'The Active Immunization against Poliomyelitis in Hungary and Its Three Years' Results', in The Control of Poliomyelitis by Live Poliovirus Vaccine. Studies on Mass Vaccinations in Hungary, in the USSR, in Czechoslovakia and the German Democratic Republic. Papers Presented at the Hungarian-Soviet Medical Conference September 24–30, 1960, 77.

[111] A report from the city of Eger states that while previously they could achieve the vaccination ration of 80% in the population, with the Sabin vaccine this number rose to 93% 'Végrehajtó Bizottsági Ülés Jegyzőkönyve.' Budapest: City Archives of Budapest, MSZMP Eger Városi Bizottsága Végrehajtó Bizottság ülései XXXV-29–3, 130. őe. (5. doboz), 1963.

[112] St. Rangelova et al., 'Epidemiological and Serological Evaluation of Results of Mass Vaccination with Live Vacine in Bulgaria', in Vaccination and epidemiology of poliomyelitis and allied diseases, new developments in the programmes of vaccination, virological and serological studies, clinical problems. VIIth symposium of the European Association against Poliomyelitis and Allied Diseases, ed. H. C. A. Lassen (Prague: Euro Assoc. Poliomyelitis and Allied Diseases, 1963).

[113] I. Spinu, Sanda Biberi Moroianu, and S. Popa, 'Considérations Épidémiologiques et la Vaccination Contre la Poliomyélite en Roumanie', [Epidemiological Considerations and the Vaccination against Poliomyelitis in Romania] ibid.

[114] M. V. Milovanovic, 'Poliomyelitis in Yugoslavia', ibid.

2 months and 20 years immunised. Vaccination with the oral vaccine became compulsory in 1961, reaching 43 per cent of the total population by 1962.[115] Other European countries started using the live vaccine in the years 1962 and 1963.[116]

The introduction of the Sabin vaccine was peppered with controversies, rivalries and delays in the case of the United States. While it took American authorities an incredible two hours to license the Salk vaccine in 1955,[117] it took over three years for the United States Public Health Service to do the same for the live vaccine.[118] The Ad Hoc Committee on Live Poliovirus Vaccines, organised under the Division of Biologics Standards in 1958, repeatedly met until 1962, when Sabin's vaccine was finally licensed. The deliberations surrounding the live poliovirus vaccine had to do in part with the widespread use of the Salk vaccine, its cultural significance in a society that marched, danced and collected its dimes for research against polio and the all too recent memories of the Cutter incident.

Reservations over the new vaccine also threw light on underlying fault lines in international vaccine research. While cooperation in live vaccine development reached over the Iron Curtain and forged cooperation that was untypical of its time and celebrated as a triumph over political dividing lines, Cold War rhetoric had the upper hand when it came to the evaluation of its results. The words of virologist David Dane from 1959 encapsulate the pervasiveness of Cold War rhetoric in live vaccine development, as he discussed the potential perils of attenuated strains:

It may be that the brain washing which these polioviruses have had in the laboratories of Drs Sabin, Cox and Koprowski have cleansed them of all their potential of indulging in un-American neurotropic activities and that they will remain as stable as the coelacanth. It may be that they will replace all deviationist particles throughout the whole world and we shall all be infected with a common but stable and harmless virus which will occupy and pass peacefully from alimentary tract to alimentary tract for ever more under the auspices of the WHO.[119]

---

[115] T. Kima and W. A. Belian, 'National Report of Immunisation Program of German Democratic Republic', in *Programs of Vaccination, encephalitis and meningitis in enteroviral infections, virological and clinical problems. VIIth symposium of the European Association against Poliomyelitis*, ed. H. C. A. Lassen (Oxford: Euro Assoc. Poliomyelitis and Allied Diseases, 1962).

[116] S. G. Drozdov. 'The Contemporary Poliomyelitis Situation in Europe.' Geneva: World Health Organization, European Symposium on Virus Diseases Control, EURO-322/8, 1966.

[117] Oshinsky, *Polio: An American Story*, 207.

[118] The Secretary of Health, Education and Welfare was responsible for giving license, acting on the recommendation of the Surgeon General. The latter was advised by the National Institutes of Health and the Division of Biologics Standards. *Polio Vaccines*, 16 March 196, 3–4.

[119] G. W. A. Dick and D. S. Dane, 'The Evaluation of Live Poliovirus Vaccines. Paper Presented at the Conference on Live Poliovirus Vaccines, Washington, 22–26 June 1959', in *Who/Polio/ 36–44* (Geneva: World Health Organization, 1959).

What Dane is referring to here is the growing role of the WHO in coordinating the evaluation and validation of the trials. While the trials were mostly
the result of the networks of individual researchers, combined with mostly
state funds and 'volunteer' subjects, the WHO became an arena in which
Cold War tensions could find relief and professional agendas could be
pushed through.

Considering the potential harm that live polio vaccines could cause, trust
became central to the evaluation of the Eastern European Sabin trials. However, in an era of suspicion of the enemy within and without, trust did not come
easily in the Cold War. Therefore the most pressing questions about this Cold
War scientific feat, primarily for the Americans, were: could the Russians be
trusted? Would their numbers lie? Did the new vaccine actually work?

To resolve the issue of scientific trustworthiness and to bridge Cold War
suspicions, the WHO, already highly interested in global disease eradication,
sent an American specialist from Yale, Dorothy M. Horstmann, to report on
the safety of the vaccine and the validity of the trials in the Soviet Union.[120]
The idea of the visit and the proposal of Horstmann actually came from the
United States: John R. Paul, renowned virologist and polio expert at Yale
University, recommended his colleague to the Division of Communicable
Diseases at the WHO[121] and to Mikhail Chumakov.[122] Since 1954, the health
agency had established a role for itself in coordinating poliomyelitis research
and aiding in the circulation of information in statistics, epidemiology, field
trials and laboratory investigation.[123] It was happy to fulfil the American
request for the validation trip.[124] Its task of scientific evaluation fitted into its
self-proclaimed role of bridging the local and global in public health issues.[125]

Between 26 August and 17 October 1959, Horstmann visited Poland,
Czechoslovakia and several republics of the Soviet Union to gather information onsite about the vaccine trials. The WHO delegate voiced overall

[120] Dorothy Horstmann, *Report on Live Poliovirus Vaccination in the Union of Soviet Socialist Republics, Poland and Czechoslovakia* (World Health Organization, 1959).
[121] A. M.-M. Payne, 'Letter to John R. Paul', New Haven: Sterling Memorial Library, Yale University, Dorothy Millicent Horstmann Papers, Box 12, Group 1700, Folder 260, 1959; John R. Paul, 'Letter to A. M.-M. Payne', ibid. Sterling Memorial Library.
[122] 'Letter to Mikhail Chumakov', New Haven: Sterling Memorial Library, Dorothy Millicent Horstmann Papers, Box 12, Group 1700, Folder 260, 1959.
[123] 'The Co-Ordinating Role of Who in Poliomyelitis Research', Geneva: World Health Organiza-tion, Executive Board, Fourteenth Session, Provisional agenda item 4, EB14/2, 1954.
[124] Payne, 'Letter to John R. Paul', New Haven: Sterling Memorial Library, Yale Univer-sity, 1959.
[125] This was not the first instance that an international health agency took on the task of validating vaccine trials. Clifford Rosenberg has recently argued that the League of Nations Health Organization issued guidelines for vaccine developers on clinical research that eventually led to the largest vaccine trial of its time: Calmette's trial of the BCG vaccine in Algiers. Rosenberg, 'The International Politics of Vaccine Testing in Interwar Algiers'.

satisfaction in her report on the Soviet Union. She saw no reason to doubt the level of surveillance of polio cases during the trial and judged the Sabin vaccine to be safe. However, Horstmann did admit that it was difficult to say how effective the vaccine was, since many of the subjects had previously received Salk vaccine and little time had elapsed since the trial to draw definite conclusions.

If scepticism about the Russian results was rooted in Western Cold War ideas of the East, Horstmann's report used a very similar set of tools to dissolve doubts and validate those same results. She drew upon two powerful notions that were connected to communist countries: the centralised, totalitarian state and its submissive citizens.

Horstmann highlighted the role of a centralised and state-operated public health system in successfully organising such a trial: a critical difference between the East and West that was frequently mobilised in Cold War rhetoric on both sides.

The scope and magnitude of the live poliovirus vaccine programmes ... are of a type peculiarly fitted to the manner in which the medical profession is organized under the Ministries of Health in these countries. For such mass programmes, it is necessary to have a Medical Service organized almost on a military basis, particularly from the epidemiologic surveillance and Public Health stand point.[126]

In the Soviet case, a state and healthcare system that was centrally controlled from top to bottom could at once be capable of organising a project on a mass scale and, at the same time, of vouching for the rigour and scrutiny that was expected from such a scientific trial. This, implied Horstmann's report, was the upside of a totalitarian communist regime.

The favourable report was followed by yet another international polio conference, this time specifically on live poliovirus vaccines, in Washington, D.C. One American scientist bluntly confronted the Soviet results, questioning the reliability of their data in the reports of Soviet epidemiological teams.[127] The Soviet delegate replied shortly: 'I would like to assure [you] of one thing, that we in the Soviet Union love our children and are as concerned for their well-being as much as people in the United States, or any other part of the world are for their children.'[128] Thus, polio became the symbol of an equaliser, pointing to the common familial bond, a bond of responsibility between parents and children all over the world. Cold War considerations, however, seemed to be more persistent.

[126] Horstmann, *Report on Live Poliovirus Vaccination in the Union of Soviet Socialist Republics, Poland and Czechoslovakia*, 99.
[127] Benison, 'International Medical Cooperation: Dr. Albert Sabin, Live Poliovirus Vaccine and the Soviets'.
[128] Ibid. 479.

The safety and efficacy of live poliovirus vaccines were fertile grounds for Cold War fears and political considerations. Not only were Sabin's and Koprowski's vaccines new, but the whole concept of the live vaccine was novel in disease prevention. The reason for this was the vaccine's potential to spread the attenuated virus to the non-vaccinated population. Virologists and public-health officials agreed that this was the attractive, and at the same time, dangerous aspect of the new polio vaccines: 'It is recognized ... that the use of a product that spreads beyond those originally vaccinated represents a radical departure from present practices in human preventive medicine.'[129]

New faith had to be created, since the existing faith was in the development of inactivated virus vaccine only. It was also not too easy to bring over to our side the indifferent and the undecided, since my associates and I were alone in this field when the work began and remained so for several years,

Koprowski recalled on the brink of the live vaccine's success in 1960.[130] In fact, the problem of creating faith in the attenuated strains remained significant throughout all phases of development, testing, evaluation and implementation of the vaccine. One of the main reasons for concern over the vaccine's safety was, as Herald Cox pointed out, the difficulty in 'predict[ing] the behavior of a virus in a human population from what is known about its behavior in the laboratory'.[131]

Following Horstmann's visit, the WHO took further steps in validating scientific results and establishing trust along the two sides of the Iron Curtain. An expert committee on poliomyelitis, comprised of leading virologists from East and West, compiled a report on the current evaluation of both the Salk and Sabin vaccines.[132] If the previous report of the committee had given a green light to large field trials and started a wave of vaccine testing all over the globe, the evaluation of those trials was the objective of the next report, published in 1960.

The committee's report on the whole was favourable, and the majority supported the introduction of live vaccines into national prevention programmes. However, since concerns over safety still persisted in the application of a vaccine that had not been used for a long time, the WHO claimed future roles in continuing to coordinate investigation:

[129] 'Summary of Conference on Live Poliovirus Vaccines', Geneva: World Health Organization, 1959.

[130] Koprowski, 'Historical Aspects of the Development of Live Virus Vaccine in Poliomyelitis', 89.

[131] 'Live Poliovirus Vaccines', ibid., no. 5193: 202–03. 202

[132] Among the members we find the names of John R. Paul from Yale University, Viktor Zhdanov Secretary of the Academy of Sciences of the USSR, S. Gard from the renowned Karolinska Institut in Sweden, and V. Skovranek from the Czechoslovak Ministry of Health. Expert Committee on Poliomyelitis, 'Expert Committee on Poliomyelitis. Third Report', 1960.

The Committee pointed out that the spread of live-virus vaccine used in large-scale trials within a given country, even though less extensive than had been anticipated, has already caused concern in neighbouring states which were not using the vaccine ... It appears, therefore, that there is need for international cooperation in these vaccination programmes between neighbouring states and for coordination in the timing of mass programmes along national borders. The Committee considered that such coordination might best be effected through the WHO.[133]

Thus, it was national concerns that warranted international cooperation. As pathogens did not heed barbed wire, watchtowers and strictly enforced border patrols, the fear of the entry of attenuated viruses provided grounds for coordinated preventive measures across national boundaries.

The history of polio vaccination in Hungary shows that the mutual and rhetorically depoliticised goal of saving children from disability and death opened spaces in domestic and foreign policies on both sides of the Iron Curtain that legitimised actions contradicting contemporary political attitudes and processes. While political agendas and Cold War divisions pervade the story of polio vaccine development, polio prevention on the whole overrode Cold War politics to unite and coordinate efforts. Polio was not seen in the West as a Red virus, nor was it perceived in the East as an imperialist cancer on society or a disease to be 'contained'. Instead, it brought about the perception of a noble enterprise in an age when millions of children on both sides of the Iron Curtain were threatened by the crippling disease.

At the same time, the accomplishment came to serve as proof of the East's superiority in caring for its citizens in terms of healthcare and economic systems. Eastern Europeans used the success of the Sabin vaccine to empha-sise their cultural, economic and moral superiority over the West, especially the United States, embroiled in its market economy and racial segregation. The prospect of polio elimination, which became associated early on with live poliovirus vaccines, gained particular Cold War political meanings and stakes. The Sabin vaccine was (and still is) at its most potent when applied using this method. Free mass vaccination was a cherished symbol of universal healthcare in which Eastern European countries took pride, but, in some parts of the Western world, it was perceived as the devil itself. As David Oshinsky points out, health officials in the United States connected this system of prevention with socialised medicine, 'one of the great bugaboos of the Cold War era'.[134] In this reading, American resistance to widespread use of the Sabin vaccine when it first appeared can partly be traced back to healthcare ideology.

Leading Hungarian virologist Tibor Bakács remembers being puzzled as to why the United States had not switched to the Sabin vaccine, when socialist countries had already done so in 1959. He posed this question to Sabin himself

---

[133] Ibid. 44.   [134] Oshinsky, *Polio: An American Story*, 241.

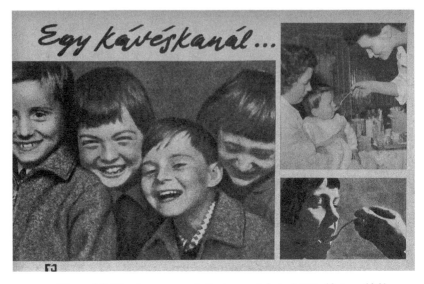

Figure 5.3 *'One teaspoon . . '. Feature article in A Hét, 18 June 1961, no. 25. 8. Credit: Arcanum Digitecha.* **This image is protected by copyright and cannot be used without further permissions clearance.**

when the professor was visiting the State Hygienic Institute in 1960. According to Bakács' memoir,

He gave a short, but thought-provoking answer: 'Sir! In the West vaccine production is mainly in private hands. These have, since 1954, since Salk has discovered his vaccine, been producing that with great capacity. They hoped to gain a huge profit from the production and distribution of this first, partially effective vaccine. Although my vaccine is more efficient, they do not produce it until there are significant Salk-vaccine supplies waiting to be sold. Until these are depleted, they will not start the mass production of the Sabin drops.' Only socialist countries chose to abandon their existing Salk-vaccine supplies. This is the reason why there were still big epidemics in the rich, Western countries in the 1960s.[135]

While Sabin's reply was most probably born out of frustration from a decade-long conflict with Jonas Salk and American funding bodies, and Bakács might have interpreted Sabin's words in a way that conformed to his own sentiments, the success of the Sabin vaccination in Hungary became a recurring example of the superiority of socialism. This narrative was reinforced by the government through newspapers as well.[136] Seven years after the

[135] Bakács, *Egy Életrajz Ürügyén*, 202.
[136] István Pintér, 'Salk És Sabin', *Népszabadság* 1959, 6–7; József Vető, 'A Sabin-Cseppek', ibid. 1960, 1.

vaccination began, Vilmos Kapos, director of the Budapest Public Health and Epidemiology Station, still felt it necessary to make a remark on the international significance of the Sabin vaccine in an internal party meeting in 1966:

> The social implications of the fight against epidemic diseases are demonstrated by the fact that while in socialist countries the occurrence of polio could be reduced to the minimum with the use of the free and effective Sabin vaccine, the results of capitalist countries, due to economic problems, do not come even close to this.[137]

The Hungarian success in polio vaccination was thus celebrated as the triumph of an entire system of political ideology, welfare and economic structure. It became the ultimate proof of the superiority of communist values and its system.

This ideological role of polio prevention was not unique to Hungary. Czechoslovakian scientists and public health officials chose to emphasise their own contribution to vaccine development and the role of the communist state in the project. Vilém Škovránek, Chief Hygienist, declared the achievement of the Czechoslovakian polio prevention strategy to be an evidence of good government: 'The success of the mass vaccination was a proof of the highly developed organising abilities of the Czechoslovak Ministry of Health and the profound understanding of our people for health problems. The vaccination campaign was accomplished without any particular troubles and the attendance of the population was very high.'[138]

Sabin vaccination thus became a particularly Eastern European project. It was through collaboration with Soviet, Czechoslovak and Hungarian virologists and public health officials that the vaccine became a powerful tool for polio prevention. As Viktor Zhdanov put it in his concluding remarks to the favourable evaluation of the Soviet field trials with the Sabin vaccine, 'a feature worthy of comment is the fruitful international cooperation on the problem of the live poliovirus vaccine ... on the basis of a wide exchange of scientific information, personal meetings, the exchange of the results of research work and mutual support'.[139] As an acknowledgement of his work

[137] Vilmos Kapos. 'Jelentés a Főváros Közegészségügyi Járványügyi Helyzetéről', Budapest: City Archives of Budapest, MSZMP Budapesti pártértekezletei 1957–1989, XXXV.1.a.2., 4. őe, 1966.
[138] V. Škovránek, 'The Organization and Results of Mass Vaccination against Poliomyelitis in CSSR', in *The Control of Poliomyelitis by Live Poliovirus Vaccine. Studies on Mass Vaccinations in Hungary, in the USSR, in Czechoslovakia and the German Democratic Republic. Papers Presented at the Hungarian-Soviet Medical Conference September 24–30, 1960*, ed. J. Weissfeiler (Budapest: Akadémiai Kiadó, 1961), 43.
[139] V. M. Zhdanov, M. P. Chumakov, and A. A. Smorodintsev, 'Large-Scale Practical Trials and Use of Live Poliovirus Vaccine in the U.S.S.R.', in *Live Poliovirus Vaccines: Papers Presented and Discussions Held at the Second International Conference on Live Poliovirus Vaccines* (Washington, D.C.: Pan American Health Organization, 1960), 576–88.587.

and collaboration with scientists in Hungary, Sabin was offered honorary membership in the Hungarian Academy of Sciences in 1965.[140] Since the late 1950s, Sabin has been seen as a great friend to the people and politics of Eastern Europe and, subsequently, his Americanness has diminished. The Sabin vaccine has been incorporated into Eastern European identity to the extent that today a number of Hungarians who grew up during the communist era believe that Sabin was in fact Russian.[141] Sabin himself was very cognisant of his vaccine being the product of international collaboration and the result of a global project, and emphasised the importance of working with colleagues across borders in interviews and talks upon his visit to Hungary in 1960.[142] He also used the story of his vaccine to champion reconciliation and urge the end of the Cold War in the 1980s with his article, 'Role of my cooperation with Soviet scientists in the elimination of polio: Possible lessons for relations between the U.S.A. and the U.S.S.R.'.[143]

The Eastern European-ness and the particular Cold War politics that the success of polio vaccination represented contributed to the erasure of this history on the Western side of the Iron Curtain, with a strong influence on current historiography and popular historical narratives. In Western narratives during the Cold War and in current historical analyses, Sabin's work is addressed mostly through his lifelong conflict and competition with Salk and his vaccine is considered to be undoubtedly American.[144] The intricate and thorough ways in which the development of the Sabin vaccine was an international project have mostly been written out of its history. Moreover, the Eastern European-ness of the Sabin vaccine disappeared altogether. In the official narrative represented by the Global Polio Eradication Initiative, for instance, it is in 1961 that 'Dr Albert Sabin develops a 'live' oral vaccine against polio (OPV), which rapidly becomes the vaccine of choice for most national immunization programmes in the world'.[145] By that time, polio epidemics had all but disappeared from several Eastern European countries through official national vaccination campaigns.

[140] István Árkus, 'Sabin Professzornak Átnyújtották a Magyar Tudományos Akadémia Tiszteleti Tagságáról Szóló Oklevelet', *Népszabadság* 1965, 4.
[141] Judit Juhász, interview by Dora Vargha, 26 October 2015.
[142] 'Albert Sabin Magyarországra Készül', *Népszabadság* 1960, 6; 'A Gyermekbénulás Elleni Küzdelemről Tárgyal a IX. Magyar-Szovjet Orvosi Konferencia', *Népszabadság* 1960, 6.
[143] Sabin, 'Role of My Cooperation with Soviet Scientists in the Elimination of Polio: Possible Lessons for Relations between the U.S.A. and the U.S.S.R.'
[144] Smallman-Raynor et al., *Poliomyelitis*; Paul, *A History of Poliomyelitis*; Charlotte DeCroes Jacobs, *Jonas Salk: A Life* (Oxford: Oxford University Press, 2015). While David Oshinsky does devote a whole chapter to Sabin's cooperation with Chumakov, vaccine development remains very much an 'American story' in his work. Oshinsky, *Polio: An American Story*.
[145] Global Polio Eradication Initiative, 'History of Polio', www.polioeradication.org/Polioandprevention/Historyofpolio.aspx.

Despite the erasure of the Eastern European history of live polio vaccine development, this socialist history should be taken into account when considering twentieth-century epidemics, international and global public health and eradication programmes. Countries like Hungary, Czechoslovakia and the Soviet Union were not only sites of scientific and technological innovation; just as in the West, virological work was embedded in a particular political ideology of what health was, who was responsible for it and how access to it should be distributed. Similarly to the ways in which particular American ideas played a substantive part in the development of and trials with the Salk vaccine, the Sabin vaccine itself is inseparable from the political, social and cultural context in which it was developed and tested in Eastern Europe. As we have seen in previous chapters, political decisions and scientific assessments regarding disease prevention shaped the development and introduction of the Sabin vaccine, and were based on experiences on a very local level. These socialist political and social structures, in turn, had a tremendous effect on the global polio eradication programme of the later twentieth and twenty-first centuries.

6   After the End of Polio

In 1963, Katalin Parádi meticulously arranged the patient files of polio patients. The girl who had emerged from a bomb shelter in 1956 to get to her physical therapy session and who had been sleeping on a makeshift bed in the early days of the Heine-Medin Hospital now had an important task to complete as polio epidemics drew to a close in Hungary. Having stayed in the hospital as an administrator, for weeks she took copies of each of the patient records, tracked down the address of every patient and sent the copies to their local health centre in the hope that at the other end a similarly meticulous administrative procedure would ensure the continued medical care of polio patients.[1] The Heine-Medin Hospital, as such, was closing down and being transformed into a general children's hospital. Polio was officially over and done with.

From as early as 1960, parents no longer needed to look for the reports on outbreaks on the back page of the newspaper, and children could freely seek relief from hot summer days in public pools and baths. In this 'second world' country with an economy of shortage, polio was, in technical terms, eradicated: not through an international programme, humanitarian aid or pressure from a superpower, but instead as something intrinsic to the country's self-identified socialist health system. The epidemic of 1959 proved to be the last in the country's history, and by the early 1960s, polio had all but disappeared from the epidemic reality of Hungary. As soon as 1962, journal articles were discussing in a matter-of-fact manner the fact that polio was no longer present in the country.[2] Between 1961 and 1990 a total of 66 new cases of polio were recorded in Hungary. Out of these cases, 56 were vaccine-derived paralytic polio (VAPP), one was an imported case and in four cases virological studies were not able to confirm the clinical diagnosis. This left five wild, domestic polio cases in the course of twenty-nine years, of which four were a cluster

---

[1] Parádi, interview by Vargha, 27 January 2010.
[2] Andor Bándi, 'A Folyamatos Oltásról', *Népegészségügy* 43, no. 5 (1962): 150–52, at 150.

outbreak in an isolated rural community in 1966 and the fifth, last case was recorded in 1969.[3]

Our story could end here as well, a dreaded epidemic going out with a bang. However, there is still much to tell about the era after the end of polio. The history of the disease in Hungary invites us to look further and reconsider the conventional take on the ways in which epidemics work. What happened to polio as a disease once it was over? What were the consequences of proclaiming the end of the disease on a global and local level? Where and for whom did polio end and who was excluded or forgotten?

What comes after the end of a disease is more often than not relegated to epilogues and usually comes up as an afterthought to the master narrative. Yet diseases are often imprinted on the bodies of survivors, societies and cultures. Epidemics may change economic structures and social interaction, and shape practices of international intervention and attitudes towards healthcare. In some cases, the proclaimed end of a disease leaves individuals or whole societies and states without resources previously guaranteed by the perceived epidemic threat. In others, the action of looking back after the end creates space for moral judgements on individuals, societies, governments and international organisations.

The course that the epidemic narrative runs is usually well-defined. Charles Rosenberg, in his classic paper, 'What is an epidemic?', stresses the episodic nature of epidemics and lays out the particular dramaturgy of the way epidemics take place. 'Epidemics start at a moment in time, proceed on a stage limited in space and duration, follow a plot line of increasing and revelatory tension, move to a crisis of individual and collective character, then drift toward closure.'[4] This narrative has been little contested since. Priscilla Wald, in a more recent work, *Contagious*, portrays a similar plotline for what she calls the outbreak narrative, which 'in its scientific, journalistic and fictional incarnations … follows a formulaic plot that begins with the identification of an emerging infection, includes discussion of the global networks throughout which it travels, and chronicles the epidemiological work that ends with its containment.'[5] While Wald's book takes important steps towards critically assessing the narrative by focusing on its consequences, stakes and cultural, scientific and political significance, the questions of how and when these narratives end are little raised. The end of the storyline in the case of epidemics and outbreaks, then, is successful containment. As such, the story of this book

[3] Elza Baranyai, 'Oltási Poliomyeitis', in *A Gyermekbénulás Elleni Küzdelem*, ed. Rezső Hargitai and Ákosné Kiss (Budapest: Literatura Medica, 1994), 162–68.

[4] Charles Rosenberg, 'What Is an Epidemic? AIDS in Historical Perspective', *Daedalus* 118, no. 2 (1989): 1–17.

[5] Priscilla Wald, *Contagious: Cultures, Carriers, and the Outbreak Narrative* (Durham, NC and London: Duke University Press, 2008), 2.

would end here, with dwindling numbers of polio cases and the disappearance of the disease.

Disability historians have been at the vanguard of moving past this narrative. As Catherine Kudlick pointed out in a recent paper on the survivors of smallpox, epidemics have a hidden history interwoven with disability and survival. Because of this, disability history has the potential to transform the way we understand the impact of epidemic disease, not just at the level of individual reactions but also at the level of social and political responses. By paying attention to survivors rather than mortality, Kudlick argues, we can reimagine epidemic scripts.[6] Along these lines, disability historians Daniel Wilson and Julie Silver's research on post-polio syndrome, oral history projects such as Polio's Legacy and memoirs point to the lingering presence of polio's imprint on bodies and societies and the resurfacing of a disease that ended long ago.[7]

Global health history can benefit noticeably from these perspectives and take the opportunity to broaden the scope of its study. By placing the 'after' into the centre of analysis, we can gain a more nuanced understanding of what epidemics are, the way we might study them and who and what gets left out of the master narrative of beginning, crisis and end. This shift of focus also highlights the narrative's shortcomings and the stakes at hand as epidemic narratives shape global and local health policies.

The Hungarian case shows us how *after* the abrupt *end* of polio, the *ending* of the disease became synonymous with particular vaccine choices and epidemic management programmes. The successful application of the Sabin vaccine in both virological and organisational terms in Hungary then became part of standardised global public health models and policies across the Iron Curtain, informing global polio eradication programmes well into the twenty-first century.

Polio, of course, did not end in Hungary, or elsewhere in the world. For the thousands of children (and adults) who had already contracted the disease, the success of the Sabin vaccine did not bring an end to their polio. It did bring the end of the state's investment of resources in their care, as specialised polio services were dispersed. Nor did people stop getting polio. While the Sabin

---

[6] Catherine Kudlick, 'Smallpox, Disability and Survival: Rewriting Paradigms from a New Epidemic Script', in *Disability Histories*, ed. Susan Burch and Michael Rembis (Urbana, Chicago and Springfield: University of Illinois Press, 2014), 185–200.

[7] J. K. Silver and Daniel J. Wilson, *Polio Voices: An Oral History from the American Polio Epidemics and Worldwide Eradication Efforts*, The Praeger Series on Contemporary Health and Living (Westport, Conn.: Praeger, 2007); Gary Presley, *Seven Wheelchairs: A Life beyond Polio* (Iowa City: University of Iowa Press, 2008); Edmund J. Sass, George Gottfried, and Anthony Sorem, *Polio's Legacy: An Oral History* (Lanham, Md.: University Press of America, 1996).

vaccine was particularly apt at eliminating disease on a population-wide scale, its drawback was the sporadic appearance of vaccine-derived paralytic cases. Some of these lingering effects of polio were integrated into the model of disease elimination, while others were mostly ignored. Hungary became particularly ideal for studying vaccine-derived polio and its effects on the population. The country, which was among the first to successfully control and eliminate polio, systematically used the same vaccination strategy and vaccine for over three decades and its internationally recognised experts published seminal works on the effects of vaccination that are still referenced in scientific publications today.

While vaccine-derived polio presented a problem for future vaccination strategies and the prospect of eradication, polio that had lingered, imprinted on the bodies of survivors, was often relegated to the realm of the past. As reminders of a bygone era of scientific uncertainties and failures in epidemic management, many people with polio found themselves pushed to the margins as funding for their care dwindled, practitioners specialising in polio care disappeared and polio was no longer a currency that could mobilise state and society. Furthermore, the unexpected survival of respiratory polio patients complicated the concept of the disease's end, as it blurred boundaries of human bodies, life, and medicine.

Polio as a disease changed drastically after epidemics ended. From an epistemic perspective, until the early 1960s, polio was a matter of virology and clinical medicine. The canon of both bodies of knowledge covered, explored and researched polio as a shared medical category. However, the clinical dimension was progressively eroded as the epidemic dimension of polio ceased to threaten the Hungarian and eventually broader populations. The knowledge of polio care was seldom discussed or further developed after the 1960s. International Poliomyelitis Conferences, with their rich discussions on both prevention and treatment, came to a stop in 1960. The European Association against Poliomyelitis integrated 'allied diseases' into its 8th Symposium programme in 1962 and meetings shifted from annual to sporadic, with the last one held in Bucharest on the epidemiology of polio in 1969.[8]

Discussions on post-polio syndrome altered this late twentieth- and early twenty-first-century perception of polio only slightly, and in limited ways. Post-polio syndrome as a term was coined in the early 1980s in the United States, as people who had contracted polio decades before began to experience

---

[8] European Association against Poliomyelitis and Allied Diseases, ed. *L'épidemiologie de la Poliomyelité. 12e Symposium, Bucharest, 4–7 May, 1969: Rapport et Discussions* (Buchuresti: Academiei Republicii Socialiste Romania, 1969); Porras, Báguena, and Ballester, 'Spain and the International Scientific Conferences on Polio.

symptoms once again. Medical research and lay activity in post-polio syndrome increased through the 1980s and 1990s, and has been declining since, most probably because the affected population is not replenished, as is the case with other chronic diseases.[9] North American experiences with post-polio syndrome point to the fact that polio as a complex disease with clinical manifestation has become a distant memory both on the individual and on the collective level. Through analyses of polio narratives, Amy Fairchild and Daniel Wilson have respectively argued that, for many, the onset of post-polio syndrome contested past experiences of conquering the disease, either through particular ideas of masculinity or through role models such as Franklin D. Roosevelt. The unexpected return of a disease experience and the frustrations it created has exposed the temporal situatedness of the meanings of polio.[10]

Despite the marked change in the meanings of the disease, polio as a global issue has remained strikingly stable since the 1950s. The particular political, social and scientific circumstances of the early Cold War that produced national and international public health programmes for preventing and treating polio may have changed over the decades, but the high priority given to the disease remained. In a way, this particular product of the Cold War outlived its own era and continues to shape global public health campaigns. Understanding these continuities and changes after the end of a disease is the focus of this chapter.

Global Significance: Eastern Europe's Role in Polio Eradication

The fact that Eastern European vaccination campaigns were successful was not lost on the international scientific community. Hungarian serological analyses and studies on vaccine-derived poliomyelitis in the decades following the end of polio in Hungary contributed to the understanding of the vaccine's risks and the refinement of its composition.[11] Moreover, successful mass vaccination campaigns with the Sabin vaccine, such as the Hungarian one, Cuba's campaigns in the 1960s and Brazil's in the 1970s came to serve as models for the current polio eradication programme.[12]

---

[9] Lauro S. Halstead, 'A Brief History of Postpolio Syndrome in the United States', *Archives of Physical Medicine and Rehabilitation* 92, no. 8 (2011): 1344–49.

[10] Fairchild, 'The Polio Narratives: Dialogues with FDR'; Wilson, *Living with Polio*.

[11] Paul E. M. Fine and Ilona A. M. Carneiro, 'Transmissibility and Persistence of Oral Polio Vaccine Viruses: Implications for the Global Poliomyelitis Eradication Initiative', *American Journal of Epidemiology* 150, no. 10 (1999): 1001–21; Victor M. Cáceres and Roland W. Sutter, 'Sabin Monovalent Oral Polio Vaccines: Review of Past Experiences and Their Potential Use after Polio Eradication', *Clinical Infectious Diseases* 33, no. 4 (2001): 531–41.

[12] Hull et al., 'Progress toward Global Polio Eradication'.

The beginnings of polio eradication are usually placed in the early 1980s following the success of the global eradication of smallpox in 1978.[13] While some veterans of the smallpox campaign, like Donald A. Henderson, argued against the launch of new global eradication programmes (and suggested 'eradicat[ing] the word eradication' instead),[14] the quest for the next disease to be globally eradicated began in 1980 at a conference held at the Fogarty International Centre, a research institute of the NIH near Washington D.C. Among the candidates were measles, schistosomiasis, yaws and poliomyelitis.[15] Through interviews and conference proceedings, historian William Muraskin tracks the emergence of polio as the ultimate candidate for eradication and suggests that the scientific community far from wholeheartedly supported the decision. Rather, it was a small group of eradicationists who pushed the agenda of polio eradication through to become a global health policy.[16] In 1988, the World Health Assembly passed a resolution to eradicate polio globally by the year 2000.[17] As of the completion of this book, the Global Polio Eradication Initiative is still an ongoing programme.

An Eastern European perspective shows, however, that polio came up as a potential object of eradication much earlier in global health politics. Soviet researchers Chumakov and Vorosilova already regarded the Sabin vaccine as a potential tool for global eradication during the phase of vaccine development, and in 1960 polio eradication became an object of serious consideration at the WHO. The concept of polio eradication was already then very much connected to smallpox eradication, although less directly than later on in the 1980s. The beginnings of smallpox eradication were tied to experiences of disease control in a socialist regime: upon the return of the Soviet Union to the World Health Organisation, it was Viktor Zhdanov, Deputy Minister of Health, who proposed the global eradication programme. Zhdanov based his proposal on smallpox control in the Soviet Union, where compulsory vaccination introduced by the revolutionary government in 1919 led to the elimination of the disease by 1936. As historian Erez Manela points out, disease control was one issue that

[13] William A. Muraskin, *Polio Eradication and its Discontents: An Historian's Journey through an International Public Health (Un)Civil War*, New Perspectives in South Asian History (New Delhi: Orient Blackswan, 2012); Nancy Stepan, *Eradication: Ridding the World of Diseases Forever?* (Ithaca, NY: Cornell University Press, 2011).
[14] D. A. Henderson, 'The Global Eradication of Smallpox: Historical Perspectives and Future Prospects', in *The Global Eradication of Smallpox*, ed. Sanjoy Bhattacharya and Sharon Messenger, New Perspectives in South Asian History (New Delhi: Orient Black Swan, 2010), 35.
[15] For the conference proceedings see Charles Stuart-Harris and Jr. DeWitt Stetten, 'Report on the International Conference on the Eradication of Infectious Diseases. Can Infectious Diseases Be Eradicated?', *Reviews of Infectious Diseases* 4, no. 5 (1982): 913–84.
[16] Muraskin, *Polio Eradication and Its Discontents*.
[17] The Forty-First World Health Assembly, 'WHA 41.28 Global Eradication of Poliomyelitis by the Year 2000' (Geneva: World Health Organization, 1988).

transcended the politics of avoiding international organisations from the early days of revolutionary Russia: the Soviet Union cooperated with the League of Nations in typhus control long before it actually joined the organisation.[18]

At the time of Zhdanov's proposal, eradication was all the rage in international public health. While efforts and ideas of eradication as absolute disease elimination can be traced back to the early twentieth century with yellow fever control,[19] eradicationism[20] took off on a global scale in the post-war era. The Malaria Eradication Programme, framed by Cold War ideas of development and Western powers' struggle against political revolution, was launched in 1955 by the WHO.[21]

It was in this international political and scientific context that the potential for eradication became a central feature of the Sabin vaccine. The WHO's Expert Committee on Poliomyelitis addressed polio eradication in more detail in their Third Report in 1960, under a section titled 'The concept of polio eradication'. After reviewing both inactivated and live virus polio vaccines, the committee stated that the possibility of eradication had emerged with the appearance of the oral vaccine.

The widespread use of potent inactivated vaccine may well lead to a substantial reduction in the numbers of cases of paralytic poliomyelitis but can do little to eliminate the causal virus from the gastro-intestinal tract of man. The possibility of eliminating poliovirus as a human pathogen has been brought much nearer by the development and application of live poliovirus vaccine. If such a goal is envisaged, the first step will be to effect the mass vaccination of the whole population, or at least of those age groups most susceptible to infection, by administration of attenuated viruses within a short period of time. Following this 'blanketing' with vaccine viruses, special studies will have to be conducted to determine the most feasible means of maintaining the resistance of the population.

The report called on more studies to explore the differences in behaviour of the virus under various climates, in different socio-economic groups and healthcare systems of various resources. Rather than an immediate plan of action, the expert committee raised the very real possibility of eradication as an avenue to pursue for the future.

The report drew its conclusions on available national experiences 'on an extensive or massive scale [in] the USSR, Poland, Czechoslovakia, Hungary,

[18] Erez Manela, 'A Pox on Your Narrative: Writing Disease Control into Cold War History', *Diplomatic History* 34, no. 2 (2010): 299–323.
[19] See Margaret Humphreys, *Yellow Fever and the South* (Baltimore, Md.: Johns Hopkins University Press, 1999).
[20] For more on eradicationism, see Stepan, *Eradication*.
[21] Packard, '"No Other Logical Choice": Global Malaria Eradication and the Politics of International Health in the Post-War Era'; Cueto, *Cold War, Deadly Fevers*; Siddiqi, *World Health and World Politics*.

certain Latin American countries, certain regions of Africa, and one area in the USA'.[22] Committee members acknowledged the magnitude of the project by declaring that 'this concept of complete eradication of poliomyelitis is a bold one and the whole problem is worthy of the closest study, not only in the field but also at the theoretical level'.[23]

The exploration of the possibility of polio eradication through studies did, in fact, begin very soon after the publication of the report. In a paper presented at a WHO training course on poliomyelitis control held in Prague in 1961, Vilém Škovránek, Czechoslovakian Minister of Health, asserted that experiences with nationwide mass vaccination campaigns with the Sabin vaccine 'justify the conclusion that in this way we shall also be able to approach most closely and most rapidly the ideal results of vaccination with live attenuated polio-viruses, i.e. the eradication of poliomyelitis'. This use of the eradication concept was much more than an empty reference to a fashionable idea of the era. In what followed, Skovranek gave a detailed description of what was required in terms of epidemiological data collection, virological examinations, rapid vaccine administration, health services and public communication for what he referred to as the 'final success'.[24]

Given the discussions among virologists from the late 1950s onwards, the WHO report and detailed plans to study the method with which polio eradication would be possible, it is striking that some twenty years later the disappearance of polio as a result of vaccination with the Sabin vaccine would be 'largely unpredicted', 'never expected' or 'a surprise' to some American researchers.[25] One explanation for this could be the limits of internationalism in public health in the Cold War, explored in the previous chapter. While, as we will see below, Eastern European experiences, methods and expertise were actively drawn upon in devising eradication strategies, at the same time they could have been rendered invisible as valid projections or theoretical consider-ations by Cold War politics. Where disease control opened one gap in the Iron Curtain, Cold War concepts closed another.

Not only did the idea of polio eradication itself emerge in the late 1950s and early 1960s, but so did criticism of the notion. Alongside enthusiasm for the possibility of ridding the world of polio, the idea was also contested in this golden age of eradicationism. Critical voices were already emerging at the

[22] Expert Committee on Poliomyelitis, 'Expert Committee on Poliomyelitis. Third Report', 51.
[23] Ibid. 30.
[24] Vilém Škovránek, 'Principles of Organization of Vaccination with Live Vaccine with Particular Reference to the Experience Assembled in Czechoslovakia. In Letter from Skovranek, Vilem to Sabin, Albert B. Dated 1961-05-13.' Cincinnatti: Albert B. Sabin Archives, Hauck Center for the Albert B. Sabin Archives, 1961, Correspondence, Unsorted, Box 02, File 04 (1961), 1961.
[25] Neal Nathanson cited by Muraskin, *Polio Eradication and Its Discontents*, 11.

beginning of the process, and some questioned whether polio eradication was a good idea at all:

Let us remember in all our discussions that the development of attenuated poliovirus vaccines was originally stimulated by the need to prevent paralytic poliomyelitis in North America. In many parts of the world poliomyelitis is both relatively and absolutely less important. It would be a pity in our enthusiasm to rid the world of poliomyelitis if in some countries we encourage a demand for poliovirus vaccines in preference for measures for preventing other diseases of greater economic and human importance.[26]

These words of 1960, from David Dane of the University of Belfast, might ring familiarly to our ears today. After an unsuccessful trial with the Koprowski vaccine, Dane became a staunch critic of live polio vaccines. His observations have not lost currency over the decades, however. Many critics of the global polio eradication programme have raised similar issues about the money and resources spent on the eradication of a disease that might not be high on the public health agenda for many societies.

At the same time, the elimination and possible eradication of polio took hold. The success of certain national strategies in the 1960s and 1970s became blueprints for the global polio eradication programme later in the twentieth century. Countries that had been among the first to eliminate polio and were consistently using and refining the same vaccination method were particularly suited for contributing to a model of polio eradication. Hungary thus, in several ways, became one of the cornerstones in shaping global polio eradication.

From the initial mass vaccination onwards, immunisation with the Sabin vaccine in Hungary continued to be executed in annual mass campaigns, maintaining the model of the first one: with monovalent vaccines (containing one strain each, Type I, followed by III, then II), each administered on a national scale to children between 2 months and 3 years of age, within a week, four to six weeks apart. The mass campaigns were organised in the winter months to avoid conflict with wild enteroviruses, which might interfere with immunity.[27] The Hungarian mass vaccination based its method on previous

---

[26] Dick and Dane, 'The Evaluation of Live Poliovirus Vaccines. Paper Presented at the Conference on Live Poliovirus Vaccines, Washington, 22–26 June 1959', in Who/Polio/36–44, at 12.

[27] Instead, it was influenza outbreaks in the winter that disrupted Sabin campaigns; therefore in 1977 the annual campaigns were pushed back to the autumn. Hungary conducted mass vaccination campaigns with the Sabin vaccine until 1992, when the vaccination method was modified and the country switched back to the inactivated vaccine. Since then, children in Hungary have been receiving polio vaccine in the form of a combined vaccine as part of their routine immunization. István Dömök, 'A Kampányoltások Időszaka', in A Gyermekbénulás Elleni Küzdelem, ed. Rezső Hargitai and Ákosné Kiss (Budapest: Literatura Medica, 1994), 169–78, at 175. Concepción F. Estívariz et al., 'Paralytic Poliomyelitis Associated with Sabin Monovalent and Bivalent Oral Polio Vaccines in Hungary', American Journal of Epidemiology 174, no. 3 (2014): 316–25.

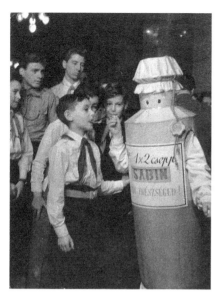

Figure 6.1 *János Jakus's postcard to Albert Sabin, 24 September 1960.*
Poliomyelitis, International Cooperation, Hungary 1959–60. Box 12. File
3.5, University of Cincinnati. Hauck Center for the Albert B. Sabin Archives.
This image is protected by copyright and cannot be used without further
permissions clearance.

field trials, most importantly the Soviet and Czechoslovakian trials. While in
the former, Soviet virologists used both monovalent and trivalent vaccines
(containing all three strains), in the trial campaigns, their Czechoslovakian
colleagues applied monovalent vaccines exclusively, each four weeks apart.[28]
By 1960, Albert Sabin referred to the monovalent vaccination at intervals of
four to six weeks as being 'regarded as optimum during the cold months of the
year in temperate zones'.[29]

Similarly to state socialist countries in Eastern Europe, the new revolutionary state in Cuba placed emphasis on the prevention of communicable

---

[28] M. P. Chumakov et al., 'Preliminary Report on Mass Oral Immunization of Population against
Poliomyelitis with Live Virus Vaccine from A.B. Sabin's Attenutated Strains', in *Live Poliovirus Vaccines: Papers Presented and Discussions Held at the First International Conference
on Live Poliovirus Vaccines* (Washington, D.C.: Pan American Sanitary Bureau, 1959),
517–29; V. Skovránek et al., 'Field Trial with Sabin's Live Poliovirus Vaccine in Czechoslovakia 1958–1959', ibid.

[29] Albert B. Sabin et al., 'Live, Orally Given Poliovirus Vaccine. Effects of Rapid Mass Immunization on Population under Conditions of Massive Enteric Infection with Other Viruses',
JAMA, no. 173 (1960): 1521–26, at 1521.

diseases, paired with the health education of the public.[30] The polio vaccination programme is perhaps the most well-known campaign of this time. National mass vaccination with the Sabin vaccine was adopted in Cuba in 1962, with active Eastern European participation, and Hungarian newspapers kept an eye on the process.[31] The vaccine arrived from the Soviet Union and Karel Zacek, a Czechoslovakian polio expert, provided support on-site in serological studies and establishing the surveillance system.[32] The Czechoslovak expert assessed incident rates in different age groups, and studied the seasonality of the disease. The vaccination programme was then designed with his recommendations in mind, immunising the population between the age of 1 month and 15 years, with the Sabin trivalent vaccine.[33] Zacek also participated in the organisation of the vaccination campaign. He held national and regional lectures on the disease and the oral polio vaccine for health professionals and zone directors, who in turn trained vaccinators, health brigade members and social organization members.[34]

Cuba became the first populous country to eradicate wild poliovirus in the Western Hemisphere.[35] Cuban experiences then became the basis for Latin American National Immunisation Days in the subsequent decades. A notable case in Latin American polio eradication was the introduction of National Immunisation Days (NIDs) in Brazil, which influenced global strategies significantly. Brazil had introduced national immunisation with the Sabin vaccine in 1973, which started with mass vaccinations and was integrated into routine vaccination programmes soon after. However, after an outbreak in 1979 prompted national authorities to change strategy, they introduced 'blanket' vaccination campaigns to be conducted in a short period of time, twice a year.[36] Similarly to the Hungarian case, the Brazilian military regime saw an opportunity in the introduction of a national polio prevention campaign to legitimate its rule, which had been marked by political and economic crises at the time.[37]

---

[30] P. Sean Brotherton, *Revolutionary Medicine: Health and the Body in Post-Soviet Cuba*, ed. Michael M. J. Fischer and Joseph Dumit, Experimental Futures: Technological Lives, Scientific Arts, Anthropological Voices (Durham Duke University Press, 2012), 69.

[31] 'A Gyermekbénulás Elleni Oltást Latin-Amerikában Elsőnek Kubában Vezetik Be', *Népszabadság* 1962, 6; 'Intézkedések Kubában a Gyermekbénulás Megelőzésére', *Népszabadság* 1962, 6.

[32] P. Más Lago, 'Eradication of Poliomyelitis in Cuba: A Historical Perspective', *Bulletin of the World Health Organization* 77, no. 8 (1999): 681–87.

[33] Beldarraín, 'Poliomyelitis and Its Elimination in Cuba: An Historical Overview'.

[34] Ibid. 34.

[35] Smallman-Raynor et al., *Poliomyelitis. A World Geography: Emergence to Eradication*, 519.

[36] Nascimento, 'Poliomyelitis Vaccination Campaigns in Brazil Resulting in the Eradication of the Disease (1961–1994)'.

[37] André Luiz Vieira de Campos, Dilene Raimundo do Nascimento, and Eduardo Maranhão, 'A História Da Poliomielite No Brasil E Seu Controle Por Imunização', *História, Ciencias, Saúde-Manguinhos* 10, no. Suppl. 2 (2003): 573–600.

NIDs as tools of polio control soon spread to Nicaragua, the Dominican Republic and other parts of Latin America. Seen as a success, the Pan American Health Organisation announced a plan of action in 1985, calling on all American countries where polio was endemic to institute NIDs by 1990.[38] The method of mass vaccination with the Sabin vaccine was then adopted by China in the early 1990s and, based on the campaign's success there, was extended to the Western Pacific region of the WHO.[39]

Experiences with the Hungarian, Cuban and Brazilian vaccination programmes thus became the basis for the eradication strategy recommended by the WHO, notably that children under 5 years were to be immunised on National Immunisation Days in two rounds, four to six weeks apart.[40] One crucial element seems to stand out from the models used in the Global Polio Eradication Initiative well into the twenty-first century: all were implemented by so-called authoritarian regimes. As the concerns surrounding the development and safety of the Sabin vaccine show, Cold War rhetoric and stereotypes regarding political systems played crucial roles in the global evaluation of the Sabin vaccine. Preoccupation with authoritarian political systems in public health management was not new. As early as 1948, at the First International Poliomyelitis Conference, leading British orthopaedist Herbert J. Seddon reflected on the status of polio at the crossroads of the post-war trauma and the progressing Cold War:

At the present time there is more than enough dictatorship in the world and we do not want to add to it. Yet there is no doubt that the cheapest and best way of dealing with poliomyelitis is to have organizations in readiness headed by men of acknowledged competence, who, for a limited time, are permitted a very large measure of authority.[41]

Seddon had every reason for phrasing the dilemma with caution. It was only very recently that Nazi Germany had applied the rhetoric and practice of control and eradication to disease and people, connecting medicine and epidemic management with genocide, as historian Paul Weindling has argued.[42] The rise of the Stalinist Soviet Union and the unfolding Cold War did nothing to appease the very real concerns over authoritarianism and disease control.

---

[38] Jean-Marc Olivé, Joao Baptista Risi, and Ciro A. de Quadros, 'National Immunization Days: Experience in Latin America', *The Journal of Infectious Diseases* 175, no. Suppl. 1 (1997): 189–93.
[39] Stepan, *Eradication: Ridding the World of Diseases Forever?*, 238.
[40] G. J. Ebrahim, 'Polio Eradication, and After. . .', *Revista Brasileira de Saúde Materno Infantil* 2, no. 2 (2002), 189–91; Harry F. Hull et al., 'Progress toward Global Polio Eradication', *Journal of Infectious Diseases* 175, no. Supplement 1 (1997): S4–S9.
[41] Herbert J. Seddon, 'Economic Aspects of the Management of Poliomyelitis', in *First International Poliomyelitis Conference* (New York: Lippincott, 1948), 35.
[42] Paul Weindling, *Epidemics and Genocide in Eastern Europe, 1890–1945* (Oxford and New York: Oxford University Press, 2000).

The merit of certain autocratic measures in successfully preventing or treating disease and its increasing connection with Cold War ideas of democracy and autocratic rule became a recurring issue in the history of polio. It played a crucial part in the evaluation of the Sabin vaccine's potency and safety based on the early and massive trials conducted in the Soviet Union by Dorothy Horstmann. Cold War stereotypes and frustrations with autocratic measures persisted until the end of the disease. After their success in actually eliminating polio quickly and effectively, Eastern European and Latin American methods transitioned into models used worldwide, seemingly without many problems, deliberations or concerns.

The models of Hungary and Cuba continued to be used in global polio eradication campaigns in other ways. The mass vaccination campaigns of these countries not only proved to be highly efficient in suddenly ending polio, but the vaccination method, along with the vaccines, continued to be constant for decades. This stability was partly guaranteed by the political system in these countries and has been drawn upon for research on polio eradication well into the twenty-first century. Moreover, once polio epidemics ended and the disease became a rarity, the monitoring system seems to have functioned reliably. This was most probably the achievement of internationally acclaimed virologist István Dömök, who started working at the virology department of the State Hygienic Institute of Hungary in 1961 and was the organisation's director from 1973 onwards. Furthermore, the rarity of polio in Hungary after 1960 permitted a system where all suspect cases could be treated centrally, and thus monitored and assessed more easily.

One of the biggest challenges for polio eradication with live poliovirus vaccines has been the presence of vaccine-associated paralytic polio (VAPP) from vaccine-derived poliovirus (VDPV), discussed in more detail in the previous chapter. As mentioned earlier, polio cases did not disappear in Hungary after the end of outbreaks: over three decades, dozens of vaccinated children became paralysed by polio contracted from the vaccine. The rate of VAPP in Hungary was high in international terms: almost seven to eight times as high as in the United States and almost three times as high as in East Germany.[43]

The country's virological and public health history thus became terrain for study in the late twentieth and early twenty-first centuries when collecting information for the endgame of the global polio eradication programme and attempting to solve the dilemma of OPVs, which were both best suited for eradication and the only tools through which polioviruses could not disappear

---

[43] Estívariz et al., 'Paralytic Poliomyelitis Associated with Sabin Monovalent and Bivalent Oral Polio Vaccines in Hungary'.

from the world. As Victor Cáceres of the CDC and Roland Sutter of the WHO Polio Eradication Campaign put it:

[T]he best data on VAPP caused by MOPV comes from Hungary, where these strains have been used the longest. Dömök described the experience in Hungary where for >20 years MOPV had been delivered through biannual mass campaigns to children between 2 and 38 months of age. These campaigns effectively eliminated indigenous transmission of wild poliovirus. Hungary had maintained an excellent surveillance system for poliomyelitis since 1966, requiring that every patient with suspected polio-myelitis be admitted to the Central Hospital for Infectious Diseases in Budapest, for thorough clinical and laboratory evaluation. Therefore, in Hungary there existed these unique conditions: (1) a largely susceptible birth cohort; (2) absence of 'confounding' protection from previous exposure to wild poliovirus strains; and (3) an excellent surveillance system.[44]

Reviewing Hungarian vaccination data and VAPP cases became important once again after 2005, as the Global Polio Eradication Initiative moved away from trivalent OPV (Sabin vaccine containing all three poliovirus strains) to monovalent (containing one strain) and bivalent (containing two strains) vaccines. Wild poliovirus Type II disappeared from circulation in 1999, and the Global Commission for the Certification of Poliomyelitis Eradication announced its global eradication. Since monovalent and bivalent (containing Type I and Type III) were found to have higher efficacy, the GPEI started shifting to the use of these vaccines.[45] The question now was the risk of monovalent polio vaccines causing VAPP. Since the monovalent Sabin vac-cine had been used in Hungary from 1961 through 1991, a team of researchers from the CDC, WHO, Bill and Melinda Gates Foundation and Hungarian public health institutes analysed Hungarian historical epidemiological and virological data, along with that of other Eastern European countries and the former Soviet Union, to assess the risks of monovalent vaccine use in the twenty-first century.[46]

The fact that the country was among the first to introduce a national mass vaccination programme, along with the abrupt end of polio that the campaign brought, the consistent use of the same vaccination method and a surveillance system that was considered to be reliable, meant that Hungary became a model for polio eradication, both in exploring potential problems, such as VAPP and VDPV, and in providing a method for efficient disease control. This model, as we will see, was restrictive. With the end of polio in Hungary, focus on

---

[44] Cáceres and Sutter, 'Sabin Monovalent Oral Polio Vaccines: Review of Past Experiences and Their Potential Use after Polio Eradication'.
[45] Chris Maher, interview by Dóra Vargha, 2012.
[46] Estívariz et al., 'Paralytic Poliomyelitis Associated with Sabin Monovalent and Bivalent Oral Polio Vaccines in Hungary'.

medicine, public health and state services shifted to prevention, which soon became the exclusive point of engagement with what was a complex disease.

Local Consequences: Endings from Below

With no new polio cases in Hungary, in 1963, just seven years after it was established, the Heine-Medin Hospital was turned into a general children's hospital. Polio patients were sent home, and the staff were retrained or disbanded. It was as Katalin Parádi had feared: the majority of patient files she had so carefully prepared were lost in the administrative jumble of state socialist Hungary.

This lack of access to their own medical history made life difficult for many children growing up with polio, since the details of their previous surgeries, orthopaedic needs and prescriptions were all lost. Fortunately, Katalin had the foresight to keep the originals in the archives of the new hospital, where she continued to work, and she was happy to make further copies for anyone who requested. This did not help the majority, some of whom were treated in other institutions and many of whom probably did not know about the central archive of records. Furthermore, access to these archives ceased long before the need for them ended: when Katalin Parádi retired, she lost control over the boxes that contained the patient files.[47] The files disappeared, leaving patients struggling with post-polio syndrome in a difficult position.

What happened to the patient files is unclear. Current hospital staff say that they were moved to a mouldy basement that is now hazardous to health and is closed off from public use. According to archivist rumour, the basement, also known as the 'spidery', is not hazardous, but records are not there. Perhaps they were destroyed during an administrative takeover of old hospital buildings in the post-socialist era. The fate of the files once more demonstrates the disorganization and ineffectiveness that coexisted with centralized and efficient structures within the socialist state, even within the sphere of public health.

The ways in which the proclaimed end of a disease can be exclusionary and the ways certain people are left out of the narrative come to light through the story of Hungarian polio survivors. As vaccination with the Sabin vaccine put an end to polio epidemics, the state lost interest in polio on the whole, treatment centres were dismantled, and the medical and educational care of children with polio withered away. As the state pulled away from polio – a disease that no longer threatened its population – patients whose lives were untouched by the benefits of vaccination found their care to be

---

[47] Parádi, interview by Vargha, 27 January 2010.

determined more by their geographic location and social status than ever before. Many children returned to their families; those with the financial means could continue physical therapy in their homes. Others, who did not have families or whose families could not or did not want to care for them, continued living in secluded institutions. Some of these children were abandoned when they were first diagnosed with polio, while others could not return to their parents, who lived in excessive poverty and often worked long hours as day labourers.[48]

Perhaps the most striking change that the end of polio caused was in the lives of children left in institutions, partly because of the excessive poverty of their families. A large group of institutionalised children with polio no longer received medical treatment. Since the state did not allocate an adequate building for their care, the large group of children was shuffled from institution to institution across the country. Similarly to the Romanian practice of housing disabled children, these sites were often castles and palaces once owned by the aristocracy. The buildings were usually in a derelict state, having been used as warehouses or stables by passing armed forces during the war. These sites were far from cities, and their location contributed to the exclusion and neglect experienced by some of the children.[49] Remembering this time, some former patients jokingly called this part of their lives the 'travelling circus'.[50]

Their life was partly determined by the location where they ended up each year. Although living in seclusion, the children forged lifelong friendships, attended beat concerts, sneaked out to parties and, in their teenage years, to each other's rooms for romantic or sexual encounters. Some institutions were worse than others: of the years of travelling year after year 'from border to border' in uncertainty,[51] the most traumatic memory was their stay in a mental asylum. Here, the children shared corridors with adult mental patients who were often restrained and 'screamed at night'.[52]

This structuring, or rather un-structuring, of polio care was a huge break with the paternalistic practice of centrally organised, institutional social and medical care. Access to specialised care ceased for children living outside the capital. Delegating specialist care to local district general practitioners, who often lacked the funds, time or expertise to care for children with polio, as well as the complete lack of any medical care in the depository institutions, deprived children of important and significant resources that had been

---

[48] Franciska Kormos, *Magánkeringő* (Budapest: Aposztróf Kiadó, 2010).
[49] Maria Roth, 'Child Protection in Communist Romania (1944–1989)', in *Social Care under State Socialism (1945–1989). Ambitions, Ambiguities and Mismanagement*, ed. Sabine Hering (Opladen and Farmington Hills: Barbara Budrich Publishers, 2009), 201–11.
[50] Julianna Bedő, Tamás Kertész and Tibor Szabó, 'Interview', Hévíz 2010.
[51] Kormos, *Magánkeringő*, 107.
[52] Bedő, Kertész and Szabó, 'Interview'. Also see Kormos, *Magánkeringő*.

available to them before polio ended. The absence of children with polio in visual representations, paired with their absence from society due to the seclusion of their treatment, then took on an even greater invisibility. Polio patients disappeared from the concerns of state healthcare and from the pages of medical journals. Their care was no longer organised and their needs – medical, social, emotional and material – were not addressed.

The end of polio in Hungary also contributed to the end of knowledge about the disease. Polio treatment was no longer taught in medical schools. Since most physicians and physical therapists who practised in the 1950s and early 1960s have died, knowledge of polio treatment can be found in a handful of publications collecting dust in the depths of the National Library of Hungary. This problem is not a local one: a recent American and British study on polio survivors notes that 'the vast majority of physicians and other healthcare professionals working in developed countries in the post-vaccine era have never encountered a case of polio and thus often lack experience and understanding of the treatment and long-term pathology of the disease'.[53]

Through interviews with people living with polio, however, it has become clear that knowledge about treatment has not entirely disappeared. Rather, its site has changed: it is the patients themselves, many battling post-polio syndrome, who are in possession of medical knowledge regarding their own treatment. They know the exact equipment (e.g. shoes, crutches, braces) they need, and some have a very clear idea of exactly what corrective surgery their limbs require. Yet the expertise and prescriptions of primary care physicians and specialists are needed for their special equipment, vouchers for physical therapy and operations. Accepting complete authority in treatment from patients is often problematic for many doctors, and some patients have recounted bitter battles with physicians and surgeons over the course of action to be taken. Others have had more positive encounters, where their expertise on polio was acknowledged and the physician was ready to take notes from them. But polio patients themselves sometimes do not have much information about their own condition. Many were small children at the time of their operations and treatment, and since many of the patient records have been lost or are unrecoverable, they have no access to knowledge of the kinds of medical interventions they were exposed to. Most polio patients first learned about post-polio syndrome at a polio convention in 2010, through translations of American brochures.

In this sense, the end of polio in Hungary is a case in agnotology: the cultural production of ignorance and forgetting, as Robert Proctor and Londa

---

[53] Nora Ellen Groce, Lena Morgon Banks, and Michael Ashley Stein, 'Surviving Polio in a Post-Polio World', *Social Science & Medicine* 107, April (2014): 171–78, at 174.

Schiebinger have described.[54] Medical knowledge and practice of the disease did not vanish because there was no need for it anymore. The elimination of polio from the country did not directly change the condition of patients who already had the disease, but it did eliminate polio from the priorities of health and population policies. Through this elimination, polio patients, their bodies and the scientific knowledge their treatment required became invisible in the eyes of the state, the public and the medical profession. Polio patients kept on living after the end of polio, a life that was now mostly determined by a disease that was no more.

One group of patients was *not* expected to keep on living, though.

Some patients – children and adults alike – saved from death by suffocation with the help of long-term mechanical ventilation during the acute phase of poliomyelitis could not be freed from the use of respirators later on either, due to the paralysis of respiratory muscles. It is through them that we could learn the concept and reality of chronic respiratory paralysis – a human condition. Our aim here is to describe this new human life form.

This is how the head of the Hungarian respiratory ward begins her habilitation thesis titled 'The fate of polio patients with respiratory paralysis kept alive by long-term mechanical ventilation'. The objects of her study were people living in or with respiratory machinery like iron lungs for decades after the epidemics of the 1950s.[55]

Since the lives of patients with respiratory paralysis were physically bound to heavy machinery, the Heine-Medin Hospital's iron lung ward was the only one that remained primarily focused on polio care after 1963. For the next few decades, access to continuous care in the framework of the socialist healthcare system, paired with lack of resources, created a community in the respiratory ward that challenged concepts of childhood, families and conventions in terms of medical knowledge and caretaker roles. Medical staff assumed parental duties, nurses worked with highly specialised medical knowledge and also doubled as technicians and children became active participants in shaping their own treatment.

In a setting where the provider role of the state overrode individual responsibilities for health and care, there was no pronounced goal of integrating respiratory polio patients in society and sending them home. Medical care was free and institutionalised. There was no financial incentive for the families of patients for home care, which would have required significantly more funds and constant family member care. Moreover, the ideology of state paternalism,

[54] Robert Proctor and Londa L. Schiebinger, *Agnotology: The Making and Unmaking of Ignorance* (Stanford, Calif.: Stanford University Press, 2008).
[55] Dr Kiss, 'Tartós Gépi Lélegeztetéssel Életben Tartott Postpoliós Légzésbénultak Sorsa'.

which significantly formed medical treatment at this time, further contributed to the lifelong hospital stay of many of these patients.

This institutionalisation also meant that the children, and later adults, who spent their lives connected to respiratory machines were viewed almost exclusively through a medical and scientific lens. The community of iron lung and respiratory patients was constantly observed by the staff, occasionally by sociologists, and their lives were the focus of medical publications and psychological studies.[56] The bodies of the patients and their coexistence with intricate machinery were perceived in terms of infections, complications, possible malfunctions and endangerment by power outages and were managed with further technological interventions such as suctioning and measuring (level of oxygen content, temperature, muscle activity, etc.). At the same time, the social and emotional care of the patients, from combing their hair to reading to them, as well as resolving conflict among room-mates over the use of the radio, also became part of the everyday tasks of the medical staff.[57] Respiratory patients thus transformed the professions of their carers. Nurses became highly skilled technicians, who could fix the machines on a whim, but also provided social and emotional work. Physicians had to reconsider their roles and their ideas of healing, as the management of these chronic patients excluded the possibility of improvement.[58] Chronic care ended with the death of the patients, many of whom had spent their entire lives from early infancy as objects of medical attention – eternal patients.

Living with respiratory technology was a wholly new experience for patients and physicians alike: 'There was no medical precedent for this. As far as we knew, these children could live one, two or three years in iron lungs or other respiratory devices', remarked the director of the ward.[59] As time went by, it became clear that these children would not only survive for a few years, but would also actually grow up with the help of respiratory technology. Thus, the concept of a 'new human life form' was created, one that did not exist without machines.

Medical professionals and parents alike were unprepared for what was to come, since nobody really knew what was to come at all. Bodies that could not be separated from machinery, at least not for a significant time, and could not exist without mechanical breathing, blurred the boundaries between machine

---

[56] Anna László, *Vaspólya* (Budapest: Szépirodalmi könyvkiadó, 1979); Ákosné Kiss, 'Légzésbénult Utókezelő Osztályon Szerzett Tapasztalataink', in *Előadások a Gyermekbénulás Rehabilitációs Problémáiról*, ed. László Lukács (Budapest: Statisztikai Kiadó, 1961), 47–53; Dr. Kiss, 'Tartós Gépi Lélegeztetéssel Életben Tartott Postpoliós Légzésbénultak Sorsa'.
[57] László, *Vaspólya*.
[58] Dr. Kiss, 'Tartós Gépi Lélegeztetéssel Életben Tartott Postpoliós Légzésbénultak Sorsa', 1989; Mészáros, interview by Vargha, 11 January 2008.
[59] Ádám Csillag, 'Gyermekbénulás II', Csillag és Ádám Film; Fórum Film, Hungary, 1995.

and man, but also between the bodies of the patients and the bodies of others. Since many of the patients were completely paralysed, every activity required another, mobile body – that of a nurse, a doctor, a relative or a visitor. The boundary between body and machine and the concept of life itself became extended to and inseparable from other bodies and lives.

This 'new life form' also challenged ideas of the life cycle.[60] At first, expected to last no more than a few weeks or months, life turned into years, extending without expectation, ending at various times. There was no 'life expectancy' set for these patients. Some lived to 60, others died from complications of minor surgery at the age of 20. The lack of a foreseeable life cycle also blurred the concepts of childhood and adulthood and questioned its definitions. Respiratory patients and physicians directing their everyday lives had different ideas about their life cycle. As respiratory polio patients got older, more and more frustrations arose in the ward. Patients complained about the strict regulation of their lives, from the use of the telephone line to their decisions about their preferences of consumption, while physicians complained about patients' disregard for their own medical conditions and their pestering of the medical staff.[61] The increasing conflict in the ward and frustration on both sides (patients and carers) points to different definitions and perceptions of where childhood ends, where adulthood begins and what adulthood, independence and decision-making means at all, for those who in life and body were extended and entangled.

In sum, the life form of iron lung patients raised questions about the definitions of human life. They contested boundaries – of bodies, machines, medicine and care, life cycles. As they were unprecedented, they also revealed the preoccupation with the upcoming unknown. In the post-war context of the terrible experience of dehumanisation in the recent past on the one hand, and a strong belief in the technological and scientific progress of the future on the other, the issue of terming polio patients living with respiratory technology new life forms is an important one.

Respiratory patients in this sense were not seen as disabled, but as humans who could not be fitted into the concept of human life as it was known. This

---

[60] Sophia Roosth and Stefan Helmreich in their article 'Life forms: A Key Word Entry' provide an analysis of the term and concept through two centuries. They describe a shift in the twentieth century in the meaning of the term from archetype to future types. Life forms become relegated to the realm of science fiction and of the future. While Roosth's and Helmreich's work focuses on the term in English language and its German origins, their observations can be useful in thinking about iron lung patients in other linguistic and cultural contexts. In the case of Hungarian respiratory patients life form was at once a present challenge, due to the cutting edge technology a stuff of science fiction, and a constant reflection on the future. Life in this form was re-evaluated and constantly gained new meanings. Sophia Roosth and Stefan Helmreich, 'Life Forms: A Keyword Entry', *Representations* 112, no. 1 (2010): 27–53.

[61] László, *Vaspólya*.

perception could simultaneously be liberating and highly discriminating. By
being termed as 'new life forms', polio patients as hybrids and cyborgs were,
at least at times, free to bend boundaries and set up whole new rules and laws
governing their own and their extensions' lives. However, the demarcation
between us and them also had grave and long-lasting consequences. Perceived
as profoundly different, patients found themselves excluded from any effort at
integration, be it finding a job, establishing a family or choosing their friends.
One patient, after earning a degree in philosophy, had to make a living by
assembling flashlight key rings. A female patient had to endure remarks from
strangers while in labour about why 'these' (not even people, not things) had to
reproduce themselves. A third patient, at the age of 50, still dreamt of becoming an engineer one day.[62]

A Civil Movement in State Socialism

Former polio patients are very much aware of the effect that the end of the
disease has had on them and society. They widely refer to themselves as
'dinosaurs, a breed that is about to become extinct'.[63] While usually spoken
in jest, this recognition of being among the last in society with the condition
is also paired with a sense of pride at belonging to a unique community.
There is reason enough for this pride, since in the early 1980s former polio
patients achieved the unthinkable in state socialism: the organisation of a
civil society that was not initiated or co-opted by the state, nor based on
political dissent.

As Eastern European disability scholars, such as Elena Iarskaia-Smirnova
and Michael Rasell, have pointed out, historical accounts of Eastern European
disabled persons have mostly discussed disability in terms of oppression and
neglect and rarely considered disabled people as active agents.[64] Even fewer
have connected disability to civil society in the Eastern Bloc.[65] Histories of
activism and grassroots organisation in Eastern Europe have exclusively
focused on political dissent, and most often on its intersections with culture:
from broader discussions of intellectual self-organisation[66] to taking samizdat
(underground publishing) and tamizdat (publishing abroad) as a starting

---

[62] Csillag, 'Gyermekbénulás II'.   [63] Bedő, Kertész, and Szabó, 'Interview'.
[64] Michael Rasell and Elena Iarskaia-Smirnova, *Disability in Eastern Europe and the Former Soviet Union: History, Policy and Everyday Life*, Basees/Routledge Series on Russian and East European Studies (London and New York: Routledge, Taylor & Francis Group, 2014).
[65] Baár, 'Disability and Civil Courage under State Socialism: The Scandal over the Hungarian Guide-Dog School'.
[66] Detlef Pollack and Jan Wielgohs, *Dissent and Opposition in Communist Eastern Europe: Origins of Civil Society and Democratic Transition* (Burlington, VT: Ashgate, 2004).

point,[67] or counterculture and flourishing underground music in the 1980s.[68] Some scholars of dissent and opposition have gone as far to argue that 'genuine' civil society did not and could not exist at all in state socialist Eastern Europe.[69]

But twenty years after mass campaigns with the Sabin vaccine brought about the disappearance of polio epidemics and, with it, the abandonment of people living with the eliminated disease, a civil society did emerge, one that was united not by political dissent, but by disability. Rather than opposition to the political system, this movement was a product of it: its birth had much to do with the particularities of state paternalism and the responsibilities and expectations shared among citizens and the state. In the eyes of the ageing polio patient generation, the communist state had not fulfilled its role and had failed to provide for them as promised.

Institutionalised children and others relegated to professions like shoe or watch repair grew up with very limited life choices. Many of them share the bitter view that the state abandoned them and destined them to poverty as adults by not providing adequate education in their youth.[70] For some, this experience prompted a realisation that they needed to become proactive, developing an attitude that was not usual in state socialism. In the late 1970s, drawing on the network developed during their long hospital stays, young adult polio patients established something unimaginable and unique in a communist state: a civil association that was wholly divorced from Party politics and from dissent. 'We realised that nobody was going to help us, so we needed to help each other',[71] recalls one of the founding members of the National Association of Disabled Societies.

The disabled adults utilised the network they had built during their long hospital stays and also took advantage of the fact that the concept of private data had not taken hold in healthcare. Volunteers, some of whom had worked in the medical profession previously, contacted hospital administrations and obtained the list of polio patients treated there in the 1950s and 1960s, along

[67] Friederike Kind-Kovács and Jessie Labov, *Samizdat, Tamizdat, and Beyond: Transnational Media during and after Socialism*, Studies in Contemporary European History (New York: Berghahn Books, 2013).

[68] Anna Szemere, *Up from the Underground: The Culture of Rock Music in Postsocialist Hungary*, Post-Communist Cultural Studies Series (University Park, Pa.: Pennsylvania State University Press, 2001). Thomas Cushman, *Notes from Underground: Rock Music Counterculture in Russia*, Suny Series in the Sociology of Culture (Albany: State University of New York Press, 1995); Trevor Hagen, 'From Inhibition to Commitment: Configuring the Czech Underground', *Eastbound*, no. Down to the Underground: Popular Music and Society in Central Europe, ed. Trevor Hagen, Tamás Tófalvy and Gábor Vályi (2012), 1–34.

[69] Matt Killingsworth, *Civil Society in Communist Eastern Europe* (Colchester: ECPR Press, 2012).

[70] Ágnes Soós, 'Interview' (Budapest 2010); Bedő, Kertész, and Szabó, 'Interview'.

[71] Kálmánné Gere, interview by Dóra Vargha, July 2007.

with their phone numbers and addresses.[72] This way, they even managed to find people who had been isolated from the polio community beforehand, and had lived their whole life alone with their disability.[73] By 1979 there were six regional associations, which established the Cooperative Committee of Disabled Associations to coordinate the associations and represent them in interactions with the state. By 1980, the number of participating associations rose to ten, and the plan was to establish an association for each of the country's nineteen counties.[74]

Getting the Party's approval for such an enterprise was a more difficult matter. The initial response from the government was total rejection and it took over two years of negotiation through political connections to receive authorisation for the founding of the national association.[75] The turning point came in 1981, which was proclaimed 'International Year of Disabled Persons' by the United Nations.[76] The General Assembly adopted the resolution of the International Year in 1976, setting the theme as 'full participation'.[77] The goal of the International Year was for disabled people 'to participate fully in the social life and development of their societies and to enjoy living conditions equal to those of other citizens, as well as an equal share in the improvements in living conditions resulting from social and economic development'.[78]

In Hungary, unsurprisingly, it was through capability to work and the functioning of social services, especially rehabilitation, that full participation was perceived.[79] Accordingly, it was the Ministry of Labour that became responsible for coordinating the International Year. Disability had not received so much attention since the end of polio epidemics. Yet the involvement of the Hungarian government in the global programme was less than enthusiastic. The Council of Ministers decided that there would be no international event organised and that keeping costs low should be a priority.[80] Socialist brigades, institutions and youth organisations raised funds for the support of the disabled in the country. Several new rehabilitation institutes were built and three holiday camps were made accessible to disabled children. There was an

---

[72] Vargha, interview by Vargha, 15 June 2008.   [73] Gere, interview by Vargha, July 2007.
[74] *Fogyatékosság-Politikai Szakismeretek* Fogyatékosságtudományi Tudásbázis (Budapest: Eötvös Loránd Tudományegyetem Bárcsi Gusztáv Gyógypedagógiai Kar, 2009).
[75] Lajos Hegedűs, interview by Dóra Vargha, April, 2010.
[76] United Nations General Assembly, 'International Year of Disabled Persons, U.N. Doc. A/Res/ 36/77 (1081)' (University of Minnesota Human Rights Library, 1981).
[77] '31/123. International Year of Disabled Persons. Resolution Adopted by the General Assembly', in *A/RES/31/123* (New York, 1976).
[78] '35/133. International Year of Disabled Persons. Resolution Adopted by the General Assembly', in *A/RES/35/133. Thirty-fifth Session, Agenda item 79* (New York, 1980).
[79] Judit Csehák, 'A Foglalkoztatási Rehabilitációról – a 'Rokkantak Nemzetközi Éve' Után', *Népegészségügy* 63, no. 3 (1982): 129–36.
[80] 'A Rokkant Személyek Nemzetközi Évéhez Kapcsolódó Feladatok.' Budapest: Magyar Nemzeti Levéltár, Minisztertanácsi Jegyzőkönyvek, 288.f.7., 604. ő.e., 1980.

increase in the representation of disabled people in television and radio as well, in order to promote the integration of the disabled into society.[81]

Most steps taken in the framework of the International Year of Disabled Persons were superficial and did not have lasting effects, save one. It was this interest generated by the United Nation's global programme that created the opportunity for polio patients to take their association to a national level. The first, founding assembly of the National Association of Disabled Societies, coordinating nineteen regional organisations, was held on 13 June 1981. The Association, whose leadership (and the majority of its membership) is still made up of former polio patients, has been a major force in pushing for disability and accessibility laws; has founded a small packaging company to provide work for members and income for the organisation; and has also fulfilled a social function in organising meetings for former patients to connect or reconnect.

The activism of polio survivors and the origins of the National Association of Disabled Societies, whose leadership is still made up primarily of people disabled by polio, were prompted by the end of epidemics and the official end of polio in Hungary. Their story is not entirely unique, however, and points to the ways in which we need to revisit our understanding of Cold War societies. Historian Monika Baár has explored the self-organisation of the blind in Hungary in the 1970s, through the story of the guide dog school. In her analysis, she shows the similar starting points of the paternalist state and the 'welfare dictatorship': an implicit social contract in which the state takes on the responsibility of providing social and economic security in return for political compliance. In this sense, welfare provisions function as a legitimation of the state's power.[82]

It was this social contract that polio patients saw was broken, which in turn prompted them to organise themselves and provide for each other, as well as to enforce the social responsibilities of the state. The examples of the National Association of Disabled Societies and the guide dog school show that on the one hand, we cannot dismiss Eastern European countries as exclusively oppressive and abusive towards the disabled, with no space for resistance, negotiations and activism. In turn, a wealth of disability history attests to exclusions, neglect and inequalities in Western societies as well. More broadly, these histories can contribute to an understanding of civil society that may work in a variety of ways, some more organised and visible, some practising direct influence, albeit tacitly.

---

[81] 'A Foglalkoztatási Rehabilitációról – a 'Rokkantak Nemzetközi Éve' Után'.
[82] Baár, 'Disability and Civil Courage under State Socialism: The Scandal over the Hungarian Guide-Dog School'.

On the one hand, the end of polio in Hungary meant the end of medical care and the beginning of abandonment for thousands and thousands of children, who were already stricken with polio at the time of disease elimination. On the other, this abandonment by the state that had built itself on the role of the provider and paternal care prompted something that had been thought to be impossible in communist countries: a grassroots civil society.

The Hungarian case tells us a much broader story about the changing meanings of the disease. One could argue that what happened in Hungary after the end of polio was merely a shift from the acute to the chronic. In many ways, that is true, and prompts the question of whether we are then talking of two different diseases (epidemic polio and polio as a condition). But there is more to it: what remains behind is the uncomfortable lingering presence of the past. In the case of polio, it is an extremely visible legacy that changes from a weapon in combating the disease to invisibility.

The end of polio in Hungary highlights the fact that global disease prevention programmes cannot be divorced from the local politics of prophylaxis, and furthermore that they also cannot be separated from disease treatment and the long-term social, cultural and political consequences of ending a disease.[83] The end of the disease in Hungary had a significant impact on the epidemic management of polio on a global scale, both in shaping international scientific debates on vaccine efficacy and safety through the results of the Salk and Sabin vaccines and in serving as a model for global eradication programmes. In turn, international cooperation in vaccine development, the speedy and successful introduction of the Sabin vaccine and Hungary becoming polio-free had profound effects on society, by making disability invisible, and on the lives of thousands who still had a full life ahead of them to live with the disease.

Hungary becoming a model both in terms of socialist public health management and in global polio eradication rested on a particular concept of the end of polio: the end of epidemic outbreaks and transmission of wild polio viruses. With the global eradication campaign stepping up in the 2000s, the image of the end of polio has been reinforced through billboards showing how close the world is to ending polio, the celebration of the eradication of Type II polio virus and the reduction of countries where wild polio is still present from 125 in 1988 to just three twenty-five years later.

The focus on disease elimination and the dominant interpretation of the end of polio also changed what polio as a disease itself was. Through the narrative of the successful end to the disease and the eradication of polio, it increasingly became reduced to a virological phenomenon. The disease's bodily

---

[83] For a Latin-American and Iberian approach to the problems raised with the end of polio, see Juan Antonio Rodríguez-Sánchez, 'Poliomyelitis after Poliomyelitis: Lights and Shadows of the Eradication. An Introduction', *Hygiea Internationalis* 11, no. 1 (2015): 7–31.

manifestation and its social, cultural and political existence have been pushed to the background, turned invisible or disappeared entirely. Accordingly, the complexity of what polio is was not incorporated into the models of the end of the disease, and polio-stricken bodies and lives have not figured in the end-game strategies of the global eradication campaign.[84]

There are broader implications. Eradication may be the ultimate 'end' to a disease, but the epidemic narrative is very much present in many other health issues, from obesity to cancer. And the dramaturgy of increasing tension, crisis and closure is seductive, especially regarding the end. We all yearn for a happy ending, or at least an ending of some sorts, when it comes to diseases that challenge our faith in medical knowledge and our political systems and tear the social fabric.

Hardly anyone would contest that eradicating smallpox was a good idea, or argue that we would rather have polio epidemics back. Furthermore, the narrative can be constructive in more than one way. Epidemics and diseases more generally leave behind not just survivors, but public health practices and structures – not everything is always forgotten or works in exclusionary ways.

At the same time, the end of disease, may it be a goal or wish, or a thing of the past, is often perceived in a particular and narrow sense. Whether it is modernist projects that do not allow for complicated and messy endings (or their lack), or certain diseases themselves that fail to map onto the narrative, endings hardly mean that the story is finished. Therefore, the epidemic narrative can be as deceptive as seductive. To add one more example, the absence of vaccine-preventable diseases and their disappearance from societies have wide-reaching and severe consequences, as the death of an eight-year-old who caught diphtheria in Spain in 2015 reminds us – not just about the rise of anti-vaccination movements, but also about the lack of therapeutic interventions in public health systems for those diseases.[85]

Epidemics may go out with a bang – or a whimper. What the Hungarian case shows us is the importance of investigating what that end is: for whom it comes and does not come; who is rendered invisible by it; what the end itself means to societies, global health policies and individual lives; and how it makes us think past the epidemic narrative.

---

[84] Olen M. Kew et al., 'Vaccine-Derived Polioviruses and the Endgame Strategy for Global Polio Eradication', *Annual Review of Microbiology* 59 (2005): 587–635; Global Polio Eradication Initiative, *Polio Eradication & Endgame Strategic Plan 2013–2018* (Geneva: World Health Organization, 2013).

[85] David Bryan and Dora Vargha, 'Los Antivacunas Y El Pasado Fascista De España', *El País*, 12 June 2015.

Conclusion: Eastern Europe in Global Health History

On 5 March 1946, Winston Churchill delivered his famous Fulton speech where he described an 'Iron Curtain' descending across the continent from Stettin in the Baltic to Trieste in the Adriatic. The term 'Iron Curtain' soon became both a powerful symbol and a structural concept in understanding post-war realities. Five years later, in a lesser-known speech at the House of Commons, Churchill further elaborated on the unfolding Cold War. In a parliamentary debate on exports to China, speaking as the MP for Woodford, his words revealed the relationship with the communist East as the following:

I could see no reason why, if we had diplomatic relations with Communist Russia, Communist Poland and other countries inside the Iron Curtain, we could not have them with China. Recognition does not mean approval. One has to recognise and deal with all sorts of things in this world as they come along. After all, vaccination is undoubtedly a definite recognition of smallpox. Certainly I think that it would be very foolish, in ordinary circumstances, not to keep necessary contacts with countries with whom one is not at war.[1]

Churchill's vaccine reference may seem out of context in a speech on trade and diplomatic relations. However, as this book has shown, ideology, vaccines, disease and cross-camp relations were inextricably linked during the Cold War. These pervasive metaphors framed the era in terms of 'containment' and 'infection', and were often mobilised when framing diplomatic and economic relations between the West and the communist East. By recognising the communist disease, Churchill hoped to develop tools that that could help curb its spread.

Churchill did not need to elaborate on his shorthand. By 1951 it was clear to all what he meant by mentioning disease and vaccine and what they meant for Cold War relations. The Eastern European story of polio shows how these concepts and policies became linked in other ways later in the decade. At that point, illness and remedy, containment and cure were no longer fixed in the

---

[1] Thanks are due to Gareth Millward, who pointed out this passage to me. Winston Churchill, 'House of Commons Debate 10 May: Exports to China' (London: HANSARD 1803–2005, 1951), 2157.

dominating metaphorical plane but had very real effects on Cold War relations and were largely translated into technologies that opened and closed holes in the Iron Curtain. The experience of a disease that affected both sides created relations of a different quality: the understanding and recognition of polio, and the development of vaccines that could contain its spread, had to be worked out on common grounds, in collaboration between East and West.

Polio also turned Churchill's assessment on its head: approval could work without recognition. In the late 1950s the Hungarian Kádár government was struggling to gain political and diplomatic recognition on the international political stage. Coming to power on the back of Soviet tanks, the new Hungarian government was persona non grata in the eyes of Western Europe and the United States. At the same time, the Hungarian state methods of epidemic control gained global approval and its researchers' expertise was not only highly rated but also sought after across blocs, through scientific collaboration.

It can now be considered a truism that Eastern European perspectives tell a very different story from conventional understandings of Cold War politics and interactions. Since the 1990s, social historians have been at the helm of breaking down entrenched Western-centric concepts in historiography, exploring the diversity of the political, social and cultural landscape of the region and pointing to interactions, negotiations and achievements within and without the Soviet Bloc. More recently historians such as Jessica Reinisch, Celia Donert and Young-Sun Hong have argued for the importance of including an Eastern European viewpoint in histories of internationalism and humanitarianism.[2] While Cold War Eastern European history in a global perspective is a field that has seen rapid growth in the past decades, the history of medicine and global public health has been slow to recognise its contributions, even as anthropologists like Adriana Petryna and Erin Koch have elucidated the centrality of the region for an understanding of contemporary global health.[3]

The Hungarian history of polio offers a vital missing context from current histories of global health, which are mainly predicated on colonial and post-colonial contexts and the histories of international institutions such as the

---

[2] Jessica Reinisch, *The Perils of Peace: The Public Health Crisis in Occupied Germany* (Oxford: Oxford University Press, 2013); '"Auntie UNRRA" at the Crossroads', *Past and Present* 218, no. Suppl 8 (2013): 70–97; Young-Sun Hong, *Cold War Germany, the Third World, and the Global Humanitarian Regime*, Human Rights in History (New York: Cambridge University Press, 2015); Celia Donert, 'Whose Utopia? Gender, Ideology and Human Rights at the 1975 World Congress of Women in East Berlin', in *The Breakthrough: Human Rights in the 1970s*, ed. Jan Eckel and Samuel Moyn (Philadelphia: University of Pennsylvania Press, 2014), 68–87.

[3] Adriana Petryna, *When Experiments Travel* (Princeton and Oxford: Princeton University Press, 2009); Erin Koch, *Free Market Tuberculosis: Managing Epidemics in Post-Soviet Georgia* (Nashville, Tenn.: Vanderbilt University Press, 2013).

Rockefeller Foundation or the World Health Organisation. This is as much of a history of everyday health management as a history of leading figures and powerful organisations. Katalin Parádi's encounters with polio over a decade encapsulate the significance of the Eastern European context in global health history by using the lens of polio epidemics to understand the global Cold War politics of epidemic management from a Hungarian perspective. This is a history of epidemic geopolitics lived on the ground in a country fully involved in the political and military conflict of the early Cold War era. Global, national and local polio politics were pinned down in daily bodily experiences, prevention strategies and international cooperation initiatives. At the same time these politics were also contested, negotiated and resisted in complex, entangled networks of power at local, national and global levels.

With its Eastern European focus, its ever-shifting scales and explorations of expert and local knowledge, this book has offered tools to address current historiographical challenges in global history more broadly[4] and in the history of medicine particularly. Among them, registers of historical analysis, the often-problematic role of the state in health, and the relationship between local and global sciences have been identified by Susan Gross Solomon, Lion Murard and Patrick Zylberman in their collection *Shifting Boundaries of Public Health* as particularly central to understanding public health.[5] In the Hungarian history of polio, the management of epidemic crises, followed by the abandonment of disabled polio victims, has revealed the ways in which responsibility was imagined, enforced and negotiated between citizens and the state; evaluation and the failure of the Salk vaccine alluded to the negotiation of sciences of the local and global; while polio treatment and access to respiratory technology highlighted the porousness of individual, national and global levels of experience and their historical study. Moreover, this analysis has explored the politics, practices and knowledge production in public health by placing an alternative political system, namely the communist state and its place in global public health, under scrutiny.

The book has shifted attention away from the two superpowers to a site that is usually considered peripheral to global politics. This strategy has exposed how medical knowledge and technology circulated in the Cold War.

---

[4] See Sarah Hodges, 'The Global Menace', *Social History of Medicine* 25, no. 3 (2012): 719–28; Warwick Anderson, 'Making Global Health History: The Postcolonial Worldliness of Biomedicine', ibid. 27, no. 2 (2014): 372–84; Mark Harrison, 'Positioning Paper', *Bulletin of the History of Medicine* 89, no. 4 (2016): 639–89; Sebouh David Aslanian et al., 'AHR Conversation: How Size Matters: The Question of Scale in History', *American Historical Review* 118, no. 5 (2013): 1432–71.
[5] Susan Gross Solomon, Lion Murard, and Patrick Zylberman, *Shifting Boundaries of Public Health: Europe in the Twentieth Century*, Rochester Studies in Medical History (Rochester, NY: University of Rochester Press, 2008).

Cooperation was present where animosity would be expected, and continuities replaced conventional watersheds. Thus, the book has contributed an understanding of what the Cold War was, among whom it was 'fought' and the ways in which it did and did not affect public health policies, research and medical treatment. Furthermore, it has explored the ways in which it was possible to operate outside the framework of the Cold War through medical practice and scientific research and the Cold War frameworks that permeated seemingly neutral spaces.

An Eastern European perspective in this work has offered a viewpoint that pierces conventional histories of internationalism in public health and medicine.[6] First, the history of polio in Hungary highlights the importance of alternative internationalisms to the hegemonic liberal model. During the country's years of absence from the World Health Organisation, Hungarian virologists, doctors, public health officials and even parents successfully drew on international resources and actively participated in the global exchange of medical equipment, specimens and treatment regimens. Some of these professional networks and practices of scientific internationalism did not map onto liberal internationalism. Rather, it was organisations such as the WHO that built policies and mapped them onto existing professional networks, such as the case of Dorothy Horstmann's visit to the Soviet Union. Moreover, a particular socialist internationalism within the Eastern Bloc and between Eastern Europe and Latin America played a crucial role in the emergence of a globally adopted vaccine and immunisation practice.[7] As Cold War concepts have been persistent in shaping historical narratives of the era to this day, much of this history has become invisible and can only be uncovered when viewed from within the socialist framework.

Going beyond an analysis of the leadership and expert personnel of international agencies, and examining them from below, has been crucial in understanding the diverse ways in which international health organisations work and interact with local and national (or colonial) realities.[8] The focus on an Eastern European country has opened up new interpretations of the ways in which organisations such as the WHO and the Red Cross worked. The Hungarian history of a global disease has challenged the common view of

---

[6] For more on this approach in the history of internationalism more broadly, see Ana Antic, Johanna Conterio, and Dora Vargha, 'Beyond Liberal Internationalism', *Contemporary European History* 25, no. 2 (2016): 359–71.
[7] On socialist internationalism, see Rachel Applebaum, 'The Friendship Project: Socialist Internationalism in the Soviet Union and Czechoslovakia in the 1950s and 1960s', *Slavic Review* 74, no. 3 (2015): 484–507; Tobias Rupprecht, *Soviet Internationalism after Stalin: Interaction and Exchange between the USSR and Latin America during the Cold War* (Cambridge: Cambridge University Press, 2015).
[8] Sanjoy Bhattacharya, 'International Health and the Limits of Its Global Influence: Bhutan and the Worldwide Smallpox Eradication Programme', *Medical History* 57, no. 4 (2013): 461–86.

the WHO as merely a site where Cold War politics played out and has shown not only the effect of international agendas on individuals, but also the ways in which local experiences and national policies fed back into international practices, shaping and informing each other in the process. Similarly, the intervention of the Red Cross in Cold War affairs is seen in a new light when we look at the role of individuals in securing aid through transnational familial and lay networks when the international organisation was slow to act.

Geographically and conceptually de-centring narratives of internationalism and global public health, especially ones tied to the Cold War, is, therefore, crucial for a nuanced understanding of the long-term trajectories of this formative era. More particularly, this book has added a new dimension to the history of polio, in which the dominant American narrative of the rivalry between Salk and Sabin has come under scrutiny. This story is most often told through prominent figures, such as President Franklin D. Roosevelt, Jonas Salk, Albert B. Sabin or Sister Kenny, and these histories' geographical focus is usually the United States. However, if we look to histories of polio in seemingly marginal places and through actors with lower profiles, a new story emerges, one that is crucial to understanding the roots of global polio eradication programmes. The well-known story of whom we can credit for the success of polio prevention was worked out in a politically fraught way. The choices of the Salk and Sabin vaccines and their development, standard-isation and implementation have revealed a process that amalgamated scientific competition with geopolitical concerns.

Equally important to understanding Eastern Europe's role in global public health is to consider what issues of healthcare and epidemic management tell us about Eastern European states themselves. Polio in Hungary has revealed an Eastern European history of medicine rich in innovation, intensive scientific exchange and political experiments in healthcare. Hungarian virologists and physicians utilised their old network in the West and their new one in the East in similar ways in order to meet the local and national needs of disease prevention and treatment. Shortage, an everyday experience for those living behind the Iron Curtain, spurred technological innovation within the field of respiratory medicine, and when paired with global scarcity, integrated countries from both sides into an international network of medical emergency aid.

It was also through the meeting of local and global scarcity that the flexibility of the Hungarian communist government became visible. Negotiating access to the new Salk vaccine revealed the inner workings of state socialist public health management, diplomacy and trade, and the surprisingly diverse ways in which an otherwise stern, post-revolutionary government reacted to epidemic challenges. Embracing the international cooperation of the Catholic Church, openly acknowledging and utilising family ties with dissident emigrants and deliberating over applying or removing Cold War tools in the vaccine diplomacy with the United States all expose a more complex, pragmatic and less ideology-driven governance than Cold War narratives usually allow.

Zooming in from the national to the individual experience, a focus on polio in Hungary has allowed me to link the intimate world of families with national and international agendas through the care for disabled children with polio. I have shown children challenging ideological concepts in their decisions about their bodies in treatment; parents seeking holes in the Iron Curtain to procure cutting-edge medical technology for their children; and parental responsibilities over children's care fluctuating between the state and individuals.

The individual experience of the disease, when considered together with national policies and international practices, then, points to global questions about who is responsible for people's health, the limits of that responsibility and the part that states, international agencies and individuals should play in protecting health and treating disease.

These issues of responsibility in health – international and national, collective and individual – created flashpoints in the postwar decades and have continued to do so long after the Cold War ended. An era built on ideological division and marked by pervasive stereotypes on both side of the Iron Curtain, the Cold War left the heritage of a lexicon that frames political understandings of responsibilities, expectations and fears relating to health and disease. But these flashpoints have also worked in other ways. Many of the critical moments and processes described in this book have shaped and contributed to how global public health problems are governed, how contemporary states organize their healthcare policies and how medical research is conducted.

The conceptual, methodological and geographical shifts that Eastern European histories of health and disease demand go beyond original historiographical interventions such as new approaches to Cold War history, the history of internationalism and the modern history of medicine. Critically assessing contagion, vaccines and political relations in their practical and rhetorical significance opens the possibility of a symmetrical analysis that takes seriously the intersection between ideology, politics and medicine on both sides of the Cold War. Moreover, Eastern European perspectives, such as the Hungarian history of polio, highlight the long-term impact that fleeting geopolitical concerns can have on personal lives, national epidemic management strategies and global health agendas.

Archives and Collections

András Pető College Mária Hári Library and Regional Resource Center

City Archives of Budapest

Hauck Center for the Albert B. Sabin Archives Digital Collection

Historical Archives of Radio Free Europe, Open Society Institute

Historical Medical Library of the College of Physicians of Philadelphia

Hungarian National Film Archive

International Committee of the Red Cross Archives

Library and Archives of the World Health Organization

National Archives of Hungary

National Library of Hungary

Semmelweis University Central Library

Wellcome Library

Yale University Library Manuscripts and Archives

Interviewees

Julianna Bedő
Domokos Boda
Tamás Kertész
Chris Maher
Elvira Mészáros
Judit Enyedi Dr Dékány Pálné
Katalin Parádi
Sándor Rádai
Ágnes Soós
Tibor Szabó
Éva Paksáné Szentgyörgyi
Erzsébet Szöllősiné Földesi
Zoltán Török
György Vargha
Irén Lázok Dr Vargháné

Bibliography

38/1958. (VI.10.) Korm. Számú Rendelet a Védőoltásokról Szóló 60/1953. (Xii.20.) M.T. Számú Rendelet Kiegészítéséről.

Ábel, Olga. 'Eddig 67 000 Gyereket Oltottak Be Salk-Vakcinával a Fővárosban Az Új Akció Kezdete Óta'. *Népszava*, 7 August 1959.

Ádám, Imre. 'Az Ifjúság Csoportos Üdültetése'. Budapest: National Archives of Hungary, Egészségügyi Minisztérium Állami Közegészségügyi Felügyeleti és Járványvédeli Főosztály, XIX-C-2-e, 54228/1957, 1957.

'Agreement between the International Committee of the Red Cross, the Hungarian Red Cross and Rädda Barnen'. Geneva: International Committee of the Red Cross Archives, Accord conclu entre Rädda Barnen, le CICR et la Croix-Rouge hongroise au sujet des envois non-Croix-Rouge acheminés par le CICR à Budapest. Signé le 3 décembre 1956, B AG 280 094–017.03, 1956.

Aladár, Kátay. 'Svájci Polio-Vaccina Használhatósága'. Budapest: National Archives of Hungary, 54047, XIX-C-2-e, 1957.

'Albert Sabin Magyarországra Készül'. *Népszabadság*, 1960, 6.

Aman, Anna-Ma Toll and Bengt. 'Letter to the Health Ministry'. Budapest: Magyar Nemzeti Levéltár, Drexler Miklós Egészségügyi Miniszterhelyettes iratai, XIX-C-2-p, 336/1957, 1957.

Aman, Bengt. 'Epidemie de poliomyelite en Hongrie. Informations communiquées par le Bureau Médico-Social, Ligue des Sociétés de la Croix-Rouge'. Geneva: International Committee of the Red Cross Archives, Epidémie de poliomyélite, B AG 280 094–031.02, 7275, 1957.

Anderson, Warwick. 'Making Global Health History: The Postcolonial Worldliness of Biomedicine'. *Social History of Medicine* 27, no. 2 (2014): 372–84.

'Annual Report, 1960'. New York: The Rockefeller Foundation, 1960.

Antic, Ana. 'Heroes and Hysterics: 'Partisan Hysteria' and Communist State-Building in Yugoslavia after 1945'. *Social History of Medicine* 27, no. 3 (2014): 349–71.

Antic, Ana, Johanna Conterio and Dora Vargha. 'Beyond Liberal Internationalism'. *Contemporary European History* 25, no. 2 (2016): 359–71.

Apor, Péter. 'Eurocommunism: Commemorating Communism in Contemporary Eastern Europe'. In *European Memory? Contested Histories and Politics of Remembrance*, edited by Malgorzata Pakier and Bo Strath, 233–47. New York and Oxford: Berghahn Books, 2010.

Applebaum, Rachel. 'The Friendship Project: Socialist Internationalism in the Soviet Union and Czechoslovakia in the 1950s and 1960s'. *Slavic Review* 74, no. 3 (2015): 484–507.

214

Arendt, Hannah. *The Origins of Totalitarianism*. Orlando: Harcourt, 1973.

Árkus, István. 'Sabin Professzornak Átnyújtották a Magyar Tudományos Akadémia Tiszteleti Tagságáról Szóló Oklevelet'. *Népszabadság*, 1965, 4.

Aronova, Elena, Karen S. Baker, and Naomi Oreskes. 'Big Science and Big Data in Biology: From the International Geophysical Year through the International Biological Program to the Long Term Ecological Research (Lter) Network, 1957-Present'. *Historical Studies in the Natural Sciences* 40, no. 2 (2010): 183–224.

Ash, Timothy Garton. 'Introductory Essay: Fourty Years On'. In *The 1956 Hungarian Revolution: A History in Documents*, edited by Csaba Békés, Malcolm Byrne and János M. Rainer, xix–xxvii. Budapest: Central European University Press, 2002.

Aslanian, Sebouh David, Joyce E. Chaplin, Ann McGrath, and Kristin Mann. 'AHR Conversation: How Size Matters: The Question of Scale in History'. *American Historical Review* 118, no. 5 (2013): 1432–71.

Assembly, United Nations General. '*International Year of Disabled Persons, U.N. Doc. A/Res/36/77 (1081)*'. University of Minnesota Human Rights Library, 1981.

'35/133. International Year of Disabled Persons. Resolution Adopted by the General Assembly'. In *A/RES/35/133. Thirty-fifth Session, Agenda Item 79*. New York, 1980.

'31/123. International Year of Disabled Persons. Resolution Adopted by the General Assembly'. In *A/RES/31/123*. New York 1976.

'Attenuated Poliomyelitis Vaccines'. *British Medical Journal* 1, no. 4961 (1956): 284.

Autio-Sarasmo, Sari, and Brendan Humphreys, eds. *Winter Kept Us Warm: Cold War Interactions Reconsidered, Aleksanteri Cold War Series*. Helsinki: University of Helsinki, 2010.

Axelsson, Per. 'The Cutter Incident and the Development of a Swedish Polio Vaccine'. *Dynamis* 32, no. 2 (2012): 311–28.

'"Do Not Eat Those Apples; They've Been on the Ground!": Polio Epidemics and Preventive Measures, Sweden 1880s–1940s'. *Asclepio. Revista de Historia de la Medicina y la Ciencia* 61, no. 1 (2009): 23–38.

Höstens Spöke. De Svenska Polioepidemiernas Historia *[in Swedish]*. Stockholm: Carlssons, 2004.

Baár, Monika. 'Disability and Civil Courage under State Socialism: The Scandal over the Hungarian Guide-Dog School'. *Past and Present* 227, no. 1 (2015): 179–203.

Baczoni, Jenő. 'Levél Sebes István Elvtársnak, a Külügyminiszter Helyettesének'. Budapest: Magyar Nemzeti Levéltár, XIX-J-1-k USA Admin 1945–1964, 57, A Salk szérum beszerzése, 3516/1, 1957.

'Salk-Szérum Beszerzése'. Budapest: Magyar Nemzeti Levéltár, XIX-J-1-k USA Admin 1945–1964, 57, A Salk-szérum beszerzése, 1–00279/957, 1957.

Bahns, Ernst. *It Began with the Pulmotor. One Hundred Years of Artificial Ventilation*. Lübeck: Dräger Medical AG & Co. KG, 2007.

Baicus, Anda. 'History of Polio Vaccination'. *World Journal of Virology* 1, no. 4 (2012): 108–14.

Bakács, Dr. Tibor. 'Az Eddigi Poliomyelitis Vaccinatio Eredményeinek Értékelése'. *Orvosi Hetilap* 101, no. 20 (1960): 685–91.

'Poliomyelitis Betegek Védőoltására Vonatkozó Adat Gyűjtés'. Budapest: MOL, Járvány és Mikrobiológiai Főosztály, 5587/1959, XXVI-C-3-e, 1959.

'Poliomyelitis Betegek Védőoltására Vonatkozó Adatgyűjtés'. Budapest: National Archives of Hungary, Országos Közegészségi Intézet Járványügyi és Mikrobiológiai Főosztályának iratai, XXVI-C-3-e/1959, 5587, 1959.

'Poliomyelitis Prophylaxis in Hungary'. *Acta Microbiologica* VII, no. 3 (1960): 329–37.

Bakács, Tibor. *Egy Életrajz Ürügyén*. Budapest: Kossuth Könyvkiadó, 1978.

'A Fertőző Betegségek Elleni Küzdelem'. *Népszabadság*, 26 August 1959.

Az Országos Közegészségügyi Intézet Működése 1927–1957. Budapest: Országos Közegészségügyi Intézet 1959.

Ballester, Rosa, and María Isabel Porras. 'La Lucha Europea contra la presencia epidémica de la poliomielitis: Una reflexión histórica'. *Dynamis* 32, no. 2 (2012): 273–85.

Balló, László. 'Salk Védőoltások a Megye Területén'. Budapest: National Archives of Hungary, Egészségügyi Minisztérium Állami közegészségügyi felügyelet és járványvédelmi főosztály iratai, XIX-C-2-e, 54099, 1957.

Bán, Éva, Pál Nádas, Andrea Okányi, and Gizella Tarnói, eds. *Száz Esztendő a Mozgáskorlátozott Gyermekek Szolgálatában*. Budapest: Nádas Pál, 2003.

Bándi, Andor. 'A Folyamatos Oltásról'. *Népegészségügy* 43, no. 5 (1962): 150–2.

Bangham, Jenny. 'Blood Groups and Human Groups: Collecting and Calibrating Genetic Data after World War Two'. *Studies in History and Philosophy of Biological and Biomedical Sciences* 47, Part A (2014): 74–86.

Baranyai, Elza. 'Oltási Poliomyeitis'. In *A Gyermekbénulás Elleni Küzdelem*, edited by Rezső Hargitai and Ákosné Kiss, 162–68. Budapest: Literatura Medica, 1994.

Bark, Evelyn. 'Letter to Monsieur Amman, International Committee of the Red Cross'. Geneva: International Committee of the Red Cross Archives, Epidémie de poliomyélite, B AG 280 094–031.02, 3096, 1957.

Barla-Szabó, Jenő. 'A Heine-Medin-Kór Kezelése Lyssa Ellenes Oltásokkal'. *Orvosi Hetilap*, no. 22 (1933): 465–66.

Barr, Robert N., Henry Bauer, Herman Kleinman, Eugene A. Johnson, Mauricio Martins da Silva, and Anne Kimball. 'Use of Orally Administered Live Attenuated Polioviruses as a Vaccine in a Community Setting'. *Journal of the American Medical Association* 170, no. 8 (1959): 893–905.

Barreto, Luis, Rob Van Exan, and Christopher J. Rutty. 'Polio Vaccine Development in Canada: Contributions to Global Polio Eradication'. *Biologicals*, no. 34 (2006): 91–101.

Baskett, Thomas F. 'Silvester's Technique of Artificial Respiration'. *Resuscitation* 74, no. 1 (2007): 8–10.

Bazeley, P. L. 'Standardization of Polio Vaccine Potency'. In *Poliomyelitis. Papers and Discussions Presented at the Fifth International Poliomyelitis Conference Copenhagen, Denmark, July 26–28, 1960*, edited by International Poliomyelitis Congress, 186–95. Philadelphia and Montreal: J. B. Lippincott Company, 1961.

Bedő, Julianna, Tamás Kertész, and Tibor Szabó. '*Interview*'. Hévíz, 2010.

Békés, Csaba. *Az 1956-Os Magyar Forradalom a Világpolitikában*. Budapest: 1956-os Intézet, 2006.

Békés, Csaba, Malcolm Byrne, and M. János Rainer. *The 1956 Hungarian Revolution: A History in Documents*. National Security Archive Cold War Readers. Budapest; New York: Central European University Press, 2002.

Beldarraín, Enrique. 'Poliomyelitis and Its Elimination in Cuba: An Historical
Overview'. *MEDICC Review* 15, no. 2 (2013): 30–6.

'Bemutatták a Gyermekparalízisről Készült Filmet'. *Népszabadság*, 9 August 1957, 9.

Benda, Gyula. 'Budapest Társadalma 1945–1970'. In *Magyarország
Társadalomtörténete III. (1945–1989)*, edited by Nikosz Fokasz and Antal
Örkény, 8–31. Budapest: Új Mandátum, 1999.

Benison, Saul. 'International Medical Cooperation: Dr. Albert Sabin, Live Poliovirus
Vaccine and the Soviets'. *Bulletin of the History of Medicine* 56, no. 4 (1982):
460–83.

'Speculation and Experimentation in Early Poliomyelitis Research'. *Clio Medica* 10,
no. 1 (1975): 1–22.

Benyó, I. 'A Humán Vírus-Osztály Átvétele. Feljegyzés Dr. Vilmon Miniszterhelyettes
Elvtárs Részére'. Budapest: National Archives of Hungary, Egészségügyi
Minisztérium iratai, XIX-C-2-e, 50.654, 1957.

'Gyermekbénulás Elleni Folytatólagos Védőoltások Szervezése'. Budapest: National
Archives of Hungary, Egészségügyi Minisztérium iratai, 53.135/1957, 1957.

'Beoltják Gyermekbénulás Ellen az 1–2 Éves Gyermekeket: Külkereskedelmi
Szerveink Már 250 000 Köbcenti Vakcinát Szereztek'. *Népakarat*, July 10 1957.

Berend, Ivan T. 'The First Phase of Economic Reform in Hungary: 1956–1957'.
Journal of European Economic History, 12. no.3 (1983): 523–71'.

*Central and Eastern Europe, 1944–1993: Detour from the Periphery to the
Periphery*. Cambridge Studies in Modern Economic History. Cambridge:
Cambridge University Press, 1996.

Berndorfer, Alfréd, Béla Egyed, Kálmán Frank, Endre Fejér, István Flesch, Kálmán
Kalocsay, György Kovács, et al. *Egészséges és Beteg Gyermek*. Budapest:
Gondolat Kiadó, 1957.

Bernstein, Frances L. 'Rehabilitation Staged: How Soviet Doctors "Cured" Disability in
the Second World War'. In *Disability Histories*, edited by Susan Burch and
Michael Rembis, 218–36. Urbana: University of Illinois Press, 2014.

'Prosthetic Promise in Late-Stalinist Russia'. In *Disability in Eastern Europe and the
Former Soviet Union: History, Policy and Everyday Life*, edited by Michael Rasell
and Elena Iarskaia-Smirnova, 42–64. London: Routledge, 2013.

Bernstein, Robin. *Racial Innocence. Performing American Childhood from Slavery to
Civil Rights*. New York: New York University Press, 2011.

'Beszámoló'. Budapest: National Archives of Hungary, Vilmon Gyula iratai,
Egészségügyi Minisztérium, XIX-C-2-o 1956–1957, 1956.

Bhattacharya, Sanjoy. 'International Health and the Limits of Its Global Influence:
Bhutan and the Worldwide Smallpox Eradication Programme'. *Medical History*
57, no. 4 (2013): 461–86.

Bicskei, Éva. '"Our Greatest Treasure, the Child": The Politics of Child Care in
Hungary, 1945–1956'. *Social Politics* 13, no. 2 (2006): 151–88.

Blume, Stuart, Paul Greenough, and Christine Holmberg, eds. *The Politics of
Vaccination: A Global History. Studies for the Society for the History of Medicine*.
Manchester: University of Manchester Press, 2017.

Boda, Domokos. '50 Years Ago: Polio Epidemics, Immunisation, and Politics'. *BMJ*
340 (2010): b5297.

'Interview'. By Dóra Vargha (18 November 2009).

Sorsfordulók. Budapest: Harmat, 2004.

Boda, Domokos, and László Murányi. *Respiratiós Therapia*. Budapest: Medicina Könyvkiadó, 1963.

Bókay, János. *Az 1926. Évi Heine-Medin-Járvány Csonka-Magyarországban*. Budapest: Pest könyvnyomda részvénytársaság, 1927.

Borbándi, Gyula. *Magyarok Az Angol Kertben*. Budapest: Mundus, 2004.

Borhi, László, *Iratok a Magyar-Amerikai Kapcsolatok Történetéhez 1957–1967*, edited by Mária and Vida Ormos, István, Iratok a Magyar Diplomácia Történetéhez (Budapest: Ister, 2002).

Brandt, Allan M. 'Racism and Research: The Case of the Tuskegee Syphilis Study'. *The Hastings Center Report* 8, no. 6 (1978): 21–9.

Brotherton, P. Sean *Revolutionary Medicine: Health and the Body in Post-Soviet Cuba*. Experimental Futures: Technological Lives, Scientific Arts, Anthropological Voices. Durham, NC: Duke University Press, 2012.

Brown, Kate. *Plutopia: Nuclear Families, Atomic Cities, and the Great Soviet and American Plutonium Disasters*. Oxford: Oxford University Press, 2013.

Brown, Theodore M., Marcos Cueto, and Elizabeth Fee. 'The World Health Organization and the Transition from "International" to "Global" Health'. In *Medicine at the Border: Disease, Globalization and Security, 1850 to the Present*, edited by Alison Bashford, 76–94. Basingstoke: Palgrave Macmillan, 2006.

Bruno, Richard L. 'Paralytic versus "Non-Paralytic" Polio: A Distinction without a Difference?'. *American Journal of Physical Medicine and Rehabilitation* 79 (2000): 1–9.

Bryan, David, and Dora Vargha. 'Los antivacunas y el pasado fascista de España'. *El País*, 12 June 2015.

Budai Gyermekkórház és Rendelőintézet. 'A Kórház Története'. www.budaigyk.hu/site.php?inc=0&menuId=5.

'Budapest Főváros Lakossága Egészségügyi Ellátásának 1956. Évi Fejlesztési Terve'. Budapest: City Archives of Budapest, Budapest Fővárosi Tanács VB Egészségügyi Osztályának iratai, XXIII. 115.a. 214. box, 1956.

'Budapest Fővárosi Tanács Végrehajtó Bizottsága Határozati Javaslata a Főváros Egészségügyi Helyzetének További Javítására'. Budapest: National Archives of Hungary, Egészségügyi Minisztérium Vilmon Gyula miniszterhelyettes iratai, XIX-C-2-p, 1959.

'Budapest Receives Canadian Polio Aid'. *New York Times*, 14 July 1957.

'Budapest Vezető Főorvosának Felhívása A Háziasszonyokhoz'. *Népakarat*, no. 136, 13 June 1957.

'Budapesten December 14–15–16-Án Kapják a Gyerekek a Gyermekbénulás Ellen Védő Sabin-Oltóanyagot'. *Népszava*, 26 November 1959, 1.

'Budapesten Nincsen Gyermekbénulási Járvány – Mondja a Tisztifőorvos. Egészségügyi Okokból Korlátozzák a Fővárosi Strandok Látogatását'. *Népakarat*, 28 June 1957, 1.

Buga, László. *Hogyan Gondoskodik Államunk a Dolgozó Anyáról és Gyermekéről* Útmutató Városi És Falusi Előadók Számára. Budapest: Művelt Nép könyvkiadó, 1953.

Byrom, Brad. 'The Progressive Movement and the Child with Physical Disabilities'. In *Children with Disabilities in America: A Historical Handbook and Guide*, edited by Philip L. Safford and Elizabeth J. Safford, 49–64. London: Greenwood Press, 2006.

Cáceres, Victor M., and Roland W. Sutter. 'Sabin Monovalent Oral Polio Vaccines: Review of Past Experiences and Their Potential Use after Polio Eradication'. *Clinical Infectious Diseases* 33, no. 4 (2001): 531–41.

Campos, André Luiz Vieira de, Dilene Raimundo do Nascimento, and Eduardo Maranhão. 'A História Da Poliomielite No Brasil E Seu Controle Por Imunizaçao' *História, Ciencias, Saúde-Manguinhos* 10, no. Suppl.2. (2003): 573–600.

Cardia, Isabelle Voneche. *Magyar Október Vörös Zászló és Vörös Kereszt Között* [*L'octobre Hongrois:* Entre Croix Rouge et Drapeau Rouge]. Budapest: sociotypo, 1998.

Chumakov, M. P. 'Letter to Albert B. Sabin Dated 1959–04–18'. Cincinnati: Hauck Center for the Albert B. Sabin Archives, Sabin, ALbert B., 1906–1993 – Correspondence, Box 3., File 09 (Soviet Union – 1959–68), 1959.

Chumakov, M. P., M. K. Voroshilova, K. A. Vasilieva, M. N. Bakina, Dobrova I. N., S. G. Drosdov, E. E. Ashmarina, *et al.* 'Preliminary Report on Mass Oral Immunization of Population against Poliomyelitis with Live Virus Vaccine from A.B. Sabin's Attenutated Strains'. In *Live Poliovirus Vaccines: Papers Presented and Discussions Held at the First International Conference on Live Poliovirus Vaccines*, edited by Pan American Health Organization, 517–29. Washington, D.C.: Pan American Sanitary Bureau, 1959.

Chumakov, M. P., M.K. Voroshilova, S. G. Drozdov, S. G. Dzagurov, V. A. Lashkevich, L. L. Mironova, N. M. Ralph, *et al.* 'Some Results of the Work on Mass Immunization in the Soviet Union with Live Poliovirus Vaccine Prepared from Sabin Strains'. *Bulletin of the World Health Organization* 25, no. 1 (1961): 79–91.

Churchill, Winston. 'House of Commons Debate 10 May: Exports to China'. cc2157–82. London: HANSARD, 1803–2005, 1951.

Classen, Albrecht, ed. *Childhood in the Middle Ages and the Renaissance*. Berlin: Walter de Gruyter, 2005.

'The Co-Ordinating Role of WHO in Poliomyelitis Research'. Geneva: World Health Organization, Executive Board, Fourteenth Session, Provisional agenda item 4, EB14/2, 1954.

Coigney, Rodolphe L. 'Letter from Rodolphe L. Coigney, Director of Liaison Office with United Nations to Dr. P. Dorolle, Deputy Director-General of the World Health Organization'. Geneva: Archives of World Health Organization N52/180/2/Hungary, 1957.

Colgrove, James. *State of Immunity: The Politics of Vaccination in Twentieth-Century America*. Berkeley: University of California Press, 2006.

Connelly, John. *Captive University: The Sovietization of East German, Czech and Polish Higher Education, 1945–1956*. Chapel Hill: University of North California Press, 2000.

Cordier, D.G. 'Methods of Artificial Respiration'. *British Medical Journal* 2, no. 4316 (1943): 381–3.

220   Bibliography

Crovari, Pietro. 'History of Polio Vaccination in Italy'. *Italian Journal of Public Health* 7, no. 3 (2010): 322–4.

Crowell, Richard L. 'Specific Viral Interference in Hela Cell Cultures Chronically Infected with Coxsackie B5 Virus'. *Journal of Bacteriology* 86, no. 3 (1963): 517–26.

Csanádi, Mária. 'Honnan Tovább? A Pártállam és Az Átalakulás'. In *Magyarország Társadalomtörténete (1945–1989)*, edited by Nikosz Fokasz and Antal Örkény, 147–73. Budapest: Új Mandátum, 1998.

Csehák, Judit. 'A Foglalkoztatási Rehabilitációról – a "Rokkantak Nemzetközi Éve" Után'. *Népegészségügy* 63, no. 3 (1982): 129–36.

Cserba, László. 'Az Egészségügy Gazdasági Helyzete 1957. Évben'. *Népegészségügy* 38, no. 4 (1957): 87–9.

Csillag, Ádám. 'Gyermekbénulás I'. edited by Ádám Csillag. Hungary: Csillag és Ádám Film; Fórum Film, 1995.

'Gyermekbénulás II'. edited by Ádám Csillag. Hungary: Csillag és Ádám Film; Fórum Film, 1995.

Csonka, Mária, ed. *Az Egészségnevelési Plakátok Üzenete*. Budapest: Budapest Főváros XVII. ker. Önkormányzat Egészségügyi Szolgálat Egészségnevelése, 2004.

Csumakov, M. P. 'Harc a Gyermekbénulás Ellen'. *Szabad Nép*, 10 April 1956, 4.

Csumakov, M. P., Vorosilova N. K., Vaszileja K. A., Bakina M. N., Asmarina E. E., Dobrova I. N., Drozdov Sz. G., *et al.* 'A Lakosság Poliomyelitis Elleni Tömeges Per Os Immunizálása a Szovjetúnióban Sabin Attenuált Törzseiből Készített Élő Vakcinával'. *Orvosi Hetilap* 101, no. 4 (1960): 109–17.

'Csütörtökön és Pénteken Kapják Az Első Védőoltást az 1–2 Éves Gyerekek'. *Népakarat*, 16 July 1957.

Cueto, Marcos. *Cold War, Deadly Fevers: Malaria Eradication in Mexico, 1955–1975*. Washington, D.C. and Baltimore: Woodrow Wilson Center Press; Johns Hopkins University Press, 2007.

Cummings, Richard H. *Cold War Radio: The Dangerous History of American Broadcasting in Europe, 1950–1989*. Jefferson, NC: McFarland, 2009.

Cushman, Thomas. *Notes from Underground: Rock Music Counterculture in Russia. Suny Series in the Sociology of Culture*. Albany: State University of New York Press, 1995.

Dalldorf, Gilbert. 'The Sparing Effect of Coxsackie Virus Infection on Experimental Poliomyelitis'. *Journal of Experimental Medicine* 94, no. 1 (1951): 65–71.

Dalldorf, Gilbert, and Robert Albrecht. 'Chronologic Association of Poliomyelitis and Coxsackie Virus Infections'. *Proceedings of the National Academy of Sciences USA* 41, no. 11 (1955): 978–82.

Dane, D. S., G. W. A. Dick, J. H. Connolly, O. D. Fischer, and F. McKeown. 'Vaccination against Poliomyelitis with Live Virus Vaccines. I. A Trial of TN Type II Vaccine'. *British Medical Journal* 1, no. 5010 (1957): 59–65.

Daniels, Lee A. 'Garret G. Ackerson, 88, Envoy in East Europe during Cold War'. *The New York Times*, 16 September 1992.

David-Fox, Michael. 'The Iron Curtain as a Semipermeable Membrane: Origins and Demise of the Stalinist Superiority Complex'. In *Cold War Crossings: International Travel and Exchange across the Soviet Bloc, 1940s–1960s*, edited by Patryk Babiracki and Kenyon Zimmer, 14–40. College Station: Texas A&M University Press, 2014.

Deák, Ernő. 'Adatok az 1956-os Menekülthullámról'. In *Magyarország Társadalomtörténete III. (1945–1989)*, edited by Nikosz Fokasz and Antal Örkény, 72–76. Budapest: Új Mandátum, 1999.

Debrődi, Gábor. 'A Mesterséges Lélegeztetés és az Újraélesztési Eljárások Története Magyarországon a Felvilágosult Abszolutizmus Korától Az 1960-as Évekig, a Hazai Modern Mentéstudomány (Oxyologia) Megszületéséig'. *Kharón* 7, no. 4 (2003): 52–76.

'December 14-én Kezdődnek a Gyermekbénulás Elleni Sabin-Féle Védőoltások'. *Népszava*, 22 November 1959, 1.

Dékány Pálné, Enyedi Judit Dr. 'Interview'. By Dóra Vargha (11 January 2008).

Deutsches Rotes Kreuz. 'Telegraph Message to M. Ammann International Committee of the Red Cross'. Geneva: International Committee of the Red Cross Archives, Epidémie de poliomyélite, B AG 280 094–031.02, 1118, 1957.

Dick, G. W. A., and D. S. Dane. 'The Evaluation of Live Poliovirus Vaccines: Paper Presented at the Conference on Live Poliovirus Vaccines, Washington, 22–26 June 1959'. In *WHO/Polio/36–44*. Geneva: World Health Organization, 1959.

'The Distribution and Use of Gamma Globulin: A Statement Issued April 20, 1953, by the Division of Medical Sciences of the National Research Council'. *Public Health Reports* 68, no. 7 (1953): 659–65.

Doleschall, Dr Frigyes, and Dr Aladár Kátay. 'Tájékoztató a Gyermekbénulásos Megbetegedésekről'. *Népszabadság*, 27 June 1957, 8.

Doleschall, Frigyes. 'A Magyar Egészségügy 1958. Évi Eredményei És 1959. Évi Terve'. Budapest: National Archives of Hungary, Doleschall Frigyes egészségügyi miniszter iratai, XIX-C-2-q, 1959.

'A Járványos Gyermekbénulás Elleni Védekezés Időszerű Feladatai. Előterjesztés a Magyar Forradalmi Munkás-Paraszt Kormányhoz'. edited by Minisztertanács. Budapest: National Archives of Hungary, 1957.

Dömök, I., Elisabeth Molnár, and Ágnes Jancsó. 'Virus Excretion after Mass Vaccination with Attenuated Polioviruses in Hungary'. *British Medical Journal* 1, no. 5237 (1961): 1410–17.

Dömök, István. 'A Hazai Járványügyi Helyzet Az Élő Poliovírus Vakcina Bevezetése Előtt'. In *A Gyermekbénulás Elleni Küzdelem. Beszámoló a Ma Már Múlttá Vált Betegség Ellen Folytatott Hősies Küzdelemről és Felszámolásának Lehetőségéről*, edited by Rezső Hargitai and Ákosné Kiss, 41-45. Budapest: Literatura Medicina, 1994.

'A Kampányoltások Időszaka'. In *A Gyermekbénulás Elleni Küzdelem: Beszámoló egy Ma Már Múlttá Váló Rettegett Betegség Ellen Folytatott Hősies Küzdelemről és Felszámolásának Lehetőségéről: A Szent László Kórház Centenáriumára Készült Összeállítás*, edited by Rezső Hargitai and Ákosné Kiss, 169–78. Budapest: Literatura Medica, 1994.

Donert, Celia. 'Whose Utopia? Gender, Ideology, and Human Rights at the 1975 World Congress of Women in East Berlin'. In *The Breakthrough: Human Rights in the 1970s*, edited by Jan Eckel and Samuel Moyn, 68–87. Philadelphia: University of Pennsylvania Press, 2014.

'Dr Doleschall Frigyes Miniszter Nyilatkozata a Népszavának Az Egészségügy Hároméves Tervéről, a Salk-Oltásokról És a Gyógyszerfogyasztásról'. *Népszava*, 17 June 1958, 1–2.

Drexler, Dr Miklós. 'Gyermekbénulás Elleni Védekezés'. Budapest: National Archives of Hungary, Drexler Miklós egészségügyi miniszter iratai, XIX-C-2-n, 369/1956, 18 August 1956.

'Dr. Ivanovics György Akadémikus Nyilatkozata a Genfi Gyermekparalyzis-Kongresszusról, a Hazánkban Folytatott Oltások Hatékonyságáról'. *Népszabadság*, 23 July 1957.

Drozdov, S. G. 'The Contemporary Poliomyelitis Situation in Europe'. Geneva: World Health Organization, European Symposium on Virus Diseases Control, EURO-322/8, 1966.

Dubinsky, Karen. 'Children, Ideology and Iconography: How Babies Rule the World'. *Journal of the History of Childhood and Youth* 5, no. 1 (2012): 5–13.

Ebrahim, GJ. 'Polio Eradication, and After . . .'. *Revista Brasileira de Saúde Materno Infantil* 2, no. 2 (2002): 189–91.

Egészségügyi Minisztérium. 'Az Egészségügyi Minisztérium Tájékoztatója az Ország 1957. Évi Március Havi Járványügyi Helyzetéről'. *Népegészségügy* 38, no. 4 (1957): 107–8.

'Egymillió Gyerek Kapott Idén Védőoltást. Megkezdődtek a Magyar-Szovjet Orvosi Napok'. *Népakarat*, 27 November 1957.

'Élet Egy Kanál Teában. Fővárosszerte Gyorsan És Szervezetten Folyik a Sabin-Oltás'. *Népszava*, 15 December 1959, 1.

'Eljött a Nap . . .'. *Heine-Medin Híradó* 1, July (1959): 2.

Emil, Grósz. 'A Rockefeller Foundation Magyarország Közegészségügyéért'. *Orvosi Hetilap* 68, no. 51 (1924): 910–1110.

Erickson, Paul. 'The Politics of Game Theory: Mathematics and Cold War Culture'. PhD thesis, University of Wisconsin, 2006.

Estívariz, Concepción F., Zsuzsanna Molnár, Linda Vencyel, Beatrix Kapusinszky, James A. Zingeser, Galina Y. Lipskaya, Olen M. Kew, György Berencsi, and Ágnes Csohán. 'Paralytic Poliomyelitis Associated with Sabin Monovalent and Bivalent Oral Polio Vaccines in Hungary'. *American Journal of Epidemiology* 174, no. 3 (2014): 316–25.

'European Association against Poliomyelitis'. *British Medical Journal* 2, no. 5257 (1961): 951–52.

European Association against Poliomyelitis and Allied Diseases, ed. *L'épidemiologie De La Poliomyelité. 12e Symposium, Bucharest, 4–7 May, 1969: Rapport Et Discussions*. Buchuresti: Academiei Republicii Socialiste Romania, 1969.

'Expert Committee on Poliomyelitis'. In *Techincal report series* edited by World Health Organization. Geneva: World Health Organization, 1958.

Expert Committee on Poliomyelitis. 'Expert Committee on Poliomyelitis: Third Report'. In *Technical Report Series*, edited by World Health Organization. Geneva: World Health Organization, 1960.

'Az Egészségügy Legégetőbb Problémái és az Egészségügyi Dolgozók Rehabilitációja'. *Népszava*, 23 October 1956.

Az Egészségügyi Miniszter 5/1958. (IX. 16) Eü. M. Számú Rendelete a Védőoltásokra Vonatkozó Jogszabályok Végrehajtásáról. 1958.

Az Egészségügyi Miniszter 8200–4/1953. Eü. M. Számú Utasítása a Fertőző Betegségek Megelőzéséről Szóló 61/1953 (XII.20) M. T. Számú Végrehajtása Tárgyában.

'Az Egészségügyi Miniszter 8200–5/1953. Eü.M. Számú Utasítása Védőoltásokról Szóló 60/1953. (XII.20.) M.T. Számú Rendelet Végrehajtása Tárgyában'. In *38/1958. (Eü. K. 19)*, edited by Egészségügyi Minisztérium. Budapest, 1958.

'Az Egészségügyi Minisztérium Heti Tájékoztatója a Gyermekbénulásos Megbetegedésekről'. *Népakarat*, 11 July 1957.

'Az Egészségügyi Minisztérium Tájékoztatója a Gyermekbénulásos Megbetegedésekről'. *Népszava*, 2 August 1959, 12.

'Az Egészségügyi Minisztérium Tájékoztatója a Gyermekbénulásos Megbetegedésekről'. *Népszava*, 21 July 1959.

'Az Egészségügyi Minisztérium Tájékoztatója a Gyermekbénulásos Megbetegedésekről És a Védekezés Módjairól'. *Népakarat*, no. 148, 27 June 1957.

'Az Egészségügyi Minisztérium Heti Tájékoztatója a Gyermekbénulásos Megbetegedésekről'. *Népakarat*, no. 172, 25 July 1957.

'Az Egészségügyi Minisztérium Tájékoztatója Az Ország 1959. Évi Augusztus Havi Járványügyi Helyzetéről'. *Népegészségügy* 40, no. 10 (1959): 279–80.

'Az Egészségügyi Minisztérium Tájékoztatója Az Ország 1959. Évi Július Havi Járványügyi Helyzetéről'. *Népegészségügy* 40, no. 9 (1959): 252.

'Az Egészségügyi Minisztérium Tájékoztatója Az Ország 1959. Évi November Havi Járványügyi Helyzetéről'. Budapest: National Archives of Hungary, Egészségügyi Minisztérium Állami közegészségügyi felügyelet és járványvédelmi főosztály iratai, XIX-C-2-e, 57370/1959, 1959.

Fainberg, Dina. 'The Heirs of the Future: Foreign Correspondents Meeting Youth on the Other Side of the Iron Curtain'. In *Winter Kept Us Warm Cold War Interactions Reconsidered*, edited by Sari Autio-Sarasmo, Brendan Humphreys and Katalin Miklóssy, 126–36. Helsinki: Aleksanteri Institute, 2010.

Fairchild, Amy L. 'The Polio Narratives: Dialogues with FDR'. *The Bulletin of the History of Medicine* 75 (2001): 488–534.

Faludi, András. '1958 Örvendetes Eredményeket Hozott a Gyermekbénulás Elleni Küzdelemben'. *Népszabadság*, 1959, 4.

'Az Élet Nevében. Látogatás a Heine-Medin Utókezelő Kórházban'. *Népszabadság*, 7 March 1958.

Fantini, Bernardino. 'Polio in Italy'. *Dynamis* 32, no. 2 (2012): 329–61.

Faragó, Jenő. 'Mindannyiunk Felelőssége'. *Népszabadság*, 24 July 1959.

Farley, John. *To Cast out Disease: A History of the International Health Division of the Rockefeller Foundation (1913–1951)*. Oxford: Oxford University Press, 2004.

Favez, Jean_Claude. *The Red Cross and the Holocaust*. Cambridge: Cambridge University Press, 1999.

Fehér, Rózsa. 'A Gyógyító Torna'. *Magyar Nemzet*, 24 January 1956.

'Ötszáznyolcvan Újabb Ágy a Heine-Medin-Kórban Megbetegedettek Utókezelésére'. *Magyar Nemzet*, 10 September 1957.

Ferenc, Péter, ed. *Gyermekbeteg-Ellátás a Rózsadombon 1956–2006*. Budapest: Tudomány Kiadó, 2006.

Ferencz, I. 'The Results of Mass Poliomyelitis Vaccination Program Carried out in 1957 in Hungary'. In *Vaccination and Immunity, Neurophysical and Neuropathological Aspects of Poliomyelitis. Vth Symposium of the European Association against Poliomyelitis*, edited by H. C. A. Lassen, 32–33. Madrid: Europ. Assoc. Poliomyelitis, 1959.

Fidelis, Malgorzata. 'Equality through Protection: The Politics of Women's Employment in Postwar Poland, 1945–1956'. *Slavic Review* 63, no. 2 (2004): 301–24.

'Fifth International Poliomyelitis Conference'. *British Medical Journal* 2, no. 5197 (1960): 533–4.

Fine, Paul E. M., and Ilona A. M. Carneiro. 'Transmissibility and Persistence of Oral Polio Vaccine Viruses: Implications for the Global Poliomyelitis Eradication Initiative'. *American Journal of Epidemiology* 150, no. 10 (1999): 1001–21.

The First Ten Years of the World Health Organization. Geneva: World Health Organization, 1958.

Fischer. 'Telegraph Message to Mr. Ammann International Red Cross Geneva'. Geneva: International Committee of the Red Cross Archives, Demandes d'aide pour secours en Hongrie, B AG 280 094–031.01, 280 (65), 1956.

Fogyatékosság-Politikai Szakismeretek Fogyatékosságtudományi Tudásbázis. Budapest: Eötvös Loránd Tudományegyetem Bárcsi Gusztáv Gyógypedagógiai Kar, 2009.

Földes, Pál, and Szeri Ilona. 'A Gamma-Globulin Prophylaxis Szerepe a Poliomyelitis Elleni Küzdelem Jelenlegi Helyzetében'. *Orvosi Hetilap* 100, no. 3 (1959): 115–17.

Forsythe, David P. *The Humanitarians: The International Committee of the Red Cross*. Cambridge: Cambridge University Press, 2005.

Foucault, Michel. *The History of Sexuality: An Introduction*. 1st edn. New York: Vintage Books, 1980.

Freyche, M. J. 'The Incidence of Poliomyelitis in the World, 1947–1949'. *Epidemiological and Vital Statistics Report* 4, no. 1 (1951): 3–18.

Freyche, Matthieu-Jean, and Johannes Nielsen. 'Incidence of Poliomyelitis since 1920'. In *Poliomyelitis*, edited by Robert Debré, 59-109. Geneva: World Health Organization, 1955.

Friede, Martin. *'Dose-Sparing by Intradermal Immunization'*. Geneva: World Health Organization, 2006.

Friedrich, Carl, and Zbigniew Brzezinski. *Totalitarian Dictatorship and Autocracy*. Cambridge, Mass.: Harvard University Press, 1965.

Frommer, Benjamin. 'Retribution as Legitimation: The Uses of Political Justice in Postwar Czechoslovakia'. *Contemporary European History* 13, no. 4 (2004): 477–92.

Gál, Dr György, László Dr Medve, and Dr Rák Kálmán. 'Az ETT Története'. Budapest: Egészségügyi Tudományos Tanács, 2015.

Gati, Charles. *Failed Illusions: Moscow, Washington, Budapest, and the 1956 Hungarian Revolt*. Cold War International History Project Series. Washington, D.C., Stanford, Calif.: Woodrow Wilson Center Press; Stanford University Press, 2006.

'Geneva Declaration of the Rights of the Child of 1924'. In *O.J. Spec.Supp. 21*, edited by League of Nations. Geneva, 1924.

Gere, Kálmánné. 'Interview'. By Dora Vargha (July 2007).

Geyer, Michael, and Sheila Fitzpatrick. 'After Totalitarianism – Stalinism and Nazism Compared'. In *Beyond Totalitarianism: Stalinism and Nazism Compared*, edited by Michael Geyer and Sheila Fitzpatrick, 1–41. New York: Cambridge University Press, 2008.

Gianone, András. '*Az Actio Catholica Története Magyarországon 1932–1948*'. PhD thesis, Eötvös Loránd Tudományegyetem, 2006.

Gille, Zsuzsa. *From the Cult of Waste to the Trash Heap of History: The Politics of Waste in Socialist and Postsocialist Hungary*. Bloomington and Indianapolis: Indiana University Press, 2007.

Glassheim, Eagle. 'Ethnic Cleansing, Communism, and Environmental Devastation in Czechoslovakia's Borderlands, 1945–1989'. *Journal of Modern History* 78, no. 1 (2006): 65–92.

Goldblum, Natan. 'Efficacy of Poliomyelitis Vaccine in Israel during the 3-Year Period 1957–1959'. In *Poliomyelits. Papers and Discussions Presented at the Fifth International Poliomyelitis Conference, Copenhagen, Denmark, July 26–28, 1960*, edited by International Poliomyelitis Congress, 138–42. Philadelphia: J. B. Lippincott Company, 1961.

Göllner, Barnabás. 'Gamma-Glonulin Felhasználása Fertőzőbetegségek Megelőzésére'. Budapest: City Archives of Budapest, Budapest Fővárosi Tanács VB Egészségügyi Osztályának iratai, XXIII.115.a/34. kisdoboz, 180788–1959, 1959.

Gould, Tony. *A Summer Plague: Polio and its Survivors*. New Haven: Yale University Press, 1995.

Goven, Joanna. 'Gender and Modernism in a Stalinist State'. *Social Politics* 9, no. 1 (2002): 3–28.

Graham, Loren R. *What Have We Learned about Science and Technology from the Russian Experience?* Stanford, Calif.: Stanford University Press, 1998.

Granville, Johanna C., and Raymond L. Garthoff. *The First Domino: International Decision Making during the Hungarian Crisis of 1956*. Eastern European Studies. *1st ed.* College Station: Texas A&M University Press, 2004.

Greene, Jeremy A. *Generic: The Unbranding of Modern Medicine*. Baltimore: Johns Hopkins University Press, 2014.

Greiner, Antal. 'Magyarország Egészségügyi Helyzete 1953. Évi Adatok Alapján'. Budapest: National Archives of Hungary, Simonovits István iratai, Egészségügyi Minisztérium, XIX-C-2-s Box 20, 7/1953, 1953.

Grimshaw, Margaret L. 'Scientific Specialization and the Poliovirus Controversy in the Years before World War II'. *Bulletin of the History of Medicine* 69, no. 1 (1995): 44–65.

Grinschgl, Gerald. 'Austria'. In *Third International Poliomyelitis Congress*, 31. Rome: J. B. Lippincott Company, 1955.

Groce, Nora Ellen, Lena Morgon Banks, and Michael Ashley Stein. 'Surviving Polio in a Post-Polio World'. *Social Science & Medicine* 107, April (2014): 171–8.

Gy., Sz. '"Most Jöjjön a Következő …'. *Népszava*, 11 February 1958.

226   Bibliography

Gyáni, Gábor; Kövér, György; Valuch, Tibor, ed. *Social History of Hungary from the Reform Era to the End of the Twentieth Century*, edited by Atlantic Studies on Society in Change. New York: Columbia University Press, 2004.

'A Gyermekbénulás Elleni Élő Oltóanyagról Tárgyal a Mikrobiológiai Kongresszus'. *Népszava*, 23 September 1959.

'A Gyermekbénulás Elleni Küzdelemről Tárgyal a Ix. Magyar-Szovjet Orvosi Konferencia'. *Népszabadság*, 1960, 6.

'A Gyermekbénulás Elleni Oltást Latin-Amerikában Elsőnek Kubában Vezetik Be'. *Népszabadság*, 1962, 6.

'Gyermekparalízis Elleni Védőoltás az 1–2 Éves Gyermekek Számára'. *Népszabadság*, 10 July 1957.

Gyurcsán, Judit. 'The ICRC's Operations in Hungary between 1956 and the 1960s'. *Miskolc Journal of International Law* 3, no. 3 (2006): 28–40.

Hagen, Trever. 'From Inhibition to Commitment: Configuring the Czech Underground'. *Eastbound*, no. Down to the Underground: Popular Music and Society in Central Europe, edited by Trever Hagen, Tamás Tófalvy and Gábor Vályi (2012): 1-34.

Hainiss, Elemér. 'A Heine-Medin-Betegség Kóreredete és Kezdeti Szakaszának Jelentősége'. *Orvosképzés*, no. 2 (1936): 109–13.

'Halálos Áldozata Van az Amerikában Felfedezett Gyermekparalízis Elleni Védőoltásnak'. *Szabad Nép*, 1 May 1955, 6.

Halász, Csilla. *'Agitáció és Propaganda a Népművelésben a Rákosi-Rendszer Idején'*. Eötvös Loránd Tudományegyetem, 2011.

Hale, J. H., M. Doraisingham, K. Kanagaratnam, K. W. Leong, and E. S. Monteiro. 'Large-Scale Use of Sabin Type 2 Attenuated Poliovirus Vaccine in Singapore during a Type 1 Poliomyelitis Epidemic'. *British Medical Journal* 1, no. 5137 (1959): 1541–48.

Halstead, Lauro S. 'A Brief History of Postpolio Syndrome in the United States'. *Archives of Physical Medicine and Rehabilitation* 92, no. 8 (2011): 1344–49.

Hamburger, László. 'Az Amerikai Fél Által Támasztott Salk-Szérum Szállítási Nehézségei. Feljegyzés Baczoni Jenő Miniszterhelyettes E.T. Részére'. Budapest: Magyar Nemzeti Levéltár, XIX-J-1-k USA Admin 1945–1964, 57, 1376/B, 1957.

Hammon, W. McD., L. L. Coriell, and P. F. Wehrle. 'Evaluation of Red Cross Gamma Globulin as a Prophylactic Agent for Poliomyelitis. IV. Final Report of Results Based on Clinical Diagnoses'. *Journal of the American Medical Association* 151, no. 11 (1953): 1272–85.

Hanebrink, Paul A. *In Defense of Christian Hungary: Religion, Nationalism, and Antisemitism, 1890–1944*. Ithaca, NY: Cornell University Press, 2006.

Haney, Lynne. *Inventing the Needy: Gender and the Politics of Welfare in Hungary*. Berkeley, Los Angeles and London: University of California Press, 2002.

Hantchef, Dr Z. S. 'An Outline of Red Cross Activities in the Fight against Poliomyelitis'. In *Fourth International Poliomyelitis Conference*, edited by International Poliomyelitis Congress, 3–6. Geneva: J. B. Lippincott Co., 1957.

'Rapport De Dr. Hantchef Directeur Du Bureau Médico-Social, Ligue Des Sociétés de la Croix-Rouge'. Geneva: International Committee of the Red Cross Archives, Epidémie de poliomyélite, B AG 280 094–031.02, 1957.

Hantos, János. *A Magyar Vöröskereszt 100 Éve. Emberiesség Háborúban és Békében*. Budapest: Akadémiai Kiadó, 1981.

'Harmincezer Iskolásgyermeket Üdültet a SZOT, Kétszázezer Gyerek Megy Úttörőtáborba'. *Népszava*, 4 June 1959.

Harrison, Mark. 'Positioning Paper'. *Bulletin of the History of Medicine* 89, no. 4 (2016): 639–89.

Harsch, Donna. 'Medicalized Social Hygiene? Tuberculosis Policy in the German Democratic Republic'. *Bulletin of the History of Medicine* 86, no. 3 (2012): 394–423.

'Határozat Az Anya- És Gyermekvédelem Továbbfejlesztéséről. 1004/1953. (II.8.) M.T'. In *A Családjogi Törvény*, edited by Jenő Bacsó, Géza Rády and Viktor Szigligeti, 365–74. Budapest: Közgazdasági és Jogi Könyvkiadó, 1955.

'Házi Feljegyzés'. Budapest: National Archives of Hungary, Zsoldos Sándor egészségügyi miniszter iratai, XIX-C-2-m, 821/v/1–16, 6 July 1956.

Hecht, Gabrielle, ed. *Entangled Geographies: Empire and Technopolitics in the Global Cold War*, edited byCambridge, Mass.: MIT Press, 2011.

Hegedűs, Dr Lajos. *The History of Human*. Budapest: HUMAN Pharmaceutical Works Co. Ltd., 2003.

'Interview'. By Dora Vargha (April 2010).

Heine, Jakob von. *Beobachtungen über Lähmungszustände der untern Extremitäten und deren Behandlung: Mit 7 Steindrucktafeln*. Stuttgart: Köhler, 1840.

Spinale Kinderlähmung: Monographie. Stuttgart: J. G. Cottascher Verlag, 1860.

'Heine Medin Híradó'. Budapest: Heine Medin Utókezelő Kórház, 1959–63.

'A Heine-Medines Mozgászavarok Utókezeléséről'. Hungary, 1957.

Hemmes, G. D. 'Netherlands'. In *Third International Poliomyelitis Conference*, 50–52. Rome: J. B. Lippincott, 1955.

Henderson, D. A. 'The Global Eradication of Smallpox: Historical Perspectives and Future Prospects'. In *The Global Eradication of Smallpox*, edited by Sanjoy Bhattacharya and Sharon Messenger, 7–35. New Perspectives in South Asian History. New Delhi: Orient Black Swan, 2010.

Henningsen, Dr. E. Juel. 'Poliovaccination in Denmark'. Paper presented at the VIth Symposium of the European Association of Poliomyelitis, Munich, 7–9 September 1959.

Henningsen, E. Juel. 'Denmark'. In *Fourth International Poliomyelitis Conference*, 29-30. Geneva: J. B. Lippincott, 1957.

'Denmark'. In *Third International Poliomyelitis Conference*, 37–39. Rome: J. B. Lippincott Company, 1955.

'A Hét Végéig Meghosszabbították a Sabin-Oltások Határidejét'. *Népszava*, 17 December 1959, 2.

'Hétfőn Kezdődik 500 000 Budapesti Gyerek Védőoltása'. *Népszava*, 11 December 1959, 2.

Heyck, Hunter, and David Keiser. 'Focus: New Perspectives on Science and the Cold War. Introduction'. *Isis* 101, no. 2 (2010): 362–66.

Heywood, Colin. *A History of Childhood*. Cambridge: Polity Press, 2001.

Higonnet, Anne. *Pictures of Innocence: A History and Crisis of Ideal Childhood*. London: Thames and Hudson, 1998.

228   Bibliography

Hodges, Sarah. 'The Global Menace'. *Social History of Medicine* 25, no. 3 (2012): 719–28.

Hoffman, Lily M. 'Professional Autonomy Reconsidered: The Case of Czech Medicine under State Socialism'. *Comparative Studies in Society and History* 39, no. 2 (1997): 346–72.

Hong, Young-sun. *Cold War Germany, the Third World and the Global Humanitarian Regime: Human Rights in History.* New York: Cambridge University Press, 2015.

Horstmann, Dorothy. *Report on Live Poliovirus Vaccination in the Union of Soviet Socialist Republics, Poland and Czechoslovakia.* World Health Organization, 1959.

Horváth, Attila. *A Magyar Sajtó Története a Szovjet Típusú Diktatúra Idején.* Médiatudományi Könyvtár. Budapest: Médiatudományi intézet, 2013.

Horváth, Sándor. 'Everyday Life in the First Hungarian Socialist City'. *International Labor and Working-Class History* 68 (2005): 24–46.

Horváth, Sándor. ed. *Mindennapok Rákosi és Kádár Korában: Új Utak a Szocialista Korszak Kutatásában.* Budapest: Nyitott Könyvműhely, 2008.

Horvath, Zsolt K., and Zsófia Frazon. 'A Megsértett Magyarország. A Terror Háza mint Tárgybemutatás, Emlékmű és Politikai Rítus'. *Regio*, no. 4 (2002): 303–47.

Hotez, Peter J. 'Peace through Vaccine Diplomacy'. *Science* 327, no. 5971 (2010): 1301.

Hounshell, David A. 'Rethinking the Cold War; Rethinking Science and Technology in the Cold War; Rethinking the Social Study of Science and Technology'. *Social Studies of Science* 31, no. 2 (2001): 289–97.

Howkins, Adrian John. 'Frozen Empires: A History of the Antarctic Sovereignty Dispute between Britain, Argentina, and Chile, 1939–1959'. PhD thesis, University of Texas at Austin, 2008.

Hull, Harry F., Maureen E. Birmingham, Bjorn Melgaard, and Jong Wook Lee. 'Progress toward Global Polio Eradication'. *Journal of Infectious Diseases* 175, no. Supplement 1 (1997): S4–S9.

Humán, Oltóanyagtermelő és Kutató Intézet. 'Kötelező Védőoltások Folyamatos Végrehajtása a Főváros Területén'. Budapest: National Archives of Hungary, Egészségügyi Minisztérium Állami közegészségügyi felügyelet és járványvédelmi főosztály iratai, XIX-C-2-e 1959, 51918, 1958.

Humphreys, Margaret. *Yellow Fever and the South.* Baltimore, Md.: Johns Hopkins University Press, 1999.

'Hungary Battle Polio'. *Washington Post and Times Herald,* 2 July 1957.

'Az Ifjúság Csoportos Nyaraltatásának Egészségügyi Szabályai'. *Népakarat,* 2 July 1957.

Illés, Sándor and Hablicsek, László. 'Az 1956-os Kivándorlás Népességi Hatásai'. *Statisztikai Szemle* 85, no. 2 (2007): 157–72.

Ingebrigtsen, Erik. 'Priviliged Origins: "National Models" and Reforms of Public Health in Interwar Hungary'. In *Imagining the West in Eastern Europe and the Soviet Union,* edited by György Péteri, 36–58. Pitt Series in Russian and East European Studies. Pittsburgh: University of Pittsburgh Press, 2010.

Initiative, Global Polio Eradication. 'History of Polio'. www.polioeradication .org/Polioandprevention/Historyofpolio.aspx

Polio Eradication & Endgame Strategic Plan 2013–2018. Geneva: World Health
    Organization, 2013.
'Intézkedések Kubában a Gyermekbénulás Megelőzésére'. *Népszabadság*, 1962, 6.
Irwin, Julia. 'Sauvons Les Bébés: Child Health and U.S. Humanitarian Aid in the First
    World War Era'. *Bulletin of the History of Medicine* 86, no. 1 (2012): 37–65.
Ivanov, Konstantin. 'Science after Stalin: Forging a New Image of Soviet Science'.
    Science in Context 15, no. 2 (2002): 317–38.
Ivanovics, G. 'Letter from Ivanovics, G. To Sabin, Albert B. Dated 1959–10–26'.
    Cincinnati: Hauck Center for the Albert B. Sabin Archives, Sabin, Albert B.,
    1906–1993 – Correspondence, Box 13, File 09 (Ivanovics, George – 1954–1960,
    1959.
Jacobs, Charlotte DeCroes. *Jonas Salk: A Life*. Oxford: Oxford University Press, 2015.
'Járványos Gyermekbénulás Elleni Védekezés'. Budapest: Budapest City Archives,
    Fővárosi Tanács Egészségügyi Osztálya, 10. doboz, B/8/2558/952.VIII.19, 1952.
'A Járványos Gyermekbénulás Elleni Védekezés Időszerű Feladatai. Vita'. Budapest:
    National Archives of Hungary, A Minisztertanács üléseinek jegyzőkönyvei,
    XIX-A-83-a. 1957.
'Javaslat a Gyermekparalízisről Szóló Sajtócikk Megjelenésére Vonatkozóan. Münnich
    Elvtárs Szóbeli Javaslata'. Budapest: National Archives of Hungary,
    Minisztertanács Iratai, M-KS 288.f/33. ő.e., 9R/81, 1957.
'Jegyzőkönyv 1959. Március 27-én Megtartott Elnökségi Ülésről'. Budapest: National
    Archives of Hungary, Vezető testületek, Elnökség ülésjegyzőkönyvek 1957–1962,
    P2130 MVK, 1959.
'Jegyzőkönyv a Folyó Évi Október 24-én Pénteken Délután 3 Órakkor Megtartott
    Járványügyi Ankéton Elhangzott Felszólalásokról'. Budapest: Budapest City
    Archives, Fővárosi Tanács Egészségügyi Osztálya, 10. doboz Tanácsi iratok
    gyűjteménye, B/8/3280/952, 1952.
'Jegyzőkönyv Felvéve Az 1957 Június 25-én Megtartott Országos Vezetőségválasztó
    Értekezletről'. Budapest: National Archives of Hungary, The papers of the
    Hungarian Red Cross, XXVIII-C-1, 1957.
Johnson, A. Ross. *Radio Free Europe and Radio Liberty: The CIA Years and Beyond*.
    Washington and Stanford: Woodrow Wilson Center Press; Stanford University
    Press, 2010.
Johnson, A. Ross, and R. Eugene Parta, eds. *Cold War Broadcasting: Impact on the
    Soviet Union and Eastern Europe*. Budapest; New York: Central European
    University Press, 2010.
Juhász, Judit. 'Email Interview'. By Dora Vargha (26 October 2015).
'Július 18. és 19-én Megkezdődik a Gyermekbénulás Elleni Védőoltás. Az
    Egészségügyi Minisztérium Hivatalos Tájékoztatója'. *Népakarat*, 14 July 1957.
'Kánikulai Jelentés a Strandokról, a Közlekedésről és a Vasárnapi Előkészületekről'.
    Népakarat, 11 July 1959.
Kapos, Vilmos. 'Jelentés a Főváros Közegészségügyi Járványügyi Helyzetéről'.
    Budapest: City Archives of Budapest, MSZMP Budapesti pártértekezletei
    1957–1989, XXXV.1.a.2., 4. őe, 1966.
'A Folyamatos Védőoltások a Fővárosban'. Budapest: National Archives of
    Hungary, Egészségügyi Minisztérium Állami közegészségügyi felügyelet és
    járványvédelmi főosztály iratai, XIX-C-2-e 1959, 51250, 1959.

'A Kötelező Védőoltások Folyamatos Végrehajtása a Főváros Területén'. Budapest:
National Archives of Hungary, Egészségügyi Minisztérium Állami
közegészségügyi felügyelet és járványvédelmi főosztály iratai, XIX-C-2-e 1959,
51453, 1958.

Karossa-Pfeiffer, József Dr. 'Megbízás'. Budapest: Budapest City Archives,
Budapest Főváros Tanácsa Végrehajtóbizottságának XII. Egészségügyi osztálya,
1956.

Kasza, László. 'A Magyar Állambiztonsági Szervezet és a Szabad Európa Rádió'.
In Közelítések a Kádárizmushoz, edited by Pál Germuska and János Rainer M.,
144–89. Budapest: 1956-os Intézet, 2008.

Kátay, Aladár. 'Vaccination against Poliomyelitis in Hungary'. Paper presented at
the Eigthth European Symposium on Poliomyelitis, Prague, 23–26 September
1962.

'The Active Immunization against Poliomyelitis in Hungary and Its Three Years'
Results'. In The Control of Poliomyelitis by Live Poliovirus Vaccine. Studies on
Mass Vaccinations in Hungary, in the Ussr, in Czechoslovakia and the German
Democratic Republic. Papers Presented at the Hungarian-Soviet Medical
Conference September 24–30, 1960, edited by J. Weissfeiler, 71-84. Budapest:
Publishing House of the Hungarian Academy of Sciences, 1961.

'Járványügyi Adatok Közlése az Egészségügyi Világszervezettel'. Budapest:
National Archives of Hungary, Egészségügyi Minisztérium Állami
Közegészségügyi Felügyelet és Járványvédelmi Főosztály iratai, XIX-C-2-e,
57370, 1959.

'Folyamatos Védőoltások a Fővárosban'. Budapest: Magyar Oszágos Levéltár,
Egészségügyi Minisztérium Állami közegészségügyi felügyelet és járványvédelmi
főosztály iratai, XIX-C-2-e 1959, 52417, 1958.

'A Humán Intézet Vírus Osztályának Átköltözése Az Oki-Ba'. Budapest: MOL,
Egészségügyi Minisztérium iratai, XIX-C-2-e 1957, 50.189/1957, 821/1/Virus/
1957. OKI, 1957.

'Járványügyi Helyzetünk és Feladataink'. Népegészségügy 8, no. 10–11 (1957):
247–58.

'Koppenhágai Tanulmányútról Jelentés'. Budapest: MOL, Egészségügyi
Minisztérium iratai, XIX-C-2-e, 51406, 1957.

'Polio-Vaccina Termelése'. Budapest: National Archives of Hungary, Dr. Vilmon
Gyula Egészségügyi Miniszter Iratai, XIX-C-2-e, 50.654/1957, 1957.

Kelly, Catriona. 'Defending Children's Rights, "in Defense of Peace": Children and
Soviet Cultural Policy'. Kritika: Explorations in Russian and Eurasian History 9,
no. 4 (2008): 711–46.

Children's World: Growing up in Russia 1890–1991. New Haven: Yale University
Press, 2007.

Kenez, Peter. 'The Hungarian Communist Party and the Catholic Church 1945–1948'.
The Journal of Modern History 75, no. 4 (2003).

Kéri, Katalin. 'Gyermekképünk Az Ötvenes Évek Első Felében'. Iskolakultúra, no. 3
(2002): 47–59.

Kertész, Tamás, and Tibor Szabó. 'Interview'. By Dora Vargha (November 2010).

'Két Érdekes Előadással Kezdődött Meg a Balatonfüredi Orvoskongresszus'.
Népakarat, 27 September 1957.

Kew, Olen M., Roland W. Sutter, Esther M. de Gourville, Walter R. Dowdle, and
    Mark A. Pallansch. 'Vaccine-Derived Polioviruses and the Endgame Strategy
    for Global Polio Eradication'. *Annual Review of Microbiology* 59 (2005):
    587–635.
Killingsworth, Matt. *Civil Society in Communist Eastern Europe*. Colchester: ECPR
    Press, 2012.
Kind-Kovacs, Friederike. 'Child Transports across and beyond the Empire: World
    War I and the Relocation of Needy Children from Central Europe'. *Revue
    d'histoire de l'enfance 'irréguliere'* 15, no. Enfances déplacées. (II) en temps de
    guerre (2013): 75–109.
Kind-Kovács, Friederike, and Jessie Labov. *Samizdat, Tamizdat, and Beyond:
    Transnational Media during and after Socialism*. Studies in Contemporary
    European History. New York: Berghahn Books, 2013.
Kiss, Ákosné. *'Tartós Gépi Lélegeztetéssel Életben Tartott Postpoliós Légzésbénultak
    Sorsa'*. Candidate thesis [kandidátusi értekezés], Semmelweis University, 1989.
    'Légzésbénult Utókezelő Osztályon Szerzett Tapasztalataink'. In *Előadások a
    Gyermekbénulás Rehabilitációs Problémáiról*, edited by László Lukács, 47–53.
    Budapest: Statisztikai Kiadó, 1961.
Kligman, Gail. *The Politics of Duplicity: Controlling Reproduction in Ceausescu's
    Romania*. Berkeley: University of California Press, 1998.
Kligman, Gail, and Katherine Verdery. 'Social Dimensions of Collectivization:
    Fomenting Class Warfare in Transylvania'. In *World Order after Leninism:
    Essays in Honor of Ken Jowitt*, edited by Vladimir Tismaneanu, Marc Morjé
    Howard and Rudra Sil, 127–48. Seattle: Herbert J. Ellison Center for Russian,
    East European, and Central Asian Studies, University of Washington, 2006.
Klinger, András. 'Magyarország Népesedése az Elmúlt Negyven Évben'. In
    Magyarország Társadalomtörténete III. (1945–1989), edited by Nikosz Fokasz
    and Antal Örkény, 45-65. Budapest: Új Mandátum, 1999.
Kluger, Jeffrey. *Splendid Solution: Jonas Salk and the Conquest of Polio*. New York:
    G. P. Putnam's Sons, 2004.
Knoll, Andor. *Az Egészséges Gyermek. Nevelési Tanácsok Szülők Részére*.
    Székesfehérvár: Magyar Vöröskereszt Egészségkultúrális Osztály, 1958.
Koch, Erin. *Free Market Tuberculosis: Managing Epidemics in Post-Soviet Georgia*.
    Nashville, Tenn.: Vanderbilt University Press, 2013.
Koch, Sándor. 'Szubjektív Virológia'. *Természet Világa* 130, no. 2 (1999): 60–62.
    'Present Status of Specific Poliomyelitis Prophylaxis in Hungary'. Paper presented at
    the VIth Symposium of the European Association of Poliomyelitis, Munich, 7–9
    September 1959.
Koch, Sándor, Gábor Veres, and Elek Farkas. 'Jelentés a Koppenhágai
    Tanulmányútunkról'. Budapest: MOL Egészségügyi Minisztérium iratai,
    XIX-C-2-e, 50.911, 821/4/Virus/1957, 1957.
Kocsis, Piroska. 'A Szövőszéktől a Miniszteri Bársonyszékig'. *Archívnet* 6, no. 4
    (2006): www.archivnet.hu/politika/a_szovoszektol_a_miniszteri_barsonyszekig
    .html (last accessed 8 June 2018).
Koonz, Claudia. 'Between Memory and Oblivion: Concentration Camps in German
    Memory'. In *Commemorations: The Politics of National Identity*, edited by John
    R. Gillis, 258–80. Princeton: Princeton University Press, 1994.

Koprowski, H. 'Preliminary Report as of September 1960 of Mass Vaccination in Poland with Koprowski's Strains of Attenuated Virus'. Geneva: World Health Organization Library, Study Group on Requirements for Poliomyelitis Vaccine (Live, Attenuated Virus), 1960.

Koprowski, Hilary. 'Historical Aspects of the Development of Live Virus Vaccine in Poliomyelitis'. *British Medical Journal* 2, no. 5192 (1960): 85–91.

Kormos, Franciska. *Magánkeringő*. Budapest: Aposztróf Kiadó, 2010.

Kósa, Ferenc. 'Az Amatőr Rádiózás Gyulai Emlékei'. *Gyulai Hírlap*, 2 July 2010.

Kostrzewski, Jan. 'Poliomyelitis in Poland'. Geneva: World Health Organization Library, World Heatlh Organization VIR/Polio/69.2, 1969.

Kovács, Mária. *Liberal Professions and Illiberal Politics: Hungary from the Habsburgs to the Holocaust* Washington: Woodrow Wilson Center Press, 1994.

Koven, Seth. 'Remembering Dismemberment: Crippled Children, Wounded Soldiers, and the Great War in Great Britain'. *American Historical Review* 99, no. 4 (1994): 1167–1202.

Központi Statisztikai Hivatal. 'Egészségügyi Helyzet 1963'. *Statisztikai időszaki közlemények*, no. 5 (1964).

'Népesség, Népmozgalom (1941–)'. Budapest: Központi Statisztikai Hivatal, 2012, www.ksh.hu/docs/hun/xstadat/xstadat_eves/i_wnt001a.html (last accessed 9 June 2018).

Krementsov, Nikolai. *The Cure: A Story of Cancer and Politics from the Annals of the Cold War*. Chicago and London: University of Chicago Press, 2002.

Krysko, Michael A. *American Radio in China: International Encounters with Technology and Communications, 1919–41*. Palgrave Studies in the History of the Media, edited byBasingstoke: Palgrave MacMillan, 2011.

Kudlick, Catherine. 'Smallpox, Disability and Survival: Rewriting Paradigms from a New Epidemic Script'. In *Disability Histories*, edited by Susan Burch and Michael Rembis, 185–200. Urbana, Chicago and Springfield: University of Illinois Press, 2014.

Kudlick, Catherine J. 'Disability History: Why We Need Another "Other"'. *American Historical Review* 108, no. 3 (2003): 763–93.

Kukowa. 'Poliomyelitis-Schutzimpfung in Der Deutschen Demokratiscen Republik'. In *Anti-Poliomyelitis Vaccinations, Physio-Pathology of the Respiratory Disorder, Poliomyelitis of the 'Very Young Child'. VIth symposium of the European Association against Poliomyelitis*, edited by H. C. A. Lassen, 52–53. Munich: Europ. Assoc. Poliomyelitis, 1960.

Külügyminisztérium. 'A Külügyminisztérium III. Osztályának Feljegyzése a Magyar-Amerikai Viszonyról'. Budapest: National Archives of Hungary, XIX-J-1-j USA 4/bd, 99/1958, 11. doboz, 1958.

Kun, Béla. *A Fiatalkorúak Támogatására Hivatott Jótékonycélú Intézmények Magyarországon*. Budapest: Wodianer F. és fiai könyvnyomdai műintézete, 1911.

Kürti, László. '"Red Csepel": Working Youth in a Socialist Firm'. *East European Quarterly* 23, no. 4 (1990): 45–68.

'Lago, P. Más. 'Eradication of Poliomyelitis in Cuba: A Historical Perspective'. *Bulletin of the World Health Organization* 77, no. 8 (1999): 681–87.

Lakos, Pál. 'Augusztus Hónapban Végzett Gyermekbénulás Elleni Védőoltásokról Jelentés'. Budapest: National Archives of Hungary, Egészségügyi Minisztérium

Állami közegészségügyi felügyelet és járványvédelmi főosztály iratai, XIX-C-2-e, 53885, 1957.

Lampland, Martha. 'The Technopolitical Lineage of State Planning in Mid-Century Hungary (1930–1956)'. In *Entangled Geographies: Empire and Technopolitics in the Global Cold War*, edited by Gabrielle Hecht, 155–84. Cambridge, Mass.: MIT Press, 2011.

Langmuir, Alexander D. 'Inactivated Virus Vaccines: Protective Efficacy'. In *Poliomyelitis: Papers and Discussions Presented at the Fifth International Poliomyelitis Conference Copenhagen, Denmark, July 26–28, 1960*, edited by International Poliomyelitis Congress, 105–13. Philadelphia and Montreal: J. B. Lippincott Company, 1961.

Lassen, H. C. A. 'The Epidemic of Poliomyelitis in Copenhagen, 1952'. *Proceedings of the Royal Society of Medicine* 47, no. 1, Section of Epidemiology and Preventive Medicine (1953): 67–71.

'Eröffnungsansprache'. In *VIth Symposium of the European Association of Poliomyelitis*, 5–7. Brussels: European Association of Poliomyelitis, 1959.

László, Anna. *Vaspólya*. Budapest: Szépirodalmi könyvkiadó, 1979.

Launius, Roger D., James Rodger Fleming, and David H. DeVorkin. *Globalizing Polar Science: Reconsidering the International Polar and Geophysical Years*. Palgrave Studies in the History of Science and Technology. 1st edn. New York: Palgrave Macmillan, 2010.

Lebow, Katherine. 'Public Works, Private Lives: Youth Brigades in Nowa Huta in the 1950s'. *Contemporary European History* 10, no. 2 (2001): 199–219.

Lebow, Katherine A. 'Public Works, Private Lives: Youth Brigades in Nowa Huta in the 1950s'. *Contemporary European History* 10, no. 2 (2001): 199–219.

'Lesz Szappan'. *Népakarat*, 7 December 1956.

'Letter from the District Public Health and Epidemiological Centre Dated 1960–1967?'. Cincinnati: Hauck Center for the Albert B. Sabin Archives, Sabin, Albert B., 1906–1993 – Correspondence, Box 02, File 09 (Hungary – 1960–1967), 1959.

'Letter to Jenő Incze Foreign Trade Minister'. Budapest: National Archives of Hungary, Egészségügyi Minisztérium Állami Közegészségügyi Felügyeleti és Járványvédeli Főosztály, XIX-C-2-e, 54304/1957, 1957.

Lindner, Ulrike, and Stuart Blume. 'Vaccine Innovation and Adoption: Polio Vaccines in the Uk, the Netherlands and West Germany, 1955–1965'. *Medical History* 50, no. 4 (2006): 425–46.

Linker, Beth. *War's Waste: Rehabilitation in World War I America*. Chicago: University of Chicago Press, 2011.

'Live Poliovirus Vaccines'. *British Medical Journal* 2, no. 5193 (1960): 202–03.

Losonczy, György, Gyula Vigh, Ottó Rudnai, and Domokos Boda. 'A Salk Vakcináció és a Poliomyelitis Klinikai Lefolyásának Összefüggése'. *Orvosi Hetilap* 101, no. 16 (1961): 733–35.

Lukács, László. 'A Budai Gyermekkórház Történetének Periódusai. 1956. 12 November.-1963. December 31'. In *Gyermekbeteg-Ellátás a Rózsadombon 1956–2006*, edited by Péter Ferenc. Budapest: Tudomány Kiadó, 2006.

'Feljegyzés a Fővárosi Heine-Medin Kórház és Rendelőintézet Alapításáról, Működéséről, Eredményeiről és Ezzel Kapcsolatos Tevékenységéről'. Budapest: Personal archives of Dr. Prof. Ferenc Péter, 1993.

'Letter to the Health Minister'. Budapest: National Archives of Hungary, XIX-C-2-d-8113/L/1–1954, 1954.

Lupkovics, György. 'A Nemzetközi Vöröskereszt Aktivistái a Magyar Forradalomban És a Kgb Fogságában'. *Betekintő*, no. 3 (2009): 1–7.

Lycke, Erik. 'Interference between Poliomyelitis Virus and Coxsackie B or Echo Viruses'. *Archives of Virology* 8, no. 3 (1958): 351–59.

'Magasabb Összeg Egészégügyre – 30 Millió Salk-Vaccinára. Az Egészségügy Hároméves Tervéről és Jövő Évi Költségvetéséről Tárgyalt az Országgyűlés Szociális és Egészségügyi Bizottsága'. *Népakarat*, 15 November 1957.

A Magyar Forradalmi Munkás-Paraszt Kormány 1027/1958 (VIII. 3.) Számú Határozata a Gyermekbénulás Elleni Védekezésről. 1958.

'A Magyar Forradalmi Munkás-Paraszt Kormány Határozata a Járványos Gyermekbénulás Elleni Védekezés Időszerű Feladatairól'. In *1062/1957/VII.6./ Korm*, 1957.

'A Magyar Népköztársaság Kormánya És a Csehszlovák Köztársaság Kormánya Között Az Egészségügyi Együttműködésre Vonatkozóan Létrejött és Budapesten 1955. Április 28. Napján Aláírt Egyezmény'. Budapest: National Archives of Hungary, A Minisztertanács üléseinek jegyzőkönyvei, XIX-A-83-a, 1957. junius 8., 1957.

A Magyar Televízió Története. Szekszárd: Babits Kiadó, 1996–2000.

Maher, Chris. 'Telephone Interview'. By Dóra Vargha (2012).

'The Main Results of the IV Scientific Conference of the Institute and the International Symposium on Live Poliovirus Vaccine and the 1st Soviet-American Discussions of Problems Relating to the Control of Poliomyelitis'. Paper presented at the IV Scientific Conference of the Institute and the International Symposium on live poliovirus vaccine and the 1st Soviet-American Discussions of Problems Relating to the Control of Poliomyelitis, Moscow, 1960.

Manela, Erez. 'A Pox on Your Narrative: Writing Disease Control into Cold War History'. *Diplomatic History* 34, no. 2 (2010): 299–323.

Marhall, Dominique. 'Children's Rights and Children's Action in International Relief and Domestic Welfare: The Work of Herbert Hoover between 1914 and 1950'. *The Journal of the History of Childhood and Youth* 1, no. 3 (2008): 351–88.

Mark, James. 'Discrimination, Opportunity Adn Middle-Class Success in Early Communist Hungary'. *The Historical Journal* 48, no. 2 (2005): 499–521.

Marks, Sarah, and Mat Savelli. *Psychiatry in Communist Europe: Mental Health in Historical Perspective*. Houndmills, Basingstoke and New York, NY: Palgrave Macmillan, 2015.

Martin, Emily. *Flexible Bodies: Tracking Immunity in American Culture-from the Days of Polio to the Age of Aids*. Boston: Beacon Press, 1994.

'Mass Immunization with the Live Poliovirus Vaccine in the Soviet Union'. *British Medical Journal* 1, no. 5187 (1960): 1729–30.

Mawdsley, Stephen E. *Selling Science: Polio and the Promise of Gamma Globulin*. Critical Issues in Health and Medicine. New Brunswick: Rutgers University Press, 2016.

Mecseky, László. 'Meteorológiai Vonatkozások a Heine-Medin-Kór Epidemiológiájában'. *Népegészségügy*, no. 14 (1941).

'Megérkezett Hazánkba az Első Vastüdő'. In *Magyar Filmhíradó*. Hungary, 1948.

'Megérkezett New Yorkba M. Csumakov Vezetésével a Szovjet Orgostudós-Küldöttség'. *Szabad Nép*, 20 January 1956, 4.

'Megkezdték a IV. Salk-Védőoltás Beadását'. *Népszava*, 31 July 1959.

Mészáros, Elvira. 'Interview'. By Dora Vargha (11 January 2008).

Mezei, Károly. ' . . . *Isten Van, Az Ember Történik'. Koch Sándor Virológussal Beszélget Mezei Károly*. Budapest: Kairosz Kiadó, 2006.

Michelson, Sig. *America's Other Voice: The Story of Radio Free Europe and Radio Liberty*. New York: Praeger, 1983.

Mikkonen, Simo, and Pia Koivunen, eds. *Beyond the Divide: Entangled Histories of Cold War Europe*. New York and Oxford: Berghahn Books, 2015.

Millward, Gareth. '"A Matter of Commonsense": The Coventry Poliomyelitis Epidemic in 1957 and the British Public'. *Contemporary British History*, 31, no. 3 (2016): 1–23.

'Minden Ötszázadik'. Hungary, 1967.

Minisztérium, Egészségügyi. 'Jelentés a Politikai Bizottsághoz Az Ország Közegészségügyi És Járványügyi Helyzetéről'. Budapest: Magyar Országos Levéltár, XIX-C-2-m, 115/1954, 1954.

Minisztertanács. 'Gyermekbénulás Elleni Szérum Behozataláról'. In *3311/1957*. Budapest, 18 July 1957.

'A Minisztertanács Indézkedései a Gyermekparalízis Megelőzése és a Betegellátás Érdekében'. *Népakarat*, 5 July 1957.

Moldován. 'Aki Még Nem Kapott – Áprilisban Jelentkezzék Gyermekbénulás Elleni Védőoltásra'. *Népszava*, 16 April 1958.

Moore, Bradley Matthys. 'For the People's Health: Ideology, Medical Authority and Hygienic Science in Communist Czechoslovakia'. *Social History of Medicine* 27, no. 1 (2014): 122–43.

'For the People's Health: Medical Authority and Marxist-Leninism in Communist Czechoslovakia, 1948–1956'. In *American Association for the History of Medicine 2011 Annual Meeting*. Philadelphia, 2011.

'Morbidity Statistics Acute Poliomyelitis'. *Epidemiological and Vital Statistics Report* 14 (1961): 91–117.

Moulin, Anne Marie. 'The Pasteur Institute's International Network: Scientific Innovations and French Tropisms'. In *Transnational Intellectual Networks. Forms of Academic Knowledge and the Search for Cultural Identities*, edited by Christophe Charle et al., 135–64. Frankfurt: Campus, 2004.

Münnich, Ferenc. 'A Magyar Forradalmi Munkás-Paraszt Kormány Határozata a Járványos Gyermekbénulás Időszerű Feladatairól Szóló 1062/1957/Vii.6./Korm Sz. Határozat Kiegészítéséről'. In *3290/1957*, 1957.

Muraskin, William A. *Polio Eradication and Its Discontents: An Historian's Journey through an International Public Health (Un)Civil War. New Perspectives in South Asian History*. New Delhi: Orient Blackswan, 2012.

Murray, Roderick. 'The Standardization of Potency of Poliomyelitis Vaccine'. In *Poliomyelitis. Papers and Discussions Presented at the Fifth International Poliomyelitis Conference Copenhagen, Denmark, July 26–28, 1960*, edited by

236   Bibliography

International Poliomyelitis Congress. Philadelphia and Montreal: J. B. Lippincott Company, 1961.

'A MVK Átszervezése és az ezzel Kapcsolatos Hatósági és Belső Vizsgálatok'. P 2130 MVK: National Archives of Hungary, The papers of the Hungarian Red Cross, 1957.

Nagler, F. P. 'Protective Efficacy of Inactivated Poliovirus Vaccines in Canada'. In *Poliomyelitis. Papers and Discussions Presented at the Fifth International Poliomyelitis Conference Copenhagen, Denmark, July 26–28, 1960*, edited by International Poliomyelitis Congress. Philadelphia and Montreal: J.B. Lippincott Company, 1961.

Nagy, Dániel. '250 000 Köbcentiméter Salk-Vakcina Érkezett. Az Egészségügyi Minisztérium Tájékoztatója'. *Népszabadság*, 14 July 1957.

Nagy, Károly. *Medical Microbiology*. Budapest: Institute of Medical Microbiology, Semmelweis University, 2008.

Nagy, László. 'Vastüdő Felhasználása Intratracheális Szakaszos-Túlnyomásos Lélegeztetésre'. *Orvosi Hetilap* 2, no. 7234 (1959): 86–87.

Nascimento, Dilene Raimundo do. 'Poliomyelitis Vaccination Campaigns in Brazil Resulting in the Eradication of the Disease (1961–1994)'. *Hygiea Internationalis* 11, no. 1 (2015): 130–44.

Nathanson, Neal, and Alexander D. Langmuir. 'The Cutter Incident Poliomyelitis Following Formaldehyde-Inactivated Poliovirus Vaccination in the United States during the Spring of 1955'. *American Journal of Epidemiology* 78, no. 1 (1964): 16–28.

National Heine-Medin Convention of the Hungarian Organization of Disabled Associations (Meosz). 6 November 2010.

Nehlin, Ann. *Exporting Visions and Saving Children: – The Swedish Save the Children Fund*. Linköping Studies in Arts and Science. Linköping: The Department of Child Studies, Linköping University, 2009.

'Nincs Gyermekbénulási Járvány: Hogyan Védekezzünk a Megbetegedések Ellen? Mikorra Várható a Hazai Oltóanyagok Termelése? Beszélgetés az Egészségügyi Minisztérium Vezetőivel'. *Szabad Nép*, 1956, 4.

'Note to the Editor of Népegészségügy'. Budapest: National Archives of Hungary, Állami közegészségügyi felügyeleti és járványvédelmi főosztály, XIX-C-2-e, 50.189, 1957.

'Number of Persons Immunized against Poliomyelitis'. *Epidemiological and Vital Statistics Report* 11 (1958): 330–31.

O'Connor, Basil. 'The Setting for Scientific Research in the Last Half of the Twentieth Century'. In *Fifth International Poliomyelitis Conference*, edited by International Poliomyelitis Congress, xxi–xxiv. Copenhagen, Denmark, 1960.

Oates-Indruchová, Libora, and Muriel Blaive. 'Border Visions and Border Regimes in Cold War Eastern Europe'. *Journal of Contemporary History* 50, no. 3 (2015): 656–59.

Offit, Paul A. *The Cutter Incident: How America's First Polio Vaccine Led to the Growing Vaccine Crisis*. New Haven: Yale University Press, 2005.

Olivé, Jean-Marc, Joao Baptista Risi, and Ciro A. de Quadros. 'National Immunization Days: Experience in Latin America'. *The Journal of Infectious Diseases* 175, no. Suppl. 1 (1997): S189–93.

Oreskes, Naomi, and John Krige, eds. *Nation and Knowledge: Science and Technology in the Global Cold War*. Cambridge, Mass.: MIT Press, forthcoming.

'Országszerte Hathatós Intézkedésekkel Küzdenek a Gyermekbénulás További Terhedésének Megakadályozásáért'. *Népakarat*, 29 June 1957.

Oshinsky, David M. *Polio: An American Story*. Oxford and New York: Oxford University Press, 2005.

Packard, Randall. '"No Other Logical Choice": Global Malaria Eradication and the Politics of International Health in the Post-War Era'. *Parassitologia* 40, no. 1–2 (1998): 217–29.

Paksáné Szentgyörgyi, Éva. 'Email Interview'. By Dóra Vargha (12 November 2010).

Palló, Gábor. 'Make a Peak on the Plain: The Rockefeller Foundation's Szeged Project'. In *Rockefeller Philanthropz and Modern Biomedicine: International Initiatives from World War I to the Cold War*, edited by William H. Schneider, 87–106. Bloomington: Indiana University Press, 2002.

'Rescue and Cordon Sanitaire: The Rockefeller Foundation in Hungarian Public Health'. *Studies in History and Philosophy of Biological and Biomedical Sciences* 31, no. 3 (2000): 433–45.

Papp, Zoltán. *A Magyar Rövidhullámú Amatőr Rádiózás Kibontakozása, Rádióamatőrök, Rádió Klubok Pécsett És Baranya Megyében*. Pécs: Zoltán Papp, 2011.

Parádi, Katalin. 'Interview'. By Dóra Vargha (27 January 2010).

Paul, John R. *A History of Poliomyelitis*. Yale Studies in the History of Science and Medicine. New Haven: Yale University Press, 1971.

'Letter to A. M.-M. Payne'. New Haven: Sterling Memorial Library, Dorothy Millicent Horstmann Papers, Box 12, Group 1700, Folder 260, 1959.

'Letter to Mikhail Chumakov'. New Haven: Sterling Memorial Library, Dorothy Millicent Horstmann Papers, Box 12, Group 1700, Folder 260, 1959.

Payne, A. M.-M. 'Letter from Payne, A. M. to Sabin, Albert B. Dated 1958–05–27'. Cincinnati: Hauck Center for the Albert B. Sabin Archives, Sabin, Albert B., 1906–1993 – Correspondence, Sabin Archives. Correspondence, OPV International. Box 02. File 03, 1958.

Payne, A. M.-M. 'Letter to John R. Paul'. New Haven: Sterling Memorial Library, Yale University, Dorothy Millicent Horstmann Papers, Box 12, Group 1700, Folder 260, 1959.

Peacock, Margaret. 'Broadcasting Benevolence: Images of the Child in American, Soviet and NFL Propaganda in Vietnam 1964–1973'. *Journal of the History of Childhood and Youth* 3, no. 1 (2010): 15–38.

Pearce, J. M. S. 'Poliomyelitis (Heine-Medin Disease)'. *Journal of Neurology Neurosurgery and Psychiatry*, no. 76 (2005): 128.

Pence, Katherine, and Paul Betts. 'Introduction'. In *Socialist Modern: East German Culture and Politics* edited by Katherine Pence and Paul Betts, 1–37. Ann Arbor: University of Michigan Press, 2008.

Perret, Françoise, 'L'Action du CICR en Hongrie en 1956'. *International Review of the Red Cross*, 78, no. 820 (1996): 449–63.

Petényi, Dr Géza. 'Új Módszerek a Gyermekbénulás Elleni Védekezésre, Több Légzőszervi, Ideg- És Bélbetegség Vírus Eredetű, Új Műszerek a Veleszületett Szívhibák Pontos Megállapítására'. *Népszava*, 16 August 1959, 5.

Péteri, György. *Nylon Curtain: Transnational and Transsystemic Tendencies in the Cultural Life of State-Socialist Russia and East-Central Europe*. Trondheim Studies on East European Cultures & Societies. Trondheim: Program on East European Cultures and Societies, 2006.

Pető, Andrea. 'Women's Rights in Stalinist Hungary: The Abortion Trials of 1952–1953'. *Hungarian Studies Review* XXIX, nos. 1–2 (2002): 49–76.

Petrilla, Aladár. 'Jelentés a Poliomyelitis Ellenes Védőoltások Előzetes Eredményeiről'. Budapest: National Archives of Hungary, Román József egészségügyi miniszer iratai, XIX-C-2-e, 1958.

'Polio Elleni Védőoltások Immunológiai Ellenőrzése'. Budapest, 5416, 1959.

The Results of Intracutaneous Poliomyelitis Vaccination in Hungary, 1957. Acta Microbiologica. Budapest: Akadémia Kiadó, 1958.

'Védőoltási Kimutatások Módosítása'. Budapest: National Archives of Hungary, Országos Közegészségi Intézet Járványügyi és Mikrobiológiai Főosztályának iratai, XXVI-C-3-e 1.d., 5331/1959, 1959.

Petryna, Adriana. *When Experiments Travel*. Princeton and Oxford: Princeton University Press, 2009.

Phillips, Sarah D. '"There Are No Invalids in the USSR!": A Missing Soviet Chapter in the New Disability History'. *Disability Studies Quarterly* 29, no. 3 (2009), www.dsq-sds.org/article/view/936/1111 (last accessed 11 June 2018).

Pintér, István. 'Salk és Sabin'. *Népszabadság*, 1959, 6–7.

Pittaway, Mark. *Eastern Europe 1939–2000*. London: Hodder Arnold, 2004.

'Introduction: Workers and Socialist States in Postwar Central and Eastern Europe'. *International Labor and Working-Class History* 68, Fall (2005): 1–8.

'The Politics of Legitimacy and Hungary's Postwar Transition'. *Contemporary European History* 13, no. 4 (2004): 453–75.

'The Reproduction of Hierarchy: Skill, Working-Class Culture and the State in Early Socialist Hungary'. *Journal of Modern History* 74, no. 4 (2002): 737–69.

'Polio Epidemic Feared'. *Washington Post and Times Herald*, 5 June 1957, 8.

Subcommittee on Health and Safety of the Committee on Interstate and Foreign Commerce. *Polio Vaccines*, First session on developments with respect to the manufacture of live virus polio vaccine and results of utilization of killed virus polio vaccine, March 16 1961.

'Poliomyelite Antérieure Aigue (Paralysie Infantile)'. Geneva: WHO Archives, European Regional Conference on Poliomyelitis, Brussels May 1948, WHO 1 484–1–2, A/Prog/40, 1948.

'Poliomyelitis Vaccine'. *The British Medical Journal* 1, no. 5078 (1958): 1053.

Poliomyelitis. Health Information Series. Vol. 74, Washington D.C.: U.S. Department of Health, Education and Welfare. Public Health Service., 1963.

'Poliomyelitis. Papers Presented at the Fourth International Poliomyelitis Conference'. Paper presented at the Fourth International Poliomyelitis Conference, Geneva, 1957.

'Poliomyelitis. Papers Presented at the Fourth International Poliomyelitis Conference'. *Fourth International Poliomyelitis Conference* (1957).

Pollack, Detlef, and Jan Wielgohs. *Dissent and Opposition in Communist Eastern Europe: Origins of Civil Society and Democratic Transition*. Burlington, VT: Ashgate, 2004.

Porras, María Isabel, María José Báguena, and Rosa Ballester. 'Spain and the International Scientific Conferences on Polio'. *Dynamis* 30 (2010): 91–118.

Presley, Gary. *Seven Wheelchairs: A Life beyond Polio*. Iowa City: University of Iowa Press, 2008.

Proctor, Robert, and Londa L. Schiebinger. *Agnotology: The Making and Unmaking of Ignorance*. Stanford, Calif.: Stanford University Press, 2008.

Przesmycki, F. 'Vaccination against Poliomyelitis in Poland'. In *Vaccination and Immunity. Neurophysical and Neuropathological aspects of poliomyelitis. Vth Symposium of the European Association against Poliomyelitis*, edited by H. C. A. Lassen, 40–41. Madrid: Europ. Assoc. Poliomyelitis, 1959.

Rádai, Sándor. 'Interview'. By Dora Vargha (5 May 2010).

Radin, Joanna. 'Serum as Sentinel: How Cold Blood Became a Resource for Population Health'. *Limn*, no. 3 (2013), https://www.limn.it/articles/serum-as-sentinel-how-cold-blood-became-a-resource-for-population-health/ (last accessed 11 June 2018).

'Unfolding Epidemiological Stories: How the Who Made Frozen Blood into a Flexible Resource for the Future'. *Studies in History and Philosophy of Biological and Biomedical Sciences* 47, Part A (2014): 62–73.

Radio Free Europe. 'Polio in Hungary: Background Report'. Budapest: Open Society Archives, RFE News & Information Service – Evaluation & Research Section, 1957.

Rádió Miskolc. '1956 Október 29, 23.54 H: Figyelem!'. In *A Forradalom Hangja. Magyarországi Rádióadások 1956. Október 23–November 9*, edited by Gyurgyák János. Budapest: Századvég kiadó és Nyilvánosság Klub, 1989.

'1956 Október 29: A Debreceni Kórház Felhívása!'. In *A Forradalom Hangja. Magyarországi Rádióadások 1956. Október 23–November 9*, edited by Gyurgyák János, 216. Budapest: Századvég kiadó és Nyilvánosság Klub, 1989.

'1956 Október 29. 22.14 H: Halló, Halló, Figyelem!'. In *A Forradalom Hangja. Magyarországi Rádióadások 1956. Október 23–November 9*, edited by Gyurgyák János. Budapest: Századvég kiadó és Nyilvánosság Klub, 1989.

Rainer, János M. 'The Road to Budapest, 1956. New Documentation on the Kremlin's Decision to Intervene'. *Hungarian Quarterly*, no. Summer (1996): 24–41.

Rainer, M. János, and Katalin Somlai. *The 1956 Hungarian Revolution and the Soviet Bloc Countries: Reactions and Repercussions*. Budapest: The Institute for the History of the 1956 Hungarian Revolution, 2007.

Rangel de Almeida, Joao. 'The 1851 International Sanitary Conference and the Construction of an International Sphere of Public Health'. PhD thesis, University of Edinburgh, 2012.

Rasell, Michael, and Elena Iarskaia-Smirnova. *Disability in Eastern Europe and the Former Soviet Union: History, Policy and Everyday Life*. Basees/Routledge Series on Russian and East European Studies. London and New York: Routledge, Taylor & Francis Group, 2014.

Reinisch, Jessica. '"Auntie Unrra" at the Crossroads'. *Past and Present* 218, no. Suppl 8 (2013): 70–97.

The Perils of Peace: The Public Health Crisis in Occupied Germany. Oxford, United Kingdom: Oxford University Press, 2013.

Reisner-Sénélar, Luise. 'The Birth of Intensive Care Medicine: Björn Ibsen's Records'. *Intensive Care Med*, no. 37 (2011): 1084–86.

'Rekordforgalom az Első Meleg Nyári Vasárnapon'. *Népszava*, 9 June 1959.

'Rendelet a Kötelező Védőoltásokról '. *Népakarat*, 17 September 1958.

Renne, Elisha P. *The Politics of Polio in Northern Nigeria*. Bloomington: Indiana University Press, 2010.

Reverby, Susan M. '"Normal Exposure" and Inoculation Syphilis: A Phs "Tuskegee" Doctor in Guatemala, 1946–1948'. *Journal of Policy History* 23, no. 1 (2011): 6–28.

Révész, Béla. 'Manipulációs Technikák a Hidegháború Korai Időszakában'. *Acta Juridica et Politica* 10 (1996): 3–90.

Rezső Hargitai, and Ákosné Kiss, eds. *A Gyermekbénulás Elleni Küzdelem: Beszámoló egy Ma már Múlttá Váló Rettegett Betegség ellen Folytatott Hősies Küzdelemről és Felszámolásának Lehetőségéről: A Szent László Kórház Centenáriumára Készült Összeállítás* Budapest: Literatura Medica, 1994.

Rodríguez-Sánchez, Juan Antonio. 'Poliomyelitis after Poliomyelitis: Lights and Shadows of the Eradication. An Introduction'. *Hygiea Internationalis* 11, no. 1 (2015): 7–31.

Rogers, Naomi. *Polio Wars: Sister Kenny and the Golden Age of American Medicine*. Oxford: Oxford University Press, 2014.

Dirt and Disease: Polio before FDR. New Brunswick, NJ: Rutgers University Press, 1992.

'A Rokkant Személyek Nemzetközi Évéhez Kapcsolódó Feladatok'. Budapest: Magyar Nemzeti Levéltár, Minisztertanácsi Jegyzőkönyvek, 288.f.7., 604. ő.e., 1980

Román, József. 'Gyermekbénulás Elleni Védekezés'. Budapest: National Archives of Hungary, Az Egészségügyi Minisztérium Iratai, XIX-C-n, 369/1956, 1956

'Román József Egészségügyi Miniszter Egészségügyünk Problémáiról'. *Népszava*, 21 October 1956.

Romsics, Ignác. *Hungary in the Twentieth Century*. Budapest: Osiris, 1999.

Magyarország Története a XX. Században. Budapest: Osiris Kiadó, 2001.

Roosth, Sophia, and Stefan Helmreich. 'Life Forms: A Keyword Entry'. *Representations* 112, no. 1 (2010): 27–53.

Rosenberg, Charles. 'What Is an Epidemic? AIDS in Historical Perspective'. *Daedalus* 118, no. 2 (1989): 1–17.

Rosenberg, Charles, and Janet Golden, eds. *Framing Disease: Studies in Cultural History*. 2nd edn. New Brunswick: Rutgers University Press, 1997.

Rosenberg, Clifford. 'The International Politics of Vaccine Testing in Interwar Algiers'. *American Historical Review* 117, no. 3 (2012): 671–97.

Ross, Jean C. 'A History of Poliomyelitis in New Zealand'. MA thesis, University of Canterbury, New Zealand, 1993.

Roth, Maria. 'Child Protection in Communist Romania (1944–1989)'. In *Social Care under State Socialism (1945–1989): Ambitions, Ambiguities and Mismanagement*, edited by Sabine Hering, 201–11. Opladen and Farmington Hills: Barbara Budrich Publishers, 2009.

Röthler, István. 'Házi Feljegyzés'. Budapest: National Archives of Hungary, XIX-C-2-d-8113/L/1, 1954.

Rothman, David J. *Beginnings Count: The Technological Imperative in American Health Care*. New York: Oxford University Press, 1997.

Rotschild, Rachel. 'Détente from the Air: Monitoring Air Pollution during the Cold War'. *Technology and Culture* 57, no. 4 (2016): 831–65.

Rudnai, Ottó. 'Az 1957. Évi Poliomyelitis Járvány. Közlemény Az Országos Közegészségügyi Intézet (Főigazgató: Bakács Tibor Dr.) Járványügyi Osztályáról (Osztályvezető: Petrilla Aladár Dr.)'. *Népegészségügy* 39, no. 5–6 (1958): 121–27.

The 1959 Poliomyelitis Epidemic in Hungary. Acta Microbiologica. Budapest: Academiae Scientiarum Hungaricae, 1960.

'Heti Fertőzőbeteg Jelentés 1959. 30. Hét'. Budapest: National Archives of Hungary, Országos Közegészségügyi Intézet iratai, XXVI-C-3-e, 5421/1959, 1959.

'Jelentés a Szabolcs-Szatmár Megyei Köjál Epidemiológiai Munkájának Ellenőrzéséről'. Budapest: National Archives of Hungary, Egészségügyi Minisztérium Állami Közegészségügyi Felügyeleti és Járványvédeli Főosztály, XIX-C-2-e, 56593/1959, 1959.

'Járványügyi Munkánk Néhány Hiányosságáról'. Budapest: Országos Közegészségügyi Intézet járványügyi osztálya, 1952.

Rudnai, Ottó, and Gyula Barsy. *The Results of Salk Vaccination in Hungary as Measured on the 1959 Poliomyelitis Epidemic*. Acta Microbiologica. Budapest: Akadémiai Kiadó, 1961.

Rupprecht, Tobias. *Soviet Internationalism after Stalin: Interaction and Exchange between the USSR and Latin America during the Cold War*. Cambridge, United Kingdom: Cambridge University Press, 2015.

Rutty, Christopher J. 'The Middle Class Plague: Epidemic Polio and the Canadian State, 1936–37'. *Canadian Bulletin of Medical History* 13, no. 2 (1996): 277–314.

Sabin, Albert. 'Epidemiologic Patterns of Poliomyelitis in Different Parts of the World'. In *Poliomyelitis: Papers and Discussions Presented at the First International Poliomyelitis Conference*, 3–33. Philadelphia: Lippincott, 1949.

'Letter from Sabin, Albert B. to Pillemer, L. Dated 1957–06–10'. Cincinnati: Hauck Center for the Albert B. Sabin Archives, Correspondence, Individual, Box 02. File 21 (Blaskovic, D. – 1957–69), 1957.

Sabin, Albert B. 'Role of My Cooperation with Soviet Scientists in the Elimination of Polio: Possible Lessons for Relations between the U.S.A. and the U.S.S.R'. *Perspectives in biology and medicine* 31, no. 1 (1987): 57–64.

'Letter from Sabin, Albert B. To Vaczi, L. Dated 1963–10–16'. Cincinnati: Hauck Center for the Albert B. Sabin Archives, Sabin Archives. Correspondence, Individual., Box 09 File 18 (Geder, Laszlo – 1963–68), 1963.

'Letter from Sabin, Albert B. To Domok I. Dated 1961–02–01'. Cincinnati: Hauck Center for the Albert B. Sabin Archives, Sabin Archives. Correspondence, OPV International, Box 02 File 09 (Hungary – 1960–67), 1961.

'Letter from Rethy, Lajos to Sabin, Albert B. Dated 1961–03–06'. Cincinnati: Hauck Center for the Albert B. Sabin Archives, Sabin Archives. Correspondence, OPV International, Box 02 File 09 (Hungary – 1960–67), 1961.

'Letter from Sabin, Albert B. To Clegg, H.A. Dated 1961–02–01'. Cincinnati: Hauck Center for the Albert B. Sabin Archives, Sabin Archives. Correspondence, OPV International, Box 02 File 09 (Hungary – 1960–67), 1961.

Manuel Ramos-Alvarez, José Alvarez-Amezquita, D.F. William Pelon, Richard
    H. Michaels, Ilya Spigland, Meinrad A. Koch, and Joan M. Barnes. 'Live, Orally
    Given Poliovirus Vaccine. Effects of Rapid Mass Immunization on Popluation
    under Conditions of Massive Enteric Infection with Other Viruses'. *JAMA*, no. 173
    (1960): 1521–26.
'Letter from Sabin, Albert B. To Ivanovics, G. Dated 1955-03-03'. Cincinnati:
    Hauck Center for the Albert B. Sabin Archives, Correspondence, Individual,
    Box 13. File 09 (Ivanovics, George – 1954–60), 1955.
'Paralytic Consequences of Poliomyelitis Infection in Different Parts of the World
    and in Different Population Groups'. *American journal of Public Health* 41, no. 10
    (1951): 1215–30.
'Sabin Oltások Eredményességének Értékelése'. Budapest: City Archives of
    Budapest, Budapest Főváros Tanács VB Egészségügyi Osztályának iratai,
    XXIII. 115.a. 215 kisdoboz, 188.197/1959, 1959.
'Salk Expects End of Polio Some Day'. *New York Times*, 9 July 1957, 3.
Sánchez, Juan Antonio Rodríguez, and Jesús Seco Calvo. 'Las Campañas De
    Vacunación Contra La Poliomielitis En España En 1963'. *Asclepio. Revista de
    Historia de la Medicina y la Ciencia* 61, no. 1 (2009): 81–116.
Sass, Edmund J., George Gottfried, and Anthony Sorem. *Polio's Legacy: An Oral
    History*. Lanham Md.: University Press of America, 1996.
Schadt, Mária. *'Feltörekvő, Dolgozó Nő'. Nők az Ötvenes Években*. Budapest:
    Pannónia, 2005.
Schweitzer, Nóra. *Polio 2.0* Budapest: Magyar Polio Alapítvány, 2016.
Seavey, Nina Gilden, Jane S. *Smith, and Paul Wagner. A Paralyzing Fear: The
    Triumph Over Polio in America*. 1st edn. New York: TV Books, 1998.
Seddon, Herbert J. 'Economic Aspects of the Management of Poliomyelitis'.
    In *First International Poliomyelitis Conference*, 34–39. New York: Lippincott,
    1948.
Serlin, David. 'The Other Arms Race'. In *The Disability Studies Reader*, edited by
    Lennard J. Davis, 49–65. New York: Routledge, 2006.
Shell, Marc. *Polio and Its Aftermath: The Paralysis of Culture*. Cambridge, Mass.:
    Harvard University Press, 2005.
Siddiqi, Javed. *World Health and World Politics: The World Health Organization and
    the Un System*. Columbus: University of South Carolina Press, 1995.
Silver, J. K., and Daniel J. Wilson. *Polio Voices: An Oral History from the
    American Polio Epidemics and Worldwide Eradication Efforts*. The Praeger
    Series on Contemporary Health and Living. Westport, Conn.: Praeger,
    2007.
Simándi, Irén. *Magyarország a Szabad Európa Hullámhosszán*. Nemzeti Téka, edited
    by Ferenc Kégli and István Monok. Budapest: Gondolat Kiadó, 2005.
Simonovits, Dr István. 'Feljegyzés Zsoldos Elvtárs Részére Lukács László Dr.
    Javaslatáról'. XIX-C-2-d-8113/L/1–1954, 1954.
Skovranek, V. 'Investigations of the Effectiveness of Inactivated Vaccine against
    Poliomyelitis in Czechoslovakia'. In *Poliomyelitis: Papers and Discussions
    Presented at the Fifth International Poliomyelitis Conference Copenhagen,
    Denmark, July 26–28, 1960*, edited by International Poliomyelitis Congress,
    124–37. Philadelphia and Montreal: J. B. Lippincott Company, 1961.

'The Organization and Results of Mass Vaccination against Poliomyelitis in CSSR. In *The Control of Poliomyelitis by Live Poliovirus Vaccine. Studies on Mass Vaccinations in Hungary, in the USSR, in Czechoslovakia and the German Democratic Republic. Papers Presented at the Hungarian-Soviet Medical Conference September 24–30, 1960*, edited by J. Weissfeiler. Budapest: Akadémiai Kiadó, 1961.

'Letter from Skovranek, V. to Sabin, Albert B. Dated 1959–01–22'. Cincinnati: Hauck Center for the Albert B. Sabin Archives, Sabin, Albert B., 1906–1993 – Correspondence, Box 02. File 03, 1959.

'Letter from Skovranek, V. to Sabin, Albert B. Dated 1959–05–10'. Cincinnati: Hauck Center for the Albert B. Sabin Archives, Sabin, Albert B., 1906–1993 – Correspondence, Box 3, File 09 (Soviet Union – 1959–1968), 1959.

Skovranek, V. 'Present State of Poliomyelitis after Nation Wide Vaccination with Live (Oral) Vaccine in Czechoslovakia'. In *Programs of Vaccination, Encephalitis and Meningitis in Enteroviral Infections, Virological and CLINICAL PROBLEMS. viiTH SYMPOSIUM of the European Association against Poliomyelitis*, ed. H. C. A. Lassen (Oxford: Euro Assoc. Poliomyelitis and Allied Diseases, 1962).

'Principles of Organization of Vaccination with Live Vaccine with Particular Reference to the Experience Assembled in Czechoslovakia. In Letter from Skovranek, Vilem to Sabin, Albert B. Dated 1961–05–13'. Cincinnatti: Albert B. Sabin Archives, Hauck Center for the Albert B. Sabin Archives, 1961, Correspondence, Unsorted, Box 02, File 04 (1961), 1961.

'Present State of Vaccination against Poliomyelitis in Czechoslovakia'. In *Vaccination and Immunity. Neurophysical and Neuropathological aspects of poliomyelitis. Vth Symposium of the European Association against Poliomyelitis*, edited by H. C. A. Lassen, 49–56. Madrid: Europ. Assoc. Poliomyelitis, 1959.

Škrovánek, Vilém and Žážek, Karel, 'Oral Poliovirus Vaccine (Sabin) in Czechoslovakia. Effectiveness of Nation-Wide Use in 1960'. *Journal of the American Medical Association* 176, no. 6 (1961).

Skovránek, V., K. Zácek, V. Vonka, E. Adam, V. Adamová, V. Burian, and H. Vojtová. 'Field Trial with Sabin's Live Poliovirus Vaccine in Czechoslovakia 1958–1959'. In *Live Poliovirus Vaccines: Papers Presented and Discussions Held at the First International Conference on Live Poliovirus Vaccines*, 530–71. Washington, D.C.: Pan American Sanitary Bureau, 1959.

Slonim, D., E. Svandova, P. Strand, and C. Benes. 'History of Poliomyelitis in the Czech Republic – Part III'. *Central European Journal of Public Health* 3, no. 3 (1995): 124–26.

Smallman-Raynor, Matthew. *Poliomyelitis: Emergence to Eradication*. Oxford Geographical and Environmental Studies. Oxford and New York: Oxford University Press, 2006.

Smallman-Raynor, M. R., A. D. Cliff, B. Trevelyan, C. Nettleton, and S. Sneddon. *Poliomyelitis. A World Geography: Emergence to Eradication*. New York: Oxford University Press, 2006.

Smith, Jane S. *Patenting the Sun: Polio and the Salk Vaccine*. New York: Morrow, 1990.

Smorodintsev, A. A., E. F. Davidenkova, A. I. Drobyshevskaya, V. I. Ilyenko, N. E. Gorev, L. M. Kurnosova, and T. E. Klyuchareva. 'Results of a Study of the

Reactogenic and Immunogenic Properties of Live Anti-Poliomyelitis Vaccine'. *Bulletin of the World Health Organization* 20 (1959): 1053–74.

Solomon, Susan Gross, Lion Murard, and Patrick Zylberman. *Shifting Boundaries of Public Health: Europe in the Twentieth Century*. Rochester Studies in Medical History. Rochester, NY: University of Rochester Press, 2008.

Solovey, Mark. 'Science and the State during the Cold War: Blurred Boundaries and a Contested Legacy'. *Social Studies of Science* 31, no. 1 (2001): 165–70.

Sólyom, Sándor. 'Augusztus Hónapban Végzett Gyermekbénulás Elleni Védőoltásokról Jelentés'. Budapest: National Archives of Hungary, Egészségügyi Minisztérium Állami közegészségügyi felügyelet és járványvédelmi főosztály iratai, XIX-C-2-e, 53935, 1957.

Sontag, Susan. *Illness as Metaphor and AIDS and Its Metaphors*. New York: Picador, 1990.

Soós, Ágnes. 'Interview'. By Dóra Vargha (7 April 2010).

'*Interview*'. By Dóra Vargha. Budapest, 2010.

Stanley, N. F. 'Attempts to Demonstrate Interference between Coxsackie and Poliomyelitis Viruses in Mice and Monkeys'. *Proceedings of the Society for Experimental Biology and Medicine*, no. 81 (1952): 430–33.

Starks, Tricia. *The Body Soviet: Propaganda, Hygiene and the Revolutionary State*. Madison, Wisc.: University of Wisconsin Press, 2008.

Stepan, Nancy. *Eradication: Ridding the World of Diseases Forever?* Ithaca, NY: Cornell University Press, 2011.

Sticchi, L., M. Alberti, C. Alicino, and P. Crovari. 'The Intradermal Vaccination: Past Experiences and Current Perspectives'. *Journal of Preventive Medicine and Hygiene* 51, no. 1 (2010): 7–14.

Stich, Zdenek. *Czechoslovak Health Services*. Prague: Ministry of Health, Czechoslovak Socialist Republic, 1962.

Sting, and Sergei Prokofjev. *Russians: The Dream of the Blue Turtles*. Santa Monica: A&M, 1985. Single.

Stuart-Harris, Charles, and Jr. DeWitt Stetten. 'Report on the International Conference on the Eradication of Infectious Diseases. Can Infectious Diseases Be Eradicated?'. *Reviews of Infectious Diseases* 4, no. 5 (1982): 913–84.

'Summary of Conference on Live Poliovirus Vaccines'. Geneva: World Health Organization, WHO/Polio/43, 1959.

Summerhayes, Colin P. 'International Collaboration in Antarctica: The International Polar Years, the International Geophysical Year and the Scientific Committee on Antarctic Research'. *Polar Record* 44, no. 231 (2008): 321–34.

Surányi, Gyula. *Egészséges Anya – Egészséges Gyermek Útmutató Városi És Falusi Előadók Számára* Budapest: Művelt nép könyvkiadó, 1953.

Szakolcai, Attila. 'Az 1956-os Magyar Forradalmat Követő Politikai Megtorlás Áldozatainak Hivatalos Névsora'. *Beszélő* 6, no. 24 (1994), http://beszelo.c3.hu/cikkek/az-1956-os-magyar-forradalmat-koveto-politikai-megtorlas-aldozatainak-hiteles-nevsora.

Székely, Ferenc. 'A Poliomyelitis Anterior Acuta (Heine-Medin) Serumtherapiájáról'. *Gyógyászat* 82, no. 32 (1942): 1–8.

Szelényi, Szonja. *Equality by Design: The Grand Experiment in Destratification in Socialist Hungary*. Stanford: Stanford University Press, 1998.

Szemere, Anna. *Up from the Underground: The Culture of Rock Music in Postsocialist Hungary*. Post-Communist Cultural Studies Series. University Park, Pa.: Pennsylvania State University Press, 2001.

Szentgyörgyi, Ákosné. 'Email Correspondence'. By Dóra Vargha (12 November 2010).

Szeri, Ilona, Pál Földes, and Szilárd Bognár. 'Adatok a Poliomyelitis Elleni Intrakután Védőoltás Kérdéséhez'. *Orvosi Hetilap* 100, no. 38 (1959): 1364–65.

Szigeti, Károly. 'Feljegyzés Ackerson Tanácsos Amerikai Id. Ügyvivő Látogatásáról'. Budapest: Magyar Nemzeti Levéltár, XIX-J-1-k USA Admin 1945–1964, 57. doboz, Amerikai segítség ajánlat gyermekbénulási gyógyszer vásárlásához, 19/3/h, 1957.

'Sajtóközlemény-Tervezet'. Budapest: Magyar Nemzeti Levéltár, XIX-J-1-k USA Admin 1945–1964, 57, Amerikai segítség ajánlat gyermekbénulási gyógyszer vásárlásához, 1957.

Szöllősiné Földesi, Erzsébet. 'Interview'. By Dóra Vargha (26 April 2010).

'Szülők, Vigyázzatok!'. Hungary: Health Ministry, 1957.

'Tájékoztató a Gyermekbénulásos Megbetegedésekről'. *Népszabadság*, 27 June 1957.

Takó, József. 'Az Országos Közegészségügyi Intézet Járványügyi Tájékoztatója 1957. Február Haváról'. Budapest: National Archives of Hungary, Állami közegészségügyi felügyeleti és járványvédelmi főosztály, XIX-C-2-e, 50.189, 1957.

Tamás, György. 'Élelmezésügyi Minisztérium Vizsgálatáról Készült Jelentés'. Budapest: National Archives of Hungary, A MVK átszervezése és az ezzel kapcsolatos hatósági és belső vizsgálatok 1957, P 2130, 1957.

The Forty-First World Health Assembly. 'Wha 41.28 Global Eradication of Poliomyelitis by the Year 2000'. Geneva: World Health Organization, 1988.

The Nobel Foundation. 'The Nobel Prize in Physiology or Medicine 1954. John F. Enders, Thomas H. Weller, Fredeick C. Robbins'. www.nobelprize.org/nobel_prizes/medicine/laureates/1954/

Timmermann, Carsten. 'Americans and Pavlovians: The Central Institute for Cardiovascular Research at the East German Academy of Sciences and Its Precursor Institutions as a Case Study of Biomedical Research in a Country of the Soviet Bloc (C. 1950–1980)'. In *Medicine, the Market and Mass Media*, edited by Virginia Berridge and Kelly Loughlin. London: Routledge, 2005.

'Tizennégy Éves Korig Minden Gyermek Kap a Gyermekbénulás Ellen Védő Új, Nagyobbhatású Gyógyszerből'. *Népszava*, 18 November 1959, 1.

'Tizennyolc Éves Korig Adnak Gyermekbénulás Elleni Védőoltást – Február 10-Én Kezdődik az Új Oltási Kampány'. *Népakarat*, 28 January 1958, 3.

Tomes, Nancy. *The Gospel of Germs: Men, Women, and the Microbe in American Life*. Cambridge, Mass.: Harvard University Press, 1998.

Török, Zoltán. 'Telephone Interview'. By Dóra Vargha (8 September 2011).

Tóth, Béla. 'Gyermekbénulás Elleni Védőoltások 1959. Március és Április Hónapban'. Budapest: City Archives of Budapest, Budapest Fővárosi Tanács VB Egészségügyi Osztályának iratai, XXIII.115.a/34. kisdoboz, 181.476, 51.070/1959 V/3., 1959.

Tóth, Eszter Zsófia. 'The Memory of the State Award in the Narratives of Women Workers'. In *Regimes and Transformations: Hungary in the Twentieth Century*, edited by István Feitl and Balázs Sipos. Budapest: Napvilág, 2005.

246   Bibliography

Tóth, Sándor. 'Gyermekbénulás Elleni Védőoltásokkal Kapcsolatos Felmerült Problémák'. Debrecen: National Archives of Hungary, Egészségügyi Minisztérium Állami Közegészségügyi Felügyeleti és Járványvédeli Főosztály, XIX-C-2-e, 53137, 1957.
'Új Gyermekbénulás-Utókezelő Intézetet Állítottak Fel'. Népszabadság, 1956, 3.
'Új Oltóanyag'. In Magyar Filmhíradó. Hungary: Magyar Filmhíradó és Dokumentumfilmgyár, 1959.
United Nations General Assembly. 'Declaration of the Rights of the Child'. In Resolution 1386(XIV). Geneva, 1959.
Urban, George R. Radio Free Europe and the Pursuit of Democracy. New Haven: Yale University Press, 1997.
'Use of Respirators in the Treatment of Poliomyelitis and Proposed Organization of a System of International Loan of These Apparatus'. In Report of the Executive Board. Fifth Session. Held in Geneva from 16 January to 2 February 1950, edited by World Health Organization. Geneva: World Health Organization, 1950.
'Use of Respirators in the Treatment of Poliomyelitis and Proposed Organization of a System of International Loan of These Apparatus. Addendum 1'. In Report of the Executive Board. Fifth Session. Held in Geneva from 16 January to 2 February 1950, edited by World Health Organization. Geneva: World Health Organization, 1950.
V. M. 'Harmincezer Iskolásgyermeket Üdültet a Szot, Kétszázezer Gyerek Megy Úttörőtáborba'. Népszava, 4 June 1959.
Vajda, Gábor. 'Visszaadják Őket Az Életnek'. Népszava, 26 March 1961.
Vámos, György, ed. A Szabad Európa Rádió és a Magyar Forradalom. Műsortükör 1956. Október 23-November 5. Vol. 7, História Könyvtár Okmánytárak. Budapest: MTA Történettudományi Intézete, 2010.
'Van Építőanyag a Kórházak Helyreállításához, Vöröskereszt Táborikonyhák Létesülnek, Szappant, Mosóport, Ddt-T Kapnak a Kerületek'. Népakarat, 21 Novembver 1956.
Vaptzarov, I., D. Bratovanov, and T. Kristev. 'La vaccination contre la poliomyélite en Bulgarie'. In Anti-poliomyelitis vaccinations, physio-pathology of the respiratory disorder, poliomyelitis of the 'very young child'. VIth symposium of the European Association against Poliomyelitis, edited by H. C. A. Lassen, 19–23. Munich: Europ. Assoc. Poliomyelitis, 1960.
Vargha, Dora, 'Between East and West: Polio Vaccination Across the Iron Curtain in Cold War Hungary', Bulletin of the History of Medicine 88, no. 2 (2014): 319–342.
Vargha, György. 'Interview'. By Dóra Vargha (15 June 2008).
Vargha Jánosné Lázok, Dr Irén. 'Interview'. By Dóra Vargha (24 June 2008).
Vastagh, Gábor. 'Az Országos Közegészségügyi Intézet Járványügyi Tájékoztatója 1959. Augusztus Hóról'. Budapest: National Archives of Hungary, Országos Közegészségügyi Intézet Járványügyi és Mikrobiológiai Osztályának iratai, XXVI-C-3-e, 5571/1959, 1959.
Vastagh, Gábor, and Ottó Rudnai. 'Jelentés a Fővárosi Poliomyelitis Elleni Védőoltások Ellenőrzéséről'. Budapest: National Archives of Hungary, Országos Közegészségi Intézet Járványügyi és Mikrobiológiai Főosztályának iratai, XXVI-C-3-e, 5450/1959, 1959.

'Védekezzünk a Fertőző Betegségek Ellen'. Hungary, n.d. [1920s].

'Végrehajtó Bizottsági Ülés Jegyzőkönyve'. Budapest: City Archives of Budapest, MSZMP Eger Városi Bizottsága Végrehajtó Bizottság ülései XXXV-29–3, 130. őe. (5. doboz), 1963.

Verdery, Katherine. 'From Parent-State to Family Patriarchs: Gender and Nation in Contemporary Eastern Europe'. *East European Politics and Societies* 8, no. 2 (1994): 225–55.

Veres, Gábor. 'Kimutatás Salk Vakcina Kiadásáról És Készletéről'. Budapest: National Archives of Hungary, Egészségügyi Minisztérium Állami közegészségügyi felügyelet és járványvédelmi főosztály iratai, XIX-C-2-e, 53137, 1957.

Vető, József. 'A Sabin-Cseppek'. *Népszabadság*, 1960, 1.

'Vigyázz!'. Hungary: Health Ministry, 1957.

Vikol, Dr János. 'Heine-Medin Utókezelő-Intézet Szervezése'. Budapest: National Archives of Hungary, Egészségügyi Minisztérium XIX-C-2-d-40.318–1957 (16. d.), 1956.

'Határozat'. Budapest: Budapest Főváros Tanácsa Végrehajtóbizottságának XII. egészségügyi osztálya, 1956.

von Magnus, Herdis. 'Present Knowledge about Duration of Sero-Immunity after Vaccination with Inactivated Polio Vaccines'. In *Poliomyelitis. Papers and Discussions Presented at the Fifth International Poliomyelitis Conference Copenhagen, Denmark, July 26–28, 1960*, edited by International Poliomyelitis Congress. Philadelphia and Montreal: J. B. Lippincott Company, 1961.

Wailoo, Keith, Julie Livingston, Steven Epstein, and Aronowitz Robert, eds. *Three Shots at Prevention: The HPV Vaccine and the Politics of Medicin'es Simple Solutions*. Baltimore: Johns Hopkins University Press, 2010.

Wald, Priscilla. *Contagious. Cultures, Carriers, and the Outbreak Narrative*. Durham, NC and London: Duke University Press, 2008.

Wallgren, Arvid. 'Some Observations Madde during a Short Visit to Poland'. Geneva: World Health Organization, Reports on Maternal and Child Health (MCH) Conditions – Poland, M3–418-2POL JKT 1, 1957.

Wang, Jessica. *American Science in an Age of Anxiety: Scientists, Anticommunism and the Cold War*. Chapel Hill and London: University of North Carolina Press, 1999.

Wang, Zuoyue. 'Transnational Science during the Cold War: The Case of Chinese/American Scientists'. *Isis* 101, no. 2 (2010): 367–77.

'Washington Conference on Live Poliovirus Vaccines'. *British Medical Journal* 2, no. 5146 (1959): 235–36.

Webb, Alban. *London Calling: Britain, the BBC World Service and the Cold War*. London: Bloomsbury Academic, 2014.

Weindling, Paul. *Epidemics and Genocide in Eastern Europe, 1890–1945*. Oxford and New York: Oxford University Press, 2000.

'Public Health and Political Stabilisation: The Rockefeller Foundation in Central and Eastern Europe between the Two World Wars'. *Minerva* 31, no. 3 (1993): 253–67.

Weinerman, Richard E., and Shirley B. Weinerman. *Social Medicine in Eastern Europe: The Organization of Health Services and the Education of Medical Personnel in Czechoslovakia, Hungary, and Poland*. Cambridge, Mass.: Harvard University Press, 1969.

Wilson, Daniel J. 'A Crippling Fear: Experiencing Polio in the Era of FDR'. *Bulletin of the History of Medicine* 72, no. 3 (1998): 464–95.

Living with Polio: The Epidemic and Its Survivors. Chicago: University of Chicago Press, 2005.

Polio. Biographies of Disease. Portsmouth: Greenwood Publishing Group, 2009.

'World Polio Cut by Salk Vaccine. Hungary Aided in Polio Fight'. *New York Times*, 10 July 1957/.

Žáček, Karel, Ervín Adam, Vlasta Adamová, Václav Burian, Dagmar Řezáčová, Eliška Skřídlovská, Nina Vaněčková, and Vladimír Vonka. 'Mass Oral (Sabin) Poliomyelitis Vaccination. Virological and Serological Surveillance in Czechoslovakia, 1958–59 and 1960'. *British Medical Journal* 1, no. 5285 (1962): 1091–98.

Zahra, Tara. *The Lost Children: Reconstructing Europe's Families after World War II.* Cambridge, Mass.: Harvard University Press, 2011.

Zhdanov, V. M., M. P. Chumakov, and A. A. Smorodintsev. 'Large-Scale Practical Trials and Use of Live Poliovirus Vaccine in the U.S.S.R'. In *Live Poliovirus Vaccines: Papers Presented and Discussions Held at the Second International Conference on Live Poliovirus Vaccines*, 576–88. Washington, D.C.: Pan American Health Organization, 1960.

Züst, Dr F. 'Note an Das I.K.R.K. Budapest, Z. Hd. Von Herrn Ch. Ammann: Poliomyelitis-Epidemie in Ungarn'. Geneva: International Committee of the Red Cross Archives, Epidémie de poliomyélite, B AG 280 094–031.02, 164, 1957.

Index

252   Index